The Philosophy and Practice of Psychiatric Nursing

Dedication
Many people taught me to value their experience, my experience of them and my experience of myself. I dedicate this book to those people, who taught me something of the real meaning of caring.

For Churchill Livingstone:

Senior Commissioning Editors: Alex Mathieson, Jacqueline Curthoys
Project Editor: Dinah Thom
Project Controller: Derek Robertson

The Philosophy and Practice of Psychiatric Nursing

Philip J Barker PhD RN FRCN

Professor of Psychiatric Nursing Practice,
University of Newcastle, UK

Foreword by

Annie T Altschul

Emeritus Professor of Nursing Studies, University of Edinburgh,
Edinburgh, UK

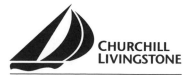
CHURCHILL
LIVINGSTONE

EDINBURGH LONDON NEW YORK PHILADELPHIA SYDNEY TORONTO 1999

CHURCHILL LIVINGSTONE
An imprint of Harcourt Brace and Company Limited

© Harcourt Brace and Company Limited 1999

⚉ is a registered trade mark of Harcourt Brace and Company Limited

The right of Phil Barker to be identified as author of this work has been asserted by him in accordance with the Copyright, Designs and Patents Act 1988

First published 1999

ISBN 0443 060045

British Library Cataloguing in Publication Data
A catalogue record for this book is available from the British Library

Library of Congress Cataloging in Publication Data
A catalog record for this book is available from the Library of Congress

The
publisher's
policy is to use
**paper manufactured
from sustainable forests**

Printed in China
NPCC/01

Contents

Commentators   *vii*
Foreword   *ix*
Preface   *xiii*

Part 1 The nature of nursing   1

1. Psychoanalysis and psychiatric nursing: a bridge too far?   3
   Commentary: Suzanne Lego

2. The philosophy of psychiatric nursing:
   the birth of the binding agent?   21
   Commentary: Hugh McKenna

3. The eye of the needle: research and the proper focus of nursing   37
   Commentaries: Colin Holmes and Ian Beech

4. The last wave? Promoting growth and development
   in community psychiatric and mental health nursing   57
   Commentary: Liam Clarke

5. Will psychiatric nurses ever offer mental health nursing?   77
   Commentary: Ann Benson

Part 2 The proper focus of nursing   97

6. Patient participation and the multiple realities of empowerment   99
   Commentary: Cheryl Waters

7. The logic of experience: developing appropriate care
   through effective collaboration   117
   Commentary: Jon Chesterson

8. Rungs on the ladder: creativity and psychic distress   133
   Commentary: Mark Radcliffe

9. Mental health in the new millenium: dreams of a new age of
   enlightenment   151
   Commentaries: Cathy Conroy and David Brandon

Part 3 Reflecting on practice   167

10. The nurse's psychotherapeutic role in caring for people
     in psychosis   *169*
     Commentary: Gloria Novel

11. An overview of clinical supervision   *183*
     Commentary: Mami Kayama

12. Where care meets treatment: common ethical conflicts
     in psychiatric nursing   *199*
     Commentary: Richard Lakeman

13. Prejudice and sexuality   *217*
     Commentary: Steve Jamieson

14. Postscript: the postcard from Gotham   *233*

Index   *249*

Commentators

Dr Suzanne Lego is a nurse psychotherapist in private practice in Pittsburgh, Pennsylvania and in Kent, Ohio, USA. She is also Editor of *Perspectives in Psychiatric Care: The Journal for Nurse Psychotherapists* and is President of the International Organization of Psychotherapists in Nursing.

Dr Hugh McKenna is Professor of Nursing and Director of the Nursing Research Unit at the University of Ulster, Jordanstown, Northern Ireland.

Dr Cheryl Waters is Senior Lecturer in the Department of Nursing at the University of Technology, Sydney, Australia.

Dr Liam Clarke is Senior Lecturer at the University of Sussex, Brighton, England

Jon Chesterson is President of the *Australian and New Zealand College of Mental Health Nurses (ANZCMHN)* and Senior Lecturer in The Department of Staff Development, The Canberra Hospital, Woden, ACT, Australia.

Ann Benson is Director of the *Institute for Psychiatric Nursing Research*, in Parkville, Victoria, Australia

Dr Gloria Novel is Professor of Psychosocial Nursing and Mental Health, and Director of the Masters Programme in Mental Health Nursing, at the School of Nursing, at the University of Barcelona, Spain.

Dr Mami Kayama is a Senior Lecturer in the Department of Community Health Nursing, School of Health Sciences and Nursing, Faculty of Medicine, University of Tokyo, Japan.

Richard Lakeman is Senior Lecturer in the Department of Nursing, Eastern Institute of Technology, Hawkes Bay, New Zealand

Ian Beech is Senior Lecturer at the School of Nursing and Midwifery, University of Glamorgan, Wales.

Dr Colin Holmes is Professor of Mental Health Nursing at the University of Western Sydney and Western Sydney Area Mental Health Service, New South Wales, Australia.

Steve Jamieson is Lecturer/Practitioner HIV–Sexual Health, Maudsley Hospital, London and Adviser for Sexual Health at the Royal College of Nursing, London, England.

Mark Radcliffe is Mental Health Editor at *Nursing Times*, London, England.

Cathy Conroy is a Mental Health Consumer Advocate in Goulburn, New South Wales, Australia

David Brandon is Professor of Community Care at the Anglia Polytechnic University, Cambridge, England

Foreword

When Phil Barker invited me to write a foreword to a collection of some of his papers, I agreed with pleasure. I anticipated a good read and the opportunity to share in the learning experience to which, until now, only a few highly privileged conference-goers had access. Now the manuscript has arrived, I am amply rewarded, but I feel extremely embarrassed to find that in several papers Phil has raised me onto a pedestal. This is an uncomfortable position from which to address a readership. I must ask you to allow me to step down, so that I can fully enter the existential world of psychiatric nurses and of those who seek their help, and so that I can invite you, the reader, to accompany Phil on his explorations.

This book is the publication of thirteen conference papers delivered between 1990 and 1996, some organised by professional people such as nurses, doctors, psychotherapists, some by those who would not regard themselves as belonging to any profession, by carers and people who are recipients of care. Some of these people have held several of these roles, simultaneously or at different periods of life. After each of the papers, one or more people add their commentary.

The joy of this book is that one can take time over each of the papers, a great advantage over being in a conference audience. On can re-read as often as one wishes, one can argue mentally with oneself, with Phil and with the commentators. With every reading one is bound to restructure one's life to some extent. With every reading one moves forward in the understanding of oneself and of others.

Of course, there is some repetition. One of the reasons people are asked to speak at conferences is that their views have become known. The conference organisers wish that these views be conveyed to the participants. Phil talks about himself, his personal background, his career path, about what he has learned from his teachers, his mentors, his family and more than anything else, from his 'patients'. His humanistic ethics, his holistic approach, his attitude to the work with people who have problems, have not changed – they have developed and matured. They are illuminated in each of the papers. However, each of the papers also introduces something new. Collectively, these papers reveal an immense range of interests and a vast domain to which Phil's work is relevant.

Phil's knowledge of art, literature, philosophy, history and anthropology, added to the depth of his mastery of psychiatric nursing, psychology and medical science, create the unique and idiosyncratic character of his work.

This collection of papers can be read as one narrative, starting at the beginning and ending with the postscript. I think readers may gain more if they tackle one paper at a time and spend at least as much effort on reflection after each paper as was spent reading. A lot might even be gained from a return to earlier papers at a later stage.

Phil's curiosity has never waned, his uncertainty has grown, his capacity for learning is infinite. Readers will, I think, find his thoughts infectious and addictive.

1999   Annie T Altschul

Preface

In loving your people and governing your state,
Are you able to dispense with cleverness?
In the opening and shutting of heaven's gate,
Are you able to play the feminine part?
Enlightened and seeing far into all directions
Can you at the same time remain detached and non-active?[1]

I am not ashamed to say that, when I entered nursing almost thirty years ago, it was by no means a career choice. It was the tail-end of the 1960s. The heightened optimism that had gripped my generation was waning fast, and many of my wild young friends were already hatching nest eggs. I remained earnest and unrealistic. Some of my friends and colleagues might say that was a feature of my personality that has not waned over the years.

My sights had been firmly set, since boyhood, on becoming a painter and sculptor. The 1960s were spent first at art school, then spliced precariously between working as a mural painter and illustrator, and in various labouring jobs: on the railway and building site, and in the factory and iron foundry. By 1969, I had been in and out of higher education and the 'university of life' and was unsure which had taught me more.

At the beginning of 1970, I was a young father, a husband and unemployed, when I was offered a job as an 'attendant at the asylum'. This turned out to be a nursing assistant's post in an old, but still proud, hospital, but such niceties meant little to the Labour Exchange clerk. So, I stepped out of the strong sunlight on a prematurely spring-like day, and stepped into the dank gloom of a long-term ward. I felt like – and probably appeared like – a creature from another world. Not only did I have some basic academic qualifications from school, unlike all the nurses who encircled me, but I had been to art school – like the Beatles!

The gulf between my new colleagues and me was as obvious as it was wide. Years later, an academic colleague would tell me how he had earned the nickname 'Professor' at his remote Scottish training asylum, on the strength of his ownership of two O-levels! I reassured myself that I was 'only passing through'. My sights remained firmly set on becoming an artist.

Although there were progressive psychiatric establishments, and there were some 'famous names' in psychiatric nursing, few of my colleagues knew, or cared for, either. They belonged to a largely closed, inward-looking order, heavily influenced by nepotism and family ties. I appeared to be the only staff member who did not have family or old friends working somewhere in the hospital. I felt on these first few days very much like Camus' *outsider* in more ways than one. Yet despite my odd background and perhaps odder ideas about life, I was warmly accepted and began to gain a feel for this thing called nursing and these people called patients.

These memories seem an appropriate place to begin this book since, thirty years on – or in the blinking of an eye – I have become the 'professor' so warmly ridiculed by my friend's asylum colleagues. I never harboured any academic pretensions in those days and, despite the challenging path I have trodden down the years, have led a most fortunate life.[2] However, in many respects I remain that wide-eyed young man who stepped out of the certain spring sunlight, into the insecure shadows of the institution. I had no idea what I would find there, but fuelled – nonetheless – by my own uncertainties, I stepped gladly from the light into the gloom. Within an hour or so, I was fascinated – what on earth was going on here? By the next day, I had become intrigued – who are these people and what has happened to them? Soon I was to become captivated. The appetite for understanding had begun to grumble deep within me. Having spent my formative years learning how to express myself, through the arts, I found myself wondering how these people might help me understand some of the meaning of their distressing lives. As I look back down those years, I appreciate only too well that my attempts to understand them were no more than vain attempts to understand myself.

Thirty years on, the hollowness of my ignorance needs constant feeding, and I remain largely unsatisfied. I remain uncertain of what it means to be 'a person' far less a 'person with any kind of mental disorder'. Having devoted so much of my life to pursuing certainty of some kind, I now appear to be comfortable at last with uncertainty. The whole chaotic order of my life, if not life in general, appears increasingly transparent to me. That said, I would not pretend that I have not gained knowledge down the years. Indeed, at various points I have misled myself into thinking that I knew either something that I did not know, or otherwise had developed – what might be called in the trade – a set of over-valued ideas. However, the ignorance, and the need to try to satisfy it, came back incessantly to haunt me, and so I became something of a philosopher.

My father and grandfather were two men who combined the warmth of nurture with the boundary of discipline. Both men had mentored me in my youth, although I had little appreciation that I had sought, far less received, their different gifts of wisdom. These two remarkable men helped me appreciate that life was an answer waiting for the right questions. It was at their feet and by their side that I became, like them, a philosopher. Perhaps not a *proper* philosopher, some would say, but, looking back, Joe and Old Phil looked like proper philosophers to me. Like them, I became a practised innocent abroad. I became someone who would end up spending much of his life asking damn, fool, silly questions. The rest of the time I would spend reflecting on what any of the answers might mean. It has been my good fortune to spend much of my life standing in god's sunlight, unlike many of those with whom I have worked. That fortune even extended to being blessed with the opportunity to earn a good living, asking damn, fool, silly questions.

These reflections serve as an apposite introduction to this book. This is a collection of some of my most recurrent questions, the earliest piece representing thoughts I had been toying with since the end of the 1980s. Ten years earlier, at the end of the 1970s. I had been focusing most of my psychiatric nursing career on learning various kinds of psychotherapy and had ended up honing my skills as a cognitive and behavioural psychotherapist. At the tail end of the 1970s I embarked on what was to become a ten-year association with women with diagnoses of psychotic depression or manic depressive psychosis. I used the experience to develop more skills in couple, group and family work and sharpened my focus on understanding better the cognitive model of depression, which I saw as 'the answer' to these women's distress. My doctoral research was built around this group of women, and I eventually completed what probably was the first randomised control trial of cognitive therapy with people with manic depression.[3] After ten years working closely with this group of women, both as therapist and researcher, I realised that I was losing my faith in the certainty of psychological models – like those underpinning cognitive therapy. I began to sense a need to gain a sense of something more fragile and diffuse than 'negative automatic thoughts' or 'dysfunctional beliefs', which appeared to unite these women in distress. In time, I was to sense this also in men who were in psychosis. I was beginning to return to the point at which I stepped from the spring sunlight into the shadows of psychiatry. In my relationships with the people in my care, or who were my 'research subjects', I was beginning to become their student, rather than their adviser.

In returning to the roots of my uncertainty, I was – once again – learning, from patients, something of what it meant to be 'in mental distress'. The lessons I have learned over the past fifteen years from the people in my care have served as the key stimulus for this book. Those people have taught me the importance of the 'uncertainty principle' and, more importantly, that the answers which we seek in mental health care are to be found in our relationships *with* the people in our care, rather than in our *delivery* to them of any therapy or care. I learned the wisdom of Harry Stack Sullivan's dictum, made in relation to working with people in psychosis, that we 'are all more alike than different'. I learned the wisdom of that lesson in my relationships with people in severe mental distress. As I write this preface I am acutely aware of the debt of gratitude I owe to those many women and men who helped me appreciate the need to journey with them, rather than simply pull them back from the jaws of madness. I thank them all for the gift so freely given.

I was privileged when Churchill Livingstone gave me the opportunity to put together the idea for this book. It was, perhaps, an unusual proposal: to publish a set of papers that, originally, were given as 'talks', adding, for good measure, brief commentaries – or reflections – by colleagues, who also are friends, from around the world.[4] For two of the chapters, I was torn between two dear friends and took the soft option of including both of them. The resulting mixture of chapters and commentaries is as diverse as, I hope, it is stimulating. Given that all the papers were written originally for 'speaking', they come in my own 'voice', which at times can be an irreverent and perhaps strident one. One of my regrets as an academic, however, is that the literature can often appear stuffy, contrived or soulless. This is unfortunate, when the human experiences – which inevitably lie at the heart of our work – are so very much alive and anarchic. I hope that these reflections on the philosophy and practice of psychiatric and mental health nursing will echo some of the reflections that have gone on in the minds of the reader. I hope that we shall come to appreciate that our philosophies of care and practice are more alike than different.

Consequently, the publication of this book is yet another chapter in my fortunate life. I thank Alex Mathieson warmly for asking me to put together these essays and for giving me the free rein to complete this work, which perhaps reflects parts of me which have not yet appeared in print. I thank him also for letting me express my confusion and uncertainty, as well as my wild ambition for the development of a human science of caring in mental health. I also thank Dinah Thom for keeping me to time and Jackie Curthoys for helping me bring the whole project, finally, to fruition.

I thank all my colleagues down the years who have helped me, in their own distinctive ways, to reach this point in my professional life. A special thanks goes to my closest colleagues at the University of Newcastle – the late Dr Phil Hearne and Drs Chris Stevenson and Shaun Parsons – for their collegiate support. I am also indebted to my academic nursing friends from around the world for challenging my thinking without challenging 'me' too harshly. Some of my current research and clinical colleagues also deserve special mention for helping keep my mind on the more practical aspects of the 'proper focus of nursing': Vanessa Black, Elsa Conway, Ben Davidson, Mike Davison, Brendan Hill, Sue Jackson, Mary Lewis, Ann McKenzie, Steven Michael, Alan Steele and Louise Walker. I also thank my many doctoral and masters students for helping me explore areas of mental health which, without their prompting, would have escaped my attention. I also thank all the conference organisers who played an invisible, yet critical part, in generating this collection of papers. Our mutual interdependence is noted with respect. A special thanks goes to the colleagues, whom I can also count as friends, from the mental health consumer, survivor and advocacy movements: Dr Irene Whitehill, Peter Campbell, Louise Pembroke and Karen Campbell from England; Sally Clay, Judi Chamberlin and Ed Manos from the USA; and Cathy Conroy and Simon Champ from Australia.

Finally, I thank my 'soulmate' Poppy who has journeyed with me down the past thirty-five years. Her contribution is deeply embedded in many of these papers. Over the years, I have picked up many a jewel fallen from her lips and swallowed it as my own. At many points in my papers can be heard echoes of her very distinctive voice. I thank her for her generosity of spirit as well as her intuitive wisdom.

I have been fortunate to meet many people down the years who have read my various published thoughts. Thankfully, not all of them agreed with what I had to say. I hope that at some point I may meet some of the readers of this book and you too might, politely, take issue with me. Until then, I thank you for taking the time to pick up my thoughts on the philosophy and practice of psychiatric and mental health nursing.

Dia dhuit[5]

1999   Phil Barker
                                                    Newport-on-Tay, Scotland

1. Lao Tzu *Tao Teh Ching* (trans J C H Wu). Shambhala, London
2. Albert Facey was described as 'Australia's pilgrim'. Facey wrote about life as if it were a journey. Along his route, crossroads offered crucial choices – in some senses his very survival was at stake – and the tracks he followed led to learning, pain and enrichment. Uneducated, he taught himself to read and write and, in his eighties, he wrote a book which integrated all his extraordinary experiences of struggle, war and great losses, and which he described as 'a fortunate life'. I am indebted to my friends Kevin and Cheryl Kellehear of Sydney for giving my wife Poppy and I a copy when last we met (Facey AB 1981 *A fortunate life*. Harmondsworth, Penguin Books.
3. Barker P 1987 *An evaluation of specific nursing interventions in the management of patients suffering from manic depressive psychosis*. Dundee Institute of Technology (University of Abertay), Scotland, unpublished PhD thesis.
4. I am grateful for the friendly, sometimes challenging, but always scholarly way my colleagues have commented on my thinking.
5. In the Gaelic greeting – 'may God be with you'.

Part 1
The nature of nursing

I have been wondering about the nature of psychiatric nursing for as long as I have been a nurse. Given the *focus* of psychiatric nursing – the call for compassion and understanding, if not also courage in the face of extreme forms of distress – I have wondered about these too, for much longer. Where psychiatric nursing came from and where it might be going, offers much potential for reflection, despite the efforts of many to suggest that the story is complete, that the formula for success is clear.

In some senses, the themes, which are traced in the first five chapters, all possess the same root: they are about history – our nursing past, our professional selves in the making and the history we might create tomorrow. They also address the context within which nursing has grown, indeed continues to grow. In particular, I wonder aloud about the possibility of ever defining *one* kind of psychiatric nursing, far less employing *one* knowledge base upon which to found a brave new profession of psychiatric caring.

In this respect I remind myself that the world of human distress is infinitely richer than any of its explanatory models and theories. In the same vein, Nasr noted that:

> 'Nature is altogether richer than the knowledge which physics arrives at through its quantitative methods which are selective in both their data and the interpretation of these data … Likewise, the very fact that its conclusions are based on experiments implies that their validity holds only within the conditions of those experiments … Physics, like all the other sciences of nature is a particular science of things, legitimate within its own assumptions and limitations, but it is not the only valid science of the natural world … That is why the application of a science which neglects these elements causes disequilibrium and brings about disorder and ugliness, especially in a world where other sciences of nature do not exist and where there is no wisdom or sapientia which could place the quantitative sciences in their proper position in the total scheme of knowledge.'

The search to establish, once and for all, the essence of nursing, and to prove its value, especially through the exercise of the scientific method, may distract us from reflecting on the virtue of diversity. It may also divert us from continuing to feed and nurture the principles of caring which are centuries old and may be the birthright of nursing as a social activity, if not a professional discipline. An over-earnest fascination with trying to narrow the definition of nursing, may dislocate us from the natural wisdom (*sapientia*), which has long infused nursing practice.

In the following chapters, I trace some of my wonderment as to the implications and foundations of the searching which goes on in nursing – a process of searching to which I have contributed some of my own energies, often to succeed only in muddying further the waters.

REFERENCE
Nasr SH 1990 *Man and nature: the spiritual crisis in modern man* Unwin, London, pp 119–120

Psychoanalysis and psychiatric nursing: a bridge too far?

Having been a psychiatric nurse for just over a quarter century, I shall use this time frame as the basis for reflecting on the history of psychiatric nursing and the place of psychoanalytic concepts within nursing. I hope that the reader will forgive me if I use this time frame both as an objective and a personal anchor. Although a tendency for self-disclosure can irritate, I hope that my blending of personal and consensual realities will not only be more acceptable here but, more importantly, might serve as a metaphor for our understanding and appreciation of the place of psychoanalytic theory and practice within psychiatric nursing.

The year of my birth – 1946 – affords a further personal and objective anchor for this chapter. Grayce Sills, the distinguished North American nurse, has described 1946 as the 'year of fulfillment' (Sills 1974). That year marked the beginning of the graduate programmes for psychiatric nurses in the USA which, at one and the same time, prepared those nurses who were to become that country's nurse leaders, and 'set the stage' for the importance of the one-to-one nurse–patient relationship. Perhaps more significantly, that 'year of fulfillment' marked the orchestrated introduction of psychoanalytic concepts into graduate nurse education. I regret to say that it has been my experience that few contemporary British psychiatric nurses appreciate that the history of the nurse as an agent of psychotherapy spans more than a decade or two. Many might be surprised to hear that nursing's history within this domain of practice is, like me, almost a half century old. Given these historical parameters, I hope that you will also forgive me if I confine myself to a brief discussion of the *nursing* consideration of psychoanalytic principles, or the application of such principles to the *practice* of psychiatric nursing. This audience may well already be conversant with the outline of this nursing history. I hope, however, to provide some detail based on my good fortune to have had personal encounters with some of the key players on this historical stage from 1946 to the present day: Peplau, Altschul, Lego, Beeber, Sills and Smoyak. Again, I hope that what may be a self-indulgent blending of personal and consensual evaluations of their contributions, will add an important dimension to our discussion of those who helped build the bridge from our therapeutic past to our present practices.

At the outset, I need to declare that the subject – 'nursing and psychoanalysis' – presents me with some problems. It would be fair to say that I am no more certain of what is, or is not, psychoanalysis, than I am certain of the definition and constituents of nursing. That said, I shall adopt the pragmatic position first mapped by Freud when he anticipated the need to:

'alloy the pure gold of analysis freely with the copper of suggestion'

noting also that whatever form this might take

> *'the most important ingredients will assuredly remain those borrowed from strict and untendentious psychoanalysis' (Freud 1919: cited by Brown and Pedder 1991).*

I need also to declare that my interest lies in exploring how psychoanalytic concepts – however pure or alloyed – might clarify our understanding of the nature and functions of psychiatric nursing. This somewhat precious interest may explain, in retrospect, the delimited nature of the history I lay before you, and my interpretation of the significance of these events.

I am a child of the 60s. I became a fine-art student in 1965 and soon was swallowed up in the heady atmosphere of the counterculture that appeared to enlighten the gloom of my post-war childhood and adolescence; a light that faded, almost as rapidly as it had begun. By the time I entered psychiatric nursing, as a second career option in 1970, I had digested all of Ronnie Laing's work which *was*, to my art school generation, rightly or wrongly, contemporary psychoanalysis. I entered a school of nursing that acted as if the 60s had never happened, a view that extended to include a denial of the existence of Laing and his fellow travellers. I mention Laing mainly as another anchoring point, since I believe that he symbolised the critical, if unacknowledged, historical linchpin for many of our contemporary ambitions in psychiatric care. Laing, as his erstwhile colleague Joe Berke observed, 'put the person back into the patient'. This was an important contribution for the 60s generation who realised, at long last, that the personal was political. I could not fail to mention, also, that Laing was a Scot. The psychiatric establishment in Britain first rejected, then vilified, Laing. His failure to maintain his reputation in later life may speak volumes for the paradoxical nature of Laing's relationship to the self and himself. My nation's difficulty with home-bred heroes is an enduring characteristic of Celtic psychopathology. Only in death do heroes ever come home applauded by all. For Laing, I suspect that belated applause may only be building.

So, I entered psychiatric nursing with the assumption that although its meanings might often be elusive, human experience was fundamentally meaningful. On reflection it would appear that much of what was passed to me as the received wisdom of psychiatric nursing involved 'explaining away' the phenomenon of the person-who-is-patient. Needless to say my school of nursing showed no evidence of having heard of Peplau – the acknowledged 'mother of psychiatric nursing' – nor any of the other great North American theorists who were beginning to dominate the nursing debate on this side of the Atlantic.[1]

'much of what was passed to me as the received wisdom of psychiatric nursing involved "explaining away" the phenomenon of the person-who-is-patient'

However, by 1970 the name of Annie T Altschul – whose contribution I shall address later – was beginning to be treated with respect. Altschul represented, in my view, the key link between the academic power of

North American psychiatric nursing and the emerging British interest in the application of interpersonal theory in nursing: arguably still the most potent alloy of the psychoanalytic method with which nurses have been associated (Barker 1995).

The psychiatric hospital outside the town in Scotland where I trained, was characterised by three features. First, it ran a small therapeutic community that, as the specialist clinical setting, was the jewel in the crown of the hospital. Second, it had a very dynamic child and adolescent service led by another *Philip Barker*, the child psychiatrist who left for Canada the year after I began training. Finally, the medical service was – like all of Scottish psychiatry at the time – greatly influenced by Adolf Meyer's psychobiology. At that time this was expressed through the clinical leadership of Sir Ivor Batchelor, the Professor of Psychiatry. I mention these three characteristics only to point to stars that faded. The therapeutic community died in that hospital at the end of the 1970s – and today is a very weak force nationally. Meyer's legacy went with the Professor's retirement – a pattern replicated no doubt with the passing of all his contemporaries; and the child and adolescent service gradually took up the peripheral position evident in most mental health services today. As we consider the discreet history of psychoanalytic influences on psychiatric nursing, we might remember that other – influential, or pivotal – features of the psychiatric service scene have been removed to the touchlines or have otherwise faded from view. We might consider whether – like some exiled monarch – they too are waiting on the opportunity to return, or merely have been starved of the critical consideration that is the lifeblood of any construct of the human condition. We might consider if this also applies to the status of the psychoanalytic method in contemporary mental health care.

The career of Hildegard Peplau will serve as the beginning and endpoint for my short historical overview. Peplau became a psychoanalyst at the William Alanson White Institute in New York in 1953. She had graduated in the late 1940s with a BA in Interpersonal Psychology, an experience which paved the way for the development of her interest in the work of Harry Stack Sullivan, whom she met at Chestnut Lodge whilst training under Frieda Fromm-Reichman's supervision. Fromm-Reichman's belief that the aloofness of patients with schizophrenia was an interpersonal defence against a repetition of the rebuffs suffered in childhood, made a great impact on Peplau. The emphasis on patience and optimism shared by Fromm-Reichman and Sullivan, and the belief that deterioration in psychotic patients was not necessarily inevitable, resulted in the development of Sullivan's emphasis on the underlying emotional and cognitive factors which promote withdrawal from interpersonal relationships. This emphasis may well be the true ancestor of today's interpersonal therapy, if not also, cognitive therapy for people with schizophrenia.[2]

Peplau recalled how, after the publication in 1952 of her book *Interpersonal Relations in Nursing*, it took nurses some time to develop the motivation and ability to study themselves as part of the patient's world (Barker 1993). It is ironic that Peplau should have published her interpersonal relations text the year before Sullivan, with whom she never enjoyed a direct working relationship, given that he was – in her words – 'pretty much anti-women'. More importantly, her use of the theory of interpersonal relations within nursing went from strength to strength, whilst Sullivan's star faded, and is perhaps only now beginning to be the subject of a realistic reappraisal.[3]

What Peplau shared with Sullivan and Fromm-Reichman was an optimistic interest in the potential of therapeutic relationships with, arguably, the most troubled people within the psychiatric hospital. I have visited Greystone Park Hospital in New Jersey where Peplau supervised her students in their one-to-one work with psychotic patients in the 1950s and 1960s. At that time the hospital had over 8000 patients, with more than a hundred to a ward on any of the five floors of the main block. It was here that Peplau took patients into broom cupboards and stairwells – anywhere which might allow the necessary space and privacy to serve as the natural boundaries for intersubjective discourse. Peplau's establishment of a theory-based process of interpersonal nursing has often been misunderstood or misrepresented (e.g. Gournay 1995) – and has been noted and commented upon by Peplau herself (Barker 1993). Such misrepresentations may well form part of the destiny of all who merit iconic status in any field. What is beyond question, is that Peplau's development of the one-to-one nursing relationship, the concept of the therapeutic milieu and her constant focus on the human experience[4] of mental distress, has become so much a part of the process of psychiatric nursing that this will surely represent her timeless legacy.

In her 86th year, Hilda Peplau continues to maintain her interest in psychotic disorders and continues to develop her appreciation of the use of interpersonal relations with this group. Last year she published a provocative argument that the five key symptoms associated with schizophrenia – anxiety, delusions, hallucinations, language-thought disorder, the self and withdrawal – should be reframed as *human responses* (Peplau 1994). Such a view may well close the loop which threads back through Laing's personal (and interpersonal) focus in the 1960s to Sullivan's dictum that 'we are all more simply human than otherwise'.

Although it has often been argued that Peplau's use of interpersonal theory is too complex, a careful reading of her work reveals not only a disarmingly clear explication of the theory but most useful practical applications. Describing the resistance of the self-system in psychosis to change, she suggested that nurses should bypass the operative system; by use of instrumental statements which address the *process* rather than the *contents* of the self-system.

> '[Such] verbal contrivances [are] most likely to evoke interest, effort and eventually the use of latent capability for self-change by patients' (Peplau 1991).

Her investigative questions, posed at the point when a problematic self-view is presented by the patient, possess a remarkable elegance – stripped of unnecessary technique – and pivot around the kind of curiosity which characterises the best examples of scientific inquiry.

'When did you get that idea?'
'What's the source of that notion about you?'
'When did you first think of yourself in that way?'
'What's the evidence for that self-reference?'
'Illustrate that!'
'Describe one time that view applied to you.'
'What do you get out of thinking that way about yourself?'
'What's the point of classifying yourself that way?'
(Peplau 1991:119)

It is interesting that many British nurses are beginning to use such lines of enquiry, *not* within an interpersonal model of therapy, but within the cognitive therapy model.[5] Many are, perhaps, blissfully unaware that Peplau first published such examples of Socratic dialogue within nursing, a decade before the formal birth of Beck's cognitive therapy within psychiatric medicine (Beck 1976). Many of today's nurses are, all too-often, obsessed with acquiring skills and technique (See Michael 1994). They may be unaware that Peplau's approach, through acknowledging the complexity of these human responses, provides an elegant means for exploring the potential for resolution that lies *within* the person *and* the person's interpersonal relations with self and others.

> 'Peplau's approach, through acknowledging the complexity of... human responses, provides an elegant means for exploring the potential for resolution that lies *within* the person *and* the person's interpersonal relations with self and others'

Peplau's approach to nursing – which she channelled initially into the one-to-one relationship and the milieu – has achieved the status of a philosophy, with its emphasis on the primary status of patients as people.[6] Unlike much contemporary rhetoric about personhood and personal needs, Peplau's philosophy is supported by a theory that affords the opportunity for experimental investigation. Peplau regrets that she did not undertake this herself, and only a small number of her students have attempted to validate the practical utility of the theory through research (e.g. Forchuk 1992).[7] It should not be forgotten, however, that Peplau did not stand alone in early 1950s America. Consider the following proposal:

> *'the nurse has to become an acute observer, who maintains an active curiosity and a habit of asking questions about her own and the patient's feelings and behaviour and an interest in developing insight into her own and other persons' stereotyped ways of thinking about and behaving with patients.'*

The same authors suggested that the 'careful observation of small changes in a patient that could be built upon and expanded is a significant part of the process'. These quotes illustrate the value of *curiosity*, especially curiosity about interpersonal relationships. Through inquiring into the nature of relating, both nurse and patient may grow more knowledgeable about what exactly is going on between them, and *within* them. With such enquiry might come the understanding both seek.

Those authors – Morris Schwartz, a sociologist, and Emmy Lanning Shockley, a nurse – published those North American views in 1956. Their book, *The Nurse and the Mental Patient*, was based upon a research project carried out between 1952 and 1953 in which the ways nurses related to patients were examined and an attempt was made to assess the effect these relationships had upon the patients' mental health. Their examples of recurring clinical problems, and the interpersonal processes common to problem situations, are disarmingly similar to those encountered today, despite the changes witnessed in the past forty years. Despite all that has changed, most important things have remained the same. That fact may be a disturbing reminder that the proper focus of psychiatric nursing remains unchanged and we may need, therefore, to return to the path from which we might have strayed (cf. Barker et al. 1995).

One of Peplau's students – Suzanne Lego – developed further the use of psychoanalytic theory in nursing practice in the 1960s. In 1974, she published an important review of the development of the concept of the one-to-one relationship, between 1946 and 1974 (Lego 1974). That review summarised neatly some of the conflicts that emerged, in the early 1960s between those nurses who believed in the potential of nurses as psychotherapeutic agents, and those who were uncomfortable with nurses dealing with unconscious material. Although nurses in the UK continue to fumble with notions of advanced nursing practice,[8] Lego's review noted that, as early as 1958, Peplau and Muller had introduced the concept of the clinical nurse specialist, prepared at master's level, who concentrated on the psychotherapeutic role. This fired the controversy over the hypothetical 'over-extension' of the nurse's role 'into the province of psychoanalysis'. In the same year, Dorothea Richter Hays conducted a survey of the nursing literature from 1946 to 1958 from which she developed suggestions for the 'clinical practice of psychiatric nurses'. Hays observed that there existed 'a dearth of interest in the psychiatric nurse's role of therapist before 1958' (Hays 1958: cited by Lego 1974). She also revealed, however, that terms such as the 'therapeutic use of self', 'therapeutic nurse–patient relationships', 'psychiatric nursing therapy', 'supportive psychotherapy' and 'nondirective counselling' all had attained some currency in the post-war years. In her review, Lego observed that it was 'fair to say that most if not all, of the published literature in the one-to-one patient relationship which has come from nursing theory', had been inspired by the work of three nurses. June Mellow had drawn on psychoanalytic theory in her work with schizophrenic patients, which emphasised the provision of a corrective emotional experience. Ida Jean Orlando had sought to help all patients 'express the specific meaning of his behaviour in order to ascertain his distress' (Lego 1974). The third was, of course, Peplau who in Lego's view was clearly the most influential figure in the late 1950s and early 1960s: a time when

> *'most psychiatric nursing text books, while emphasizing the nurse–patient relationship, base nursing action on* non-nursing theory, *particularly psychoanalytic or sociocultural theory' (Lego 1974: emphasis added).*

The contributions of Mellow, Orlando and especially Peplau took psychiatric nursing into a new realm, where the pure gold of psychoanalysis was alloyed specifically with the discrete processes of psychiatric nursing. This involved clarification of, firstly, the physical intimacy between nurse and patient and, later, the social milieu managed by the nursing team.

By the beginning of the 1960s, North American psychiatric nurses had begun to refine further their appreciation of the discrete processes involved in the one-to-one relationship: from Shirley Smoyak's examination of non-verbal behaviour to Dorothea Hays' concept of *waiting*, which she developed as a specific therapeutic technique (Hays 1963). It would be inappropriate here to do other than isolate some key themes emergent from Lego's review of that period, which may have some bearing on our situation today. Notably, Lego observed that one half of all the 166 papers she reviewed from that 18 year period were written by students and faculty colleagues of Hilda Peplau, suggesting that an enclave of sorts existed. More importantly, she noted that nurses who wrote about 'a specific topic rarely review nursing literature on the subject, although they often do review non-nursing theory'. This suggested that 'psychiatric nurses still do not respect one another sufficiently to examine and build upon one another's work' (Lego 1974). I find this observation reassuring, since before I discovered the North American literature, I had believed that the over-respectful references to the medical and psychological literature, often found in this country's nursing literature, signified a British disease. If the bridge between psychoanalysis and nursing is shaky in Britain, this may be due, in part, to our failure to strengthen the structure through the proper collegiate mentality. At the risk of mixing my metaphors, such collegiality would require us to explore and document the unique nursing progeny that might issue from such relationships.

The North American nurses of the post-war era also began to report increasingly on their work with groups (Nakagawa 1974) and their use of milieu therapy (Sills 1974). In the period before the widespread introduction of psychotropic drugs, nurses began to write about the importance of developing congruence between the work of the nurse and the doctor, and later the social worker (Gregg 1954). The interest in ways of encouraging patient participation in the nurse-controlled milieu, led indirectly to various *patient government* projects. Notable among these was the Boston Psychopathic Hospital in the early 1950s, which made an invisible link – through Maxwell Jones – to some British nurses, like Annie Altschul, and the concept of the therapeutic community. The precocious talent of North American psychiatric nurses was to find a new outlet in those post-war years in the development of family therapy. I am aware that a psychoanalytic audience may well view family therapy almost as a base metal. However, Shirley Smoyak's review (1974) of this development in the USA illustrates clearly the lineage that extended from intrapsychic theory, through interpersonal theory to systems theory. By 1968 Smoyak had observed that nurses had ceased describing their role merely as a referring agent, but had begun to illustrate their discrete role as a family therapist (Rohde 1968), especially within the province of child and adolescent psychiatry. Smoyak displayed her incisive intelligence in this review when she noted that family therapy could, however, become an ideology: 'Surely', she noted:

'there must be instances when the appropriate treatment is of the subsystem rather than the total. Too little thought has been given to identifying the appropriate therapeutic modality based on specific criteria. Family may not always be the most relevant system for an individual' (Smoyak 1974).

We may well face the same challenge today in choosing between ideologies of treatment provision – whether these are politically or institutionally driven. Perhaps the consideration of when and where the gap between psychoanalysis and nursing *can* or *should* be bridged, will be one of the emergent questions from contemporary debate.

So far, this has been wholly an American tale. But what was the situation in Britain within the same era? How deep are the roots of the relationship between psychoanalysis and psychiatric nursing in the UK? Gary Winship has observed, correctly in my view, that it is only within recent years that a psychoanalytic approach has been articulated in the teaching of nurses (Winship 1995). I think by that he means *formal* teaching, with a formal curriculum, since even my generation of students had some teaching, although it was diluted, often to homeopathic levels. The nursing literature that addresses psychoanalytic themes specifically, is limited indeed. The earliest significant report in the British literature – Elizabeth Barnes' editing of the studies from the Cassel Hospital, *Psychosocial Nursing* – was compiled as a tribute to Tom Main, the medical director of the hospital. This tribute, of itself, may well help us understand the nature of the relationship between nursing and psychoanalysis in the UK, and may offer some reasons why it has taken so long for nursing to establish any kind of identity within the broad church of psychoanalysis.[9] It is of course also interesting that the story of psychosocial nursing at the Cassel also had its origins in the year of 1946, when Main took up his directorship: that magical year in which the story related here began.

Elizabeth Barnes' book highlights two main differences between the British and North American experiences of psychoanalysis. As noted earlier, Peplau was able to observe Sullivan's work, but not to work *with* him. This may have fostered her natural independence, from which developed an independent nursing theory of interpersonal relations, and a very autonomous school of nurses who were influenced by psychoanalysis, but which did not *belong* to psychoanalysis. The English nurses' affectionate regard for Main, who explicated the importance of the nurse–patient relationship *on behalf of nurses*, comes through most clearly in the writing of the Cassel nurses in Barnes text. Main may well have been (unwittingly?) the *symbolic* father figure of psychosocial nursing. We should not forget, however, that he was not *of* nursing, and the potential dependency on Main and his influence may well be a significant part of the resulting history. Peplau, by contrast, was both a nurse and a psychoanalyst and was later rightly recognised as the *actual* 'mother of psychiatric nursing'. The symbolism attached to these respective relationships will hardly be lost on psychoanalysts.

The other difference lay in the differing foci of Main and Peplau. The Cassel dealt mainly with people described as neurotic. As I have noted, many North American nurses had explored the application of psycho-analytic approaches across the whole range of patients and situations. Peplau's interest had begun in 1946, however, with people at the more severe end of the mental illness spectrum: people in psychosis. Those early experiences were to set the tone for much of what was to follow. As a result, the North American nurses possess a burgeoning literature describing the focus on the patient in psychosis, whereas in Britain this interest is only beginning to be explored at last in print.

A recent paper by Gary Winship teases out some of the psychoanalytic influences within the family tree of nursing. As he observed, appropriately, it is possible to trace the development of psychoanalysis within *psychiatry* from the beginning of this century. However, judging how and when psychoanalytic influences were felt in British nursing is difficult, if not impossible. This situation is, clearly, a reflection of the paucity of the literature, as Winship noted. Indeed it is not until the early 1970s, when Eileen Skellern moved to the Maudsley, and built on her earlier experience of working with Maxwell Jones at the Henderson Hospital, that a psycho*dynamic*, if not entirely psycho*analytic* approach to psychiatric nursing appeared to emerge with any clarity. The outcome of Skellern's influence is only now beginning to be reported, and Winship's recent work summarises some of the important source references.

It has been my good fortune to have enjoyed a relationship with both Hilda Peplau and Annie Altschul, both having served as mentors. This has allowed me to compare the respective influences of Peplau and Altschul on American and British psychiatric nursing. My tentative conclusion is that, whereas Peplau's legacy is clearly described in the American literature, the British have not yet clarified the importance of the contribution made by Altschul to the development of all forms of psychosocial nursing in the UK. This includes the accommodation of psychoanalytic ideas.

Annie Therese Altschul was a young Jewish student when she fled to London from Austria in 1937. Her intention was always to return home once the Nazi threat abated. After working in various menial positions – as nanny or housemaid – she began training as a general nurse but was seduced by her experiences in psychiatry, and the rest is history. Altschul's training was completed towards the end of the Second World War and she was evacuated from the Maudsley Hospital, along with her patients, to Mill Hill, a boarding school on the outskirts of London. It was here that she first worked with Maxwell Jones, who was only beginning to develop his notions of the milieu and therapeutic community. In Altschul's view, the therapeutic system of nursing at Mill Hill in 1944 was farther advanced than any system of nursing she has seen since (Barker 1995). The presence of a military wing meant that any patients who proved particularly difficult were controlled by military discipline. As a result, the nurses had a free hand to try any kind of therapeutic approach which they saw fit. Altschul's fascination with the Mill Hill experience was curtailed when everyone was

'[Altschul] has maintained to this day her belief that a therapeutic system where the *whole life* of the patient is accommodated, is the most appropriate way to be of genuine help to the mentally ill'

returned to the Maudsley. However, she has maintained to this day her belief that a therapeutic system, where the *whole life* of the patient is accommodated, is the most appropriate way to be of genuine help to the mentally ill.

Altschul's description of her early experiences at the Maudsley with people experiencing severe psychosis – long before the advent of the phenothiazines – is both interesting and significant within the context of this history. Describing her experience of working with such people she observed that she:

> '*attempted to understand what people were trying to say ... perhaps they were not expressing in the sort of words which were easily understood but there was some meaning behind what they were trying to say*' (Barker 1995).

In that sense she was reflecting Orlando's theoretical position mentioned earlier. It is also worth noting that her reading outside nursing heightened Altschul's fascination with the language of psychosis.

> '*I recall working with a very crazy woman – one of the craziest women I ever met, then or since. At the time I was trying to read James Joyce in the evenings and I remember one day thinking how both of them appeared to be speaking in much the same kind of a language. I didn't know what that meant but it interested me*' (Barker 1995).

Altschul's interest in – and direct experience of – people in psychosis, and the 'meaning behind what they were trying to say', was developed greatly in her own teaching. This interest and experience has not, however, been reported adequately.[10] I hope, by suggesting some of the theoretical parameters of her territory of influence, to remedy this to some extent.

Unlike our North American cousins, British nurses were aware that they were the subject of some influence from the psychoanalytic paradigm, but were largely ignorant of the individuals – like Altschul – who served as the medium for such influences.

It is interesting also to note that Altschul went to the USA in the early 1960s and studied under Peplau at Rutgers, where she had been Professor of Nursing, for almost a decade. Altschul is without doubt the *grande dame* of British psychiatric nursing. In much the same way that Peplau shrinks back from the title of 'mother of psychiatric nursing', I suspect that Altschul would be uncomfortable with the accolade of the British 'grande dame of psychiatric nursing'. Such modesty, however, may only increase, rather than diminish, her importance.

I have often noted that Hilda Peplau, Annie Altschul and my other dear friend Shirley Smoyak all originated from within a hundred miles of one another: on the fringes of the old Austro-Hungarian Empire.[11] It does not seem any accident to me that the psychoanalytic *message* should have been carried, so ably, by three people whose very 'selves' were shaped by the genetic and cultural influences of the geographical cradle of modern psychiatry and psychoanalysis. It may be premature to observe that – like the European intellectual tradition – we may not see their likes again. I hope that I am wrong.

Before concluding, I should bring this delimited history in some way up to date. I need to ask, to what extent has anything changed over the past twenty years, especially in the USA which, if we have any sense, we shall use as a model for our professional, if not also our intellectual development. Many of the threads of psychiatric nursing development which began in the USA in 1946 were updated last year at a conference in Ohio when reviews of the last twenty years within each of the emergent modalities of nursing practice were conducted. Linda Beeber noted that the pioneering work of Peplau – expressed especially through her specification of the stages in the therapeutic relationship – has finally been examined empirically, especially by Carol Forchuk (1992). Beeber cautioned that more research, on both quantitative and qualitative fronts, is necessary to refine the theory and develop it for more effective use in practice. She also noted that the two other stars of the 1950s, June Mello and Ida Jean Orlando, had fared less well. In particular, the demise of the 'nursing therapy clinical laboratory' established by Mellow at Boston was attributed to the lack of respect for the mundane, yet vital, nature of the 'women's work' involved in many one-to-one relationships. This may well strike a chord here today, since so many nurses want to become therapists (in the consulting-room sense) that one wonders if the wider world of therapy, envisaged by Altschul as the lifeblood of change, will collapse as a result. My own research (and practice) has drifted from an early interest in the human content of mental distress, through various systems and models for therapeutically managing such distress, to a revival of interest in the human (phenomenological) experience of distress. My work may be reflecting a rejection of the masculine world view in favour of a rediscovery of the 'proper focus of nursing', which may involve an appreciation of the importance of valuing the mundane (feminine) nature of caring.

At the level of maximum provocation I would ask: do the dilemmas we face involve choosing between following the lead of 'mothers' like Peplau and Altschul, or 'fathers' like Tom Main – a choice between nursing or 'medicine', perhaps the ultimate father-figure?

'do the dilemmas we face involve choosing between following the lead of "mothers" like Peplau and Altschul, or "fathers" like Tom Main – a choice between nursing or "medicine", perhaps the ultimate father-figure?'

Today, nurses in the UK face much the same challenge as their North American cousins. Although it may be difficult to accept, the influence of biological reductionism is even greater in the USA than in the UK. This has had an influence on the developing role of the nurse, seen, not least, in initiatives like the pursuit and acquisition by nurses of prescribing privileges, and increased involvement in medical (as opposed to nursing) diagnosis. These scenarios have had a major impact on the development of services, and clearly have disadvantaged traditional systems of nursing, like the milieu. We have added insult to injury through the development of approaches such as the 'nursing process' – which Altschul resisted vigorously when it was introduced into Britain in the mid 1970s and which she still dismisses as an aberration. Our recent focus on 'primary nursing' and 'keyworkers' has, unfortunately, not led to the fulfilment of Peplau's dream:

'scheduled 50-minute talking sessions with five patients, three days each week, with clinical-data supervisory sessions with a psychiatric nurse specialist some time every week' (Peplau 1994).

Instead, patients who once had to wait for an appointment with the doctor (but at least had the nurses on hand) now enjoy the experience of waiting for appointments with their primary nurses.[12] The result may be the collapse of anything approaching the definition of the milieu, and the fostering of a care-planning process that emphasises *planning* more than anything approximating *care*.

The big question may well not be: *is* it possible to bridge the divide between psychoanalysis and psychiatric nursing, but *how* might psychoanalysis be accommodated within the kind of nursing which will emerge from the deconstruction of our traditional roles and functions? British psychiatric nursing – if my brief and selective history is in any way truthful – does not possess the depth and the tradition in psychotherapeutic theory and practice evident in psychiatric nursing in the USA. Instead, we have a highly developed tradition of behavioural and cognitive therapists,[13] who have capitalised on the British resistance to acknowledge the complexity of mental life. Their success in helping many people to manage the human evidence of their mental distress is self-evident. What remains to be done, however, is to develop models of nursing, beyond the millennium, which might address further the meaning of mental distress (Speedy 1993). When we come closer to understanding others, we may be approaching some kind of understanding of ourselves. Such putative models of psychotherapeutic nursing might benefit from a reappraisal of the history of psychoanalysis within psychiatric nursing. Indeed, such a reappraisal might help us to appreciate that the extension of our roles needs little more than an extension of the span of the bridge that has linked psychiatric nursing and psychoanalysis for the past half century. The bridge, which we might build to reach at least some aspects of our future appears, already, to be firmly anchored in the heritage of our past.

NOTES

This chapter is based on a paper presented to the conference: 'Crossing the Divide Between Nursing and Psychoanalysis' at the Tavistock Clinic, London on 28 October 1995.

1. The most remarkable revolution which has occurred in my professional lifetime, has been the renaissance of interest in the 'person' who is the patient. Peplau's original and continued interest in 'personhood' contributed greatly to this revolution.
2. There exist also links with Arieti's understanding of the relationship between cognition and volition (the cognitive-volitional model) (Arieti & Bemporad 1980).

3. See Podvoll (1991).
4. The intrinsic humanism of much of Peplau's writing may well link her strongly to Fromm (1986) and May (1990) and others within the 'humanistic movement'.
5. See Barker (1982), Barker & Fraser (1985).
6. Even to the untutored eye this looked like a most elegant exposition of personhood within 'madness'.
7. See Barker (1998a) – special 'Peplau' issue in the Journal of Psychiatric and Mental Health Nursing.
8. See Barker (1998b).
9. A new text, exploring the legacy of the Cassel, has just been published.
10. The oral tradition that exists, however, may in part reflect Altschul's capacities as a storyteller and listener. I shall edit a special edition of *The Journal of Psychiatric and Mental Health Nursing* in 1999, dedicated to Altschul's work.
11. Another notable addition to this list is my friend, the psychiatrist Tom Szasz.
12. This view is based on an observation made to me by a 'long-term user of psychiatric services' at a psychiatric audit conference in 1994.
13. I take some responsibility for fostering this 'movement' in the UK. Mea culpa!

REFERENCES

Arieti S and Bemporad J 1980 Severe and mild depression: the psychotherapeutic approach. Tavistock, London
Barker P 1982 Behaviour therapy nursing. Croom Helm, London
Barker P 1993 The Peplau legacy. Nursing Times 89:89–91
Barker P 1995 An interview with Annie T Altschul (audio tape available from the author)
Barker P 1998a The future of the Theory of Interpersonal Relations? A personal reflection on Peplau's legacy. Journal of Psychiatric and Mental Health Nursing 5 *(in press)*
Barker P 1998b Advanced practice in mental health nursing: developing the core. In: Rolfe G, Fulbrook P (eds) Advanced nursing practice. Butterworth-Heinemann, Oxford
Barker P, Fraser D 1995 The nurse as therapist: a behavioural model. Croom Helm, London
Barker P, Reynolds W, Ward T 1995 The proper focus of nursing: a critique of the 'caring' ideology. International Journal of Nursing Studies 32(4): 386–397
Beck AT 1976 Cognitive therapy and the emotional disorders. New English Library, New York
Brown D, Pedder J 1991 An introduction to psychotherapy. Routledge, London
Forchuk C 1992 The orientation phase of the nurse–client relationship: testing Peplau's theory. Doctoral dissertation, Wayne State University, Detroit, MI
Fromm E 1986 Man for himself. Ark Paperbacks, London
Gournay K 1995 New facts about schizophrenia. Nursing Times 91(25): 32–33
Gregg D E 1954 The psychiatric nurse's role. American Journal of Nursing 54:848–851

Hays D R 1963 Suggested clinical practices of psychiatric nurses recorded in the literature between 1946–58: a summary. In: Huey F L (ed) Psychiatric nursing 1946–74: a report on the state of the art. (ed) Mosby Yearbook, St Louis

Lego S 1974 The one-to one nurse–patient relationship. In: Anderson C A (ed) [1995] Psychiatric nursing 1974–1994 – a report on the state of the art. Mosby Year Book, St Louis

May R 1990 The cry for myth. W W Norton, New York

Michael S 1994 Invisible skils: how recognition and value need to be given to the 'invisible skills' frequently used by mental health nurses, but often unrecognised by those unfamiliar with mental health nursing. Journal of Psychiatric and Mental Health Nursing 1(1):56–57

Nakagawa H 1974 Group therapy in nursing practice. In: Anderson C A (1995) op. cit.

Peplau H E 1991 Interpersonal relations: theoretical constructs and applications in psychiatric nursing practice. In: Cormack D, Reynolds W (eds) Psychiatric and mental health nursing: theory and practice. Chapman and Hall, London

Peplau H E 1994 Psychiatric nursing: challenge and change. Journal of Psychiatric and Mental Health Nursing 1(1):3–7

Podvoll E 1991 The seduction of madness: a compassionate approach to recovery at home from psychosis. Century, London

Rohde IM 1968 The nurse as family therapist. Nursing Outlook 16: 49–52

Sills G 1974 Use of milieu therapy. In: Anderson C A (1995) op. cit.

Smoyak S 1974 Family therapy. In: Anderson C A (1995) op. cit.

Speedy S 1993 The search for meaning in caring for mentally ill people. Australian Journal of Mental Health Nursing 2(4):170–182

Winship G 1995 Nursing and psychoanalysis – uneasy alliances? Psychoanalytic Psychotherapy 9:289–299

Commentary

Suzanne Lego RN, PhD, CS, CGP, FAAN

Professor Barker's excellent paper concerning the integration of psycho-analytic concepts into psychiatric nursing leaves little or no room for dispute. As a nurse psychoanalyst who, like Professor Barker, has practised for over a quarter century, I have watched the two professions' slow courtship. Though Dr Hildegard Peplau married them in the early 1950s, the value of this prolific marriage has faded in the eyes of some American psychiatric nurses. Psychiatric nursing has, it seems, divorced psychoanalysis, having fallen in love with a new muse, neurobiology. This courtship was encouraged, and has flourished under the parental influence of organised psychiatry and the pharmaceutical industry. These watchful parents have also produced a new progeny, the primary care nurse.

Advanced practice psychiatric-mental health (PMH) nurses in America, those holding Masters degrees or above, now fall into two practice cate-gories: clinical nurse specialist (CNS) or, the new progeny, psychiatric nurse practitioner (NP). The CNS programmes, begun in the 1950s, have prepared nurse psychotherapists for forty years. Peplau's students were prepared in this way and were the first to open private practices in the early 1960s. In 1990, Columbia University School of Nursing opened the first psychoanalytic programme for nurses (Varcarolis 1994) Thousands of Masters-prepared PMH nurses practice psychotherapy today in the USA.

However, the 1990s 'Decade of the Brain' began a seduction that has resulted in graduate programmes preparing PMH nurses as nurse practi-tioners: that is, primary care providers who have advanced preparation in PMH nursing. This defection from psychotherapy/psychoanalysis was economically driven. Health care agencies, wanting to save money, decided that PMH nurses who could also do physical examinations, provide primary care, prescribe drugs, make hospital rounds, and take night call were a pretty good buy. Federal funding became available for primary care nurses, and programme directors rushed to cash in on this way to sustain their graduate programmes. Some graduate programmes have managed to retain the solid graduate-level content from their CNS programmes, sometimes by simply lengthening the programme to add primary care courses. Others, however, eliminated the psychotherapy courses (some of which were drawn from psychoanalytic theory) and concentrated on pri-mary care as it applied to psychiatric patients (see Dyer et al 1997)

Organised psychiatry's move toward neurobiology, accompanied by the enormous resources of the pharmaceutical industry, proved irresistible to nursing. And so in the USA, we have come full circle, back to the point when Professor Barker was a student trying to 'explain away' the phenomenon of the 'person-who-is-patient'. Today, the person is a 'brain-in-need-of-a-chemical'. The person has become a psychiatric disorder. Elsewhere (Lego 1996), I have written about the unfortunate woman who was hospitalised by her husband, a professional, who was clearly fed up with his middle-aged stay-at-home wife's depression. Her nurse told me the patient had been abusing laxatives. I asked why, meaning for constipation or to purge to lose weight? The nurse answered, 'Because she has an Abusive Personality Disorder!' Once these labels are applied and held in such high regard, there is no hope of the person making an appearance!

Professor Barker raises the question of whether psychoanalytic principles and milieu therapy have been exiled with the possibility of future return, or whether they are gone for good. In the USA, it is clear that economic factors have hastened the exile. Outpatient psychotherapy, now controlled by managed care organizations, is restricted to 20 sessions or less, spawning a preponderance of brief therapy models, though in the end this may not even be economically sound (Lego 1998). However, psychoanalytic concepts have indeed permeated the culture and are here to stay. For example, nearly all patients who come to me for therapy are acquainted with the notion that their childhoods play a role in their current problems. Milieu therapy, on the other hand, has virtually vanished from sight (Delaney 1997). The average length of stay on an inpatient psychiatric unit in the USA is 7 days (Sawyer 1996).

Psychoanalytic concepts are still used by followers of Peplau, and by nurses who have completed psychoanalytic training themselves. Though it is rare, some of these nurses continue to work with the seriously mentally ill (Thelander 1997). These nurses are able to see symptoms such as delusions and hallucinations arising from interpersonal situations, though biochemical changes may result. I have found it useful to visualise these occurrences as shown in Figure 1.1.

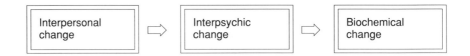

As PMH nurses we, in turn, intervene to produce a new favourable interpersonal change, through the therapeutic relationship, which in turn, leads to intrapsychic change, and then to biochemical change for the better. For example, a doctoral student who had been diagnosed schizophrenic when he had a psychotic break years ago, was now in therapy owing to the stresses of doctoral study. One day he reported hearing voices. It was the week of his final oral exams and he was feeling particularly stressed. As he was running across a street to get to a class, he began to hear voices saying 'Stupid!'. His nurse psychotherapist calmly asked him to describe the situation, using the Peplau techniques described in this chapter. Together they reached the conclusion that the symptom was merely a result of his high anxiety, and he left the office with relief, and with no further symptoms.

This brings us to the very important point Professor Barker makes about the Peplau method, addressing the phenomena arising from within the patient, rather than from without. Cognitive-behavioural therapy, rather popular today, might on the other hand be considered 'antipersonal' as opposed to 'interpersonal'. For, rather than exploring that which is in the patient, it discourages this introspection, and rather encourages the person to stop bad thoughts. These injunctions are antipersonal also in that they apply to every patient without regard to individual uniqueness.

Is the gap between psychoanalysis and psychiatric nursing too wide for reconciliation? A medical sociologist I know is currently researching the acceptance of the neurobiological revolution in America by both psychiatry and psychiatric nursing. His findings suggest that while organised PMH nursing seems by and large to accept the biological or genetic explanations for the cause of mental illness and chemical treatment, in practice, in the privacy of their own consultation rooms, they continue to use psychodynamic theory.

Research continues to reveal that drugs alone are not the answer to treating mental illness any more than counting up symptoms and teaching patients to cope with the illness is a substitute for theory-driven psychotherapy. When PMH nursing's affair with neurobiology ends, nurses will realise their marriage to psychodynamic theory has endured.

REFERENCES

Delaney K R 1997 Milieu therapy, a therapeutic loophole. Perspectives in Psychiatric Care. The Journal for Nurse Psychotherapists 33(2):19–29

Dyer G D, Hammill K, Regan-Kubinski M J, Yurick A, Kobert S 1997 The psychiatric-primary care nurse practitioner: a futuristic model for advanced psychiatric-mental health nursing. Archives of Psychiatric Nursing 9(1):2–12

Lego S 1996 Women's issues in psychiatric-mental health nursing. In: Lego S (ed) Psychiatric nursing: a comprehensive reference Lippincott, Philadelphia, ch 73, p 580

Lego S 1998 Editorial: Managed care of outpatient psychotherapy—a new twist. Perspectives in Psychiatric Care. The Journal for Nurse Psychotherapists 35(I):1

Sawyer P 1996 Designing an inpatient psychiatric unit. In: Lego S (ed) Psychiatric nursing: a comprehensive reference Lippincott, Philadelphia, ch 46, p 383

Thelander B 1997 The psychotherapy of Hildegard Peplau in the treatment of people with serious mental illness. Perspectives in Psychiatric Care. The Journal for Nurse Psychotherapists 33(3):24–32

Varcarolis E M 1994 Foundations of psychiatric mental health nursing, 2nd edn. Saunders, Philadelphia

The philosophy of psychiatric nursing: the birth of the binding agent?

AN EXISTENTIAL CRISIS?

This appears to be an era of indecision and, paradoxically, also a time for decision-making. Mental health nurses increasingly spend time considering whether or not they should aim to become the team-leader, case-manager or keyworker in community mental health services. Although this sense of ambition, if not a sense of place, within the service, is an important issue, the questions being begged are, in my view, receiving premature consideration. The biggest issue facing psychiatric nursing is intellectual promiscuity. Fearing that they might not exist, nurses borrow promiscuously from anything which might pass for academic credibility, or respectable ideology, in an effort to bolster their fragile professional egos.

Surveys in the USA have reported more than four hundred so-called psychotherapies (Karasu 1986). In an effort to help psychiatric nursing make its own therapeutic mark, some nurse educators in the UK are trying to squeeze each and every one of these schools and models of therapy into the syllabus. More may ultimately turn out to be less.

Nurses also try to fill their professional vacuum by borrowing philosophies from other disciplines. Having built their discipline around traditional psychiatric medicine, many nurses now look to social work and psychology for answers to their identity crisis. Like some sexual relationships, this may involve more taking than sharing. If an existential vacuum does exist, it may be a metaphor for the absence of an appropriate philosophy of psychiatric nursing.

What such a philosophy of psychiatric *and* mental health nursing might be is an intriguing question (Barker 1989). What is the binding agent which makes cohesive the activity of nurses in their efforts to help people in their care with psychiatric problems? In this paper, I anticipate the birth, or perhaps rebirth, of a philosophy of psychiatric nursing: the birth of the binding agent. I believe that four questions underpin such a philosophy: questions about the why, rather than the what, of nursing. Just as the limits of our language define the limits of our world (Kenny 1973), so does our psychiatric language define its world – too narrowly in my view. The world-view of psychiatric nursing needs to be examined if nurses are to develop a clear knowledge of *why* they exist. Nurses need to establish these answers before they can decide their position within the clinical team.

> 'What is the binding agent which makes cohesive the activity of nurses in their efforts to help people in their care with psychiatric problems?'

The first question is:

• 'How do nurses describe the *person* who becomes the patient?' This might be cast as the health problem.

• Secondly, 'How do we describe the patient who represents the person?' This might be cast as the illness problem.

• Thirdly, 'What is the *target population* which psychiatric nursing serves?' This might be cast as the class problem.

• And finally, we might ask: 'Does sex matter?' This might be cast as the identity problem.

Increasingly, psychiatric nurses are becoming mental health workers. Mental health has become the head of an ever-spinning coin, whose tail is engraved with the old bogey, mental illness. Often we lapse into archaic vernacular, talking about treatment, therapy or, in these days of quality assurance, *clinical* excellence. The young, upwardly mobile mental *health* nurse, however, is more likely to be overheard talking of promoting mental health within the context of an ecologically viable – and of course holistic – person-centred conceptual framework. But what exactly is this thing called 'mental health'? Is it self-actualisation or simply the relative absence of mental illness? And, if so, does this mean that mental illness is simply the relative absence of mental health? In this philosophical frame of mind we might ask: 'Do nurses know what they are talking about, or are they only playing with words?'. First, let us consider the people who become patients.

PERSONHOOD AND PATIENTHOOD: TERRORISM BY LANGUAGE

How we describe people suggests something of our relationship to them. In the game of describing and being described, some of us become unwilling victims, terrorised by the power of language and language games (Wittgenstein 1980). These games are to be found also in the relations between nurses and patients.[1] The history of psychiatry offers some fine examples of the use of language to control the less fortunate (see, for example, Scheff 1975). This was true of the theological perspective of Tuke's moral rearmament of psychiatry, through psychoanalysis and behaviourism to today's complex, reductionist biophysical models. In an apparent effort to escape these dogmas the infant *mental health* has been fostered, cast perhaps from the same mould as the humanistic corruption of the concept of *gestalt*: the idea that all people are greater than the sum of their parts. That idea was certainly more attractive than the idea that people are swallowed, without trace, by disorders, which consume them invisibly, like some remake of the 'Invasion of the Body-Snatchers'. In unashamedly clinical, scientific or research circles, adult neurotics, brittle psychotics, personality disorders and psychogeriatrics may be valid currency. Outside these conversations, such terms claim that some people are *less* than the sum of their parts. Those who take the 'mental health' pledge are clearly altruistic. By a simple turn of phrase they can restore dignity to a disenfranchised people. My own service took the pledge some years ago. In a gesture of false naivety we decreed that the recipients of our service should not be called patients, clients, users, consumers, or residents, but just people.[2] Humanising by reverse labelling is, however, no more than a token gesture. Reinvesting people with full dignity – or more correctly establishing the conditions under which people can have access to their own dignity – requires action which may be difficult to sustain.

Restoring dignity is a thorny process since it is likely to involve a puncturing of the professional ego. Acknowledging the person who is the patient is easy if we also try to avoid the political consequences. The concept of *patienthood* in psychiatry has been developing over at least the past two hundred years. Among the various stimuli for the concept might have been the need to:

- restrict choice in otherwise autonomous individuals
- create an underclass in a capitalist economy
- reduce anxiety over human rights violations, or
- promote the hedonistic philosophy of most Western cultures – patients aren't happy, therefore they must be a different form of the human species.

An analysis of the political obstacles to the use of genuine rehabilitation or normalisation principles is not appropriate here. However, three points which appear central to the concept of personhood are noted here.

The person-who-is-patient is represented by three elements – individual choice, service provision and service providers – which are meshed together in a sociopolitical web that nets a huge economic spider. Even the supporters of normalisation may have miscalculated the implications of providing a truly *human* service within the capitalist ethic (cf. Baldwin 1986). Special labels guarantee 'patients' essential services; their absence often makes such access difficult if not impossible. In these increasingly politically correct times, we should not forget that some people with 'mental illness', and their relatives or advocates, are reassured by the status which patienthood confers. We might care to ask, however, what would happen if patients were given full control over the services they needed by, for example, individualised funding? What would be the effect on nurses – and nursing – if people were truly free to choose from a range of wards, day hospitals, and community nurses, any one or any combination of which might conceivably meet their needs? How might such a scenario affect the language game between nurses and *their* (sic) patients?

Nurses may have relied too much upon role theory to explain how disadvantaged people can attain an improved quality of life. Role theory is the most spurious and weakening assumption of the normalisation principle. Any service based upon the capitalist ethic with its enormous inequalities of resource distribution, needs more than the artificial creation of socially valued roles, if at-risk groups are to experience the effects of long-term social change (Baldwin 1986).

Trying to treat patients as people will always be problematic, especially where the reasons for distinguishing between one and the other are unclear. If, as we claim, patients are fundamentally different from those who are not, we split the world into patients and people (non-patients), and endorse an illness model. If patients are, first and foremost, people, then we acknowledge that humankind is united, at least nominally, and the concept of mental health is endorsed. How nurses address *and* act towards people in their care is no academic trifle: it is an ethical and moral issue of considerable scale. Considering how we should address those in our care will influence the design of the service, the future education of all staff, and will trigger economic and political ripples that may cause a cultural tidal wave. What kind of a concept of humanity binds us, as nurses, to the people in our care? Will this binding agent bind us all together, as one humankind albeit with some internal differences; or will it bind us separately, keeping nurses and those in their care apart? Before exploring this question further, let us consider briefly the concept of *mental illness*: the seed bed upon which most of us in Psychiatric nursing were raised. The following may represent an apposite metaphor for the world of mental illness and our way of conceptualising and responding to it, through care and treatment (Barker 1988). Consider to what extent our current concept of mental health nursing is indebted to this metaphor.

THE FAMILY OF PSYCHIATRY

The Psyches are my next-door neighbours. They can trace their family tree as far back as the ancient Greeks, but are most proud of their English ancestors who developed the asylum tradition around the time of the Enlightenment. Of their three children, Psychoanalysis was the eldest. He had promised much in his youth but now his parents saw him as something of an underachiever. Strong, yet distant, Psychoanalysis was not a good mixer and tended to be hostile in company. You've probably seen him riding the bus to work, reading Kafka and making a virtue of silence. His mother had such a hard time with him that they adopted their second child, Behaviourism. He is about the same age as Psychoanalysis and he gave his folks a lot of trouble with his demands for attention, exhaustive displays of logic and his obsession for planning and recording his every function.

Like most kids, he went through phases but sometimes he changed so much that his folks didn't recognise him. They often hanker for the simple, straightforward Behaviourism they used to know. Now he's taken to mixing in bad company, hanging about street corners with the Sociology gang, making cracks about the neighbours and their cultural practices.

Life was beginning to be a big disappointment for the Psyches. They often looked enviously at the Rogers family who lived across the street with their triplets, Warmth, Empathy and Genuineness. They never seem to have any problems and when they did they just sat down and 'shared them' and that was that.

Just when they were settling into middle-age, along came little Neuroscience, the unplanned baby. They never saw such a bright kid, a human computer. As he grows up, he talks as though there is nothing he can't do. And, of course, because he is the youngest he is the favourite, and this causes a lot of bad feeling. Psychoanalysis has tried to lose some of his aloofness and has even started dating one of the Rogers kids. Behaviourism has changed quite a bit too, and is even starting to think before he acts, even talking about how his thoughts might influence his feelings. But the word on the street says it's probably too late for them. To old Ma and Pa Psyche, little Neuro is still the apple of their eye. He is the future, they say, although often they have absolutely no idea what he is talking about and old Grandad Psyche says he is a heartless little sod.

This story of everyday folks seems to serve as an icon for the various stories that we have woven into the history of modern psychiatry. Among the many functions they have served, these stories have told of our various struggles to understand some of the more curious aspects of the Family of Man. Through our attempts to define others, we have, perhaps unwittingly, defined something of ourselves.

The *Psyches* remind us that all of our critical concepts are metaphorical in origin: especially our concepts of health, illness, disease and death. Are mental illnesses things-in-themselves, – entities determined by their intrinsic nature – or are they simply ideas we have fashioned: shaped by the very concepts which we have used to define them? Some concepts are difficult to refute, like gravity, for example, which gives us very direct feedback whenever we try to challenge its existence. The relationship between social theory and human behaviour is quite different. Down the ages it has been noted that if people define situations as real, they are real in their consequences. The *World Health Organization* study of schizophrenia conducted in 1973 and 1979 provided a sobering illustration of this dictum (Eisenberg 1986). Patients who had been given a first-episode diagnosis of schizophrenia were identified in nine countries chosen for their differing cultures. At follow-up, patients in developing countries (the 'third world') showed a more favourable course than did patients in the industrialised (or 'modern') world. This suggested that people developed 'schizophrenia' in most countries of the world, but recovered more readily in the poorest parts of the world.

Although attempts have been made to explain away this phenomenon on the grounds that 'third world' countries have simpler cultures, this is a discredited hypothesis. It could be argued that the demands arising from caste, kinship, religion, sex and age variables, make these societies even more complex than those, like our own, in the industrialised nations. An alternative explanation might be found in the social explanation of disorders like schizophrenia: how the phenomenon is understood – or 'constructed' – within different cultures. In peasant societies, disorders that we might call schizophrenia, are explained by spirit possession, something *extrinsic* to the patient. This explanation allows for the possibility that the person can be exorcised, and returned to his or her former self. In western societies we have long believed that schizophrenia – if not all forms of true madness – is *intrinsic* to the person, whose only chance of change lies in remission, rather than resolution.

CLASH OF THE MODEL-MAKERS

Different cultures construct different models to explain their world of experience, each becoming real in its consequences. This is not to say that schizophrenia *per se* does not exist (Szasz 1970, 1986), merely that such a phenomenon can be interpreted in several ways. Each 'model' of schizophrenia influences how we might respond to the phenomenon. Nurses who are looking for the 'one true model' of schizophrenia – or indeed of anything – might be in for a disappointment. Eisenberg has suggested that: 'those who search for the mind in the machine will find at the end of their journey what Gertrude Stein said about her trip to a nondescript town: "When you get there, you find there's no *there* there"' (Eisenberg 1986).

Perhaps unlike rock, water and other characters in the physical world, people are a *function* of the world in which they live. If nothing else, our minds are a function of society. Anything which is wrong with our minds, must involve the society – and its cultures – which contributed to the definition of *mind* in the first place. What goes on *inside* people is important, but much of what we *assume* goes on inside us, is socially constructed.

'Anything which is wrong with our minds, must involve the society – and its cultures – which contributed to the definition of *mind* in the first place'

Although we may be uncertain of where 'the World' begins and ends, that World plays a significant role in all the affairs of men (sic). Perhaps it is time that nursing – another socially constructed phenomenon – considered the role of the social world in its own construction and deconstruction.

What has all of this to do with psychiatric nursing? I was trained, like many readers of my vintage, in the 'illness' model of mental disorder which saw all experimental disturbance as a mental equivalent of diabetes or dropsy. Mind and body were distinct although the same approach was used to study both. Despite the apparent sophistication of the 1990s we remain under the influence of Galileo, Descartes and Newton. Psychiatry has become so obsessed with rational knowledge, objectivity and quantification, that it has become insecure in dealing with human values and experiences (*cf.* Capra 1983). It may be suffering from a surfeit of *yang* – too much closing in, too much structure, order and control; and not enough *yin* – opening out, exploration, freedom.

'Psychiatry has become so obsessed with rational knowledge, objectivity and quantification, that it has become insecure in dealing with human values and experiences'

Alternative, though no less metaphorical, explanations of experiential distress have emerged in recent years. The nursing literature increasingly manipulates systemic, cognitive, interpersonal, political, psychobiological, and even spiritual, models to explain much the same phenomena, much the same human experiences. Many professions, especially nursing, are beginning to talk about holistic health care, although this, of itself, is a tautology. *Health* cannot exist unless all aspects of the person and the person's world are invoked. Health means whole.

Nurses need to be careful they are not swallowed whole, by the 'black hole' of holism. Health and illness are like yin and yang: if nurses desert the search for a proper definition of illness, they may end up merely mouthing platitudes about health. We might ask ourselves again, in the health-related context: 'What is nursing's concept of mental illness and disorder?' Is it something that binds nurses to the people in their care; or does it bind those 'patients' up, to be put away, keeping them apart from those who care for them?

PEOPLE, PATIENTS AND POPULATIONS

The idea of population takes these concerns a stage further. Psychiatry is the mother field from which mental illness, mental handicap and psychogeriatrics[3] developed. But if psychiatric nursing is about the care of people with mental disorder whatever its origins, distinctions between mental handicap and mental health nurses – if not also elderly care nurses – confuse the issue. The arbitrary distinction between the mentally ill (sic) and the mentally handicapped is particularly vexing, although I recognise that it is probably a lost cause.

For fifteen years I have tried to teach nurses to work with people with problems of living,[4] ignoring primitive diagnoses. However, even the best of nurses appear to need to cling to the idea that these groups of people are different. Perhaps there is a basic (human) need to see patients as people with two heads. Of course, when people become patients they do appear to become different, although some of this difference is attributable to social construction: we help create the patient the person becomes. However, the only things that patients have in common are problems of living they share with other people. So what are these 'problems of living' which appear to unite people-as-patients?

People are disabled, restricted or otherwise handicapped by many things. Problems of adjustment, or coping, irrational fears, disturbance of mood, relationship difficulties, emotional crises, like anger or frustration, dependency on drugs or alcohol, or dependency on people, and even the feeling that they are alone and isolated in an alien world. All these are *people problems*: the tracks of our human tears. For generations, nurses, and others, denied that people with mental handicaps had these experiences. This was a Nazi philosophy of personhood: the denial of human status of which all nurses should be ashamed. One might say that mental handicap care was the veterinary branch of psychiatry, were it not for the fact that animals often are treated much more respectfully. Now, as people with mental handicaps are beginning to be treated more like *persons*, we risk sliding back into our old ways of thinking about people in mental illness – believing that they *are* their illness, rather than *persons* with problems of adjustment, coping, fearing, loving, feeling and so on. Apropos the old mental handicap scenario, we might well ask: 'What is going to be the veterinary branch of tomorrow's mental health service?' Which subpopulation will we dismiss or disparage as somehow unworthy of recognition as a human problem of human magnitude?

My emotive language should not disturb nurses. They might, however, consider being disturbed by the illogical practice of segregating people into subpopulations through the nosological apartheid of diagnostic classification. A decade ago it was noted that since people with a mental handicap do not represent a homogenous clinical group, their educational, social and medical needs should be met by extensions of the services available to ordinary people (see Carr et al 1980). Are not the 'mentally ill' just as heterogenous? What do young articulate people with an existential depression have in common with old, near-mute people, grounded by dementia? In the city where I work, former long-stay patients (some 'mentally ill', some 'mentally handicapped', some with 'mental disabilities' arising from recent neurological damage) participate in basic education classes alongside 'ordinary' members of the community (by which we mean people with an even less certain mental status). A mutual support group for women with recurrent and severe depression and manic depression, which I helped establish, meets in a centre for the unemployed in the city centre, where the women's group is viewed as 'just another one of the resource centre's groups'. These examples of normalisation question the basic value of such subclasses. Special cases, like people with a mental handicap, or psychogeriatrics, are part of the politico-economic web referred to earlier. Perhaps they represent the prejudices of advocacy groups. Perhaps 'ginger groups' need to emphasise how the needs of different people are different, at the end of the day. However, when nurses consider how they might target people with the greatest need, the definition of such needs should be in human, rather than diagnostic terms. Discovering that someone felt all alone in the world might be an illuminating discovery. It might suggest that the person *needed* company, support or reassurance. Discovering that someone has a specific form of schizophrenia, or possesses a certain level of intellectual impairment, or has a certain kind of dementia, is interesting. I remain uncertain of what I – as a nurse – might do with such information.

> 'Discovering that someone felt all alone in the world might be an illuminating discovery. It might suggest that the person *needed* company, support or reassurance. Discovering that someone has a specific form of schizophrenia, or possesses a certain level of intellectual impairment, or has a certain kind of dementia, is interesting. I remain uncertain of what I – as a nurse – might do with such information'

OBFUSCATION BY LABELS

People with different needs do exist; I am arguing that these human needs are masked, if not distorted by the traditional labels of psychiatry. The English word 'pest' means a destructive and annoying animal or insect. It comes from the French word for plague. When we have too much of a minor pest it is often seen to be 'plaguing' us. The language we used to classify things which annoy us, but which, like the plague (*la peste*), we also fear, provided us with terms like mental handicap and mental illness. It is time to abandon these meaningless classifications so that we can embrace a humanistic ethic.

In recent years, we have begun to identify 'patients' who do not fit the traditional classifications: people distressed by homelessness, disfigurement, stress, domestic abuse, or 101 other so-called psychosocial problems. Is it to our credit that such people have been defined as the 'worried well'? One of my colleagues has remarked that all the people he sees, in this so-called category, are 'worried sick'.[5] David Smail has argued that human distress occurs for reasons which make it incurable by therapy, but which are not beyond the powers of human beings to influence (Smail 1987). People suffer pain because they do damage to one another. They will continue to suffer as long as they continue to do the damage. We alleviate and mitigate distress by *taking care of the world and the people in it*, not by treating them.

This is a tall order, but may be one which has its humble beginnings in my questions about the process of classifying patients. Shall we share the distress of the people in our care, acknowledging that these people are hurting like us, but either only more so, or in a different voice? Or shall we distance ourselves from those whom we describe as one of '57 varieties' of mental illness, each of which is in itself a mixture? Shall we bind ourselves to the philosophy of helping those with mental distress, arising from whatever source? Or shall we bind patients up into bundles, each with their own class mark; each being offered a different class of care, if indeed they are offered any?

GENDER, SEX AND PERSUASION

I have left sexuality to the end of this reflection, perhaps because this is the aspect of personhood I understand least. Gender identity is important, but I am not confident I know why. Most of my career as a nurse psychotherapist has been spent with women with longstanding mental illness. Some of these women accepted me into their company and later into their hearts, who might have had good reason for seeing all men as Jonahs. It is greatly to their human credit that they found the wherewithal to forgive my sex. My own experiences lend support to the view that some truly awful human experiences – like severe depression – can be clarified by looking at the social world of the sufferer. This certainly seems to be the case when one considers the social world of depressed women.[6] Having worked with men who are depressed, I have reached the conclusion that they use a similar emotional language to describe a quite different phenomenon. In full awareness of the danger of stereotyping, I believe that depressed women see themselves as failures: failures as mothers, mistresses, cooks or cleaners. Men, on the other hand, see themselves as a different kind of failure: failing to be providers, profiteers, one of the boys, or a sexual magnet for women. I have also worked closely with gay men and women and have been struck by the ordinariness of their relationships. All too many men I have known have been misogynists, and spend much effort seeking the company of other men. Many women I have known, on the other hand, have been less obnoxious about their sexism. Apart from the odd few who paraded their heterosexuality in public, I have had to assume that these men and women did indeed have heterosexual private lives. Beyond procreation, heterosexuality seems to be a quiet commodity.

Homophobia has always been a symbol for me of the fear of being different. Until the 1960s, homosexuality's main function was to generate fear between the homosexual and those who assumed they were 100% heterosexual. Homosexuality also served a useful function in maintaining the anxious relationship between the homosexual and himself. Following our sexual reawakenings in the 1960s we tried to adopt a more relaxed attitude towards sex. This ranged from our accommodation of transexualism as a valid ambition for some people and the publication of encyclopaedic sex manuals as necessary bedside reading for every novice lover.

Today, we are encouraged to return to the cautious, anxious kind of sexuality which characterised my generation, for quite different reasons. Although we are often flippant and facetious about sex, we can hardly afford this luxury. We need to think about sex seriously, even if only to ask that important question, in what way does sex matter? Or I could ask, 'shall we be one or shall we be many?'. Are we all fundamentally of the same sex, but divided biologically to propagate the species? Or are we derived from a range of gender types, which are more complicated than those found in other sections of the animal kingdom? I believe that this has a bearing upon how we work with the people who are our patients. How do we help them to clarify their sexual position in their own human lives, and how might they use such knowledge to relate to or influence others around them?

Such issues are important for nurses, if not also for nursing. Without such a knowledge how shall we know how to respond to sexism within our work setting, or to the sexual dimension of child-rearing practices of the people in our care, or the sexual dimension of families and other groups, or the alienation which people experience when they are uncertain of how sexuality colours their lives?

We might consider whether people who talk a lot about sex are intrigued by sex or frightened of it? We might ask is sex a sport, a recreation or a pastime? And if so, what might love be – a religion? And what of sex as a public phenomenon, where once it was kept private or confined to the more shadowy recesses of our lives? Is the public face of sex an oppression? Has our sexual openness exalted people or merely served to intimidate them further? I have to confess that I have not found any useful answers to any of these questions. However, even within the territory of sexuality, people in my care continue to ask me: 'Should I be one or should I be many?'.

This identity crisis is not exclusive to the patient body. Nurses themselves continued to anguish over the ways and means of identifying *who* should be the team leader, the keyworker, the therapist or the case manager; and *what* should be their distinguishing characteristics. The power attached to these various roles seems still to be worth squabbling over. Despite all our efforts to promote normalisation, to empower our various clientele, to make more transparent our relationships with the people in our care, being a psychiatric patient still largely involves the process of relinquishing power (Bell 1990). Although this varies across different settings, disempowerment is the commonest denominator of treatment. We might ask ourselves, should we be contesting power when such a power differential exists between us and those in our care?

BEGINNING OF THE END – OR END OF THE BEGINNING?

The four issues I have addressed here set what I consider to be the moral agenda of the philosophy of psychiatric nursing. Nurses continue to collude with the main, traditional, aim of psychiatry, which is to reshape and return patients to the lives they *had* or *should have had*. These aims are determined by conventional values and the asserted morality of psychiatry. At the same time, nurses claim to promote growth and development (through their espousal of the mental *health* nursing ethic) but appear frightened to embrace fully the humanistic ethic, since this would challenge the social norms which support, if not actually cause, much psychiatric distress. Nurses appear to pretend not to know this, by focusing their attention on mythical illness notions, or magical therapy potions. It is argued, of course, that many people accept these notions of illness, or even seek medical labels or treatment to explain and correct their 'dis-ease'. Perhaps this serves only to illustrate further the powerlessness and negative self-view engendered by the process of becoming a patient. We might care to ask whether nurses should be contesting power – for example, by enhancing their professional status – when those in their care are so transparently powerless?

Care is often viewed as something we do for people, rather than *with* people. This is an unashamedly paternalistic view. This kind of care infantilises people: maintaining them in a state of dependency. Although we appear to have made great strides in making psychiatry more accessible, it still trades in misinformation (or dysinformation). Although we have talked loudly about personhood and the humanistic values attached to it, much of our service provision is predicated on stereotyping. Psychiatric care is still about maintaining the social status quo. True *care* is about joining with the person who is patient, not separating ourselves off from the person by use of language, labels, uniforms, titles, badges and all the impediments of traditional nursing. *Care*, as Robert Pirsig observed, happens when we are not separated from what we are working on. Caring involves a feeling of identification with what one is doing (Pirsig 1976). Caring for people is a revolutionary process: giving power back to the people or helping them to realise their own power in diverse ways. This revolution is also the first stage in resolution: acknowledging patients as people; acknowledging their complementary status to ourselves.

This is not to suggest that some people do not become distressed for highly complex reasons, which can include factors within their biological, psychological and social selves. However, the more distressed such 'cases' are, the more they are at the mercy of the psychiatric professions. We miss the point by debating which of the various disciplines within the mental health team should wield the power within the clinical team. Perhaps everyone already has too much power.

I have said elsewhere that mental health nursing should be 'trephotaxic': this is a Greek neologism meaning 'the necessary conditions for the promotion of growth and development' (Barker 1989). This is a new spin on an old Nightingale concept, when she talked of nursing providing the conditions for the patient to be healed, by Nature or by God. True nursing is about helping people consolidate their experience of themselves, their own lives, the pleasure and the pain. True nursing involves helping people

> 'Care is often viewed as something we do for people, rather than *with* people. This is an unashamedly paternalistic view. This kind of care infantilises people: maintaining them in a state of dependency'

to need nurses much less. Psychiatric nurses may be the only group willing to help people in distress unconditionally. In early 16th Century Portugal, Joao Cuidad set up a shelter for the mentally ill and social outcasts, having previously been confined as a lunatic following a religious experience (Cross & Livingstone 1986). Cuidad, who was later canonised as St John of God, may be a more wholesome icon for psychiatric nurses than Nightingale, although her contribution to the development of 'modern nursing' is beyond dispute. Cuidad's work personified empathy, empowerment, direct action and direct engagement with patients. These qualities appear still alive and kicking in the social model of mental health care operating in parts of Italian psychiatry. By contrast, Nightingale's embrace of a military metaphor for nursing in the fight against sickness, stimulated, albeit unintentionally, the emergence of the starchy, interpersonally distant nurse (especially Nursing Sister) that nursing continues to try to bury. The contrast between Cuidad and Nightingale exemplifies the gulf between psychiatric nurses and their general colleagues, and may emphasise the distinctive position of mental health nursing in the whole geography of health care.

As the 20th century ends, the curtains begin to close on many of the false gods which have dominated recent history. Extreme right- and left-wing political ideologies, as well as extremist economic, industrial and religious movements, are all part of the declining culture: they are in a process of disintegration (Capra 1983). At the same time, the social movements which were born in the 1960s are now gaining a second wind. It seems ironic that humanity should seek its rebirth as the planet itself is in danger of dying. The immediate future seems likely to be characterised by conflict, as the declining culture fights to hold its position of power and supremacy. We are, according to Capra, at the 'turning point' (Capra 1983). Now is the time to re-examine the main premises and values of the nursing culture. Now is the time to reject concepts which have outlived their usefulness. Now is the time to recognise the value of ideas discarded by previous generations. The Nightingale legacy may be a symbol of our declining culture. Perhaps the selfless caring of Cuidad represents one of the discarded values psychiatric nurses need to re-examine, where direct engagement and identification *with* those in the care of nurses asumes a higher priority. Certainly, it seems time for us to gather both our thoughts, and ourselves, together. To this end I have employed the 'binding' metaphor: it reflects what we need to do, and what will be the function of our immediate tasks – the 'greening' of psychiatric nursing.

On occasions like this it is all too easy to drift into 'visionary' mode. It is all too easy to talk of 'having a dream'. I hope that I have avoided both of these traps and have offered no more, or less, than suggestions: suggesting that a new philosophy of psychiatric and mental health nursing practice might be fashioned out of some age-old precepts concerning the experience of, response to, and management of, human distress. For nursing this might result in the birth of a binding agent, and within psychiatric nursing, the turning of the tide. What our ancestors would have called signs from heaven, or the gods, will bring nurses together to share and to bind such concerns into a viable philosophy. Now is the time to act. I hope that psychiatric nurses can seize the time.

NOTES

This chapter is based on a paper presented to the International Psychiatric Nursing Conference 'Clinical Excellence' at the Civic Centre, Newcastle upon Tyne, in April 1990.

1. I am acutely conscious that the term 'patient' has assumed a new significance in this post-politically-correct world.
2. On reflection, this emphasis on 'the person' was probably an exercise in philosophical purism on my part, as team leader.
3. These terms have now largely been replaced by even vaguer concepts such as 'learning disability (or difficulty) and 'older people with mental health problems'.
4. The contribution made by Thomas Szasz (1970) to clarifying this concept cannot be overlooked.
5. I am indebted to my former colleague, John Swan, for this piece of wisdom.
6. See also Brown & Harris (1979).

REFERENCES

Baldwin S 1986 Wolf in sheep's clothing: impact of normalisation teaching on human services and service providers. International Journal of Rehabilitation Research 8(2):131–142

Barker P 1988 Reasoning about madness: the long search for the vanishing horizon (Part 2). Community Psychiatric Nursing Journal 8(5):14–19

Barker P 1989 Reflections on the philosophy of caring in mental health. International Journal of Nursing Studies 26(2):131–141

Bell L 1990 How and why psychiatry does not heal. Changes 8(1):57–62

Brown G, Harris T 1979 The social origins of depression: a study of psychiatric disorder in women. Tavistock, London

Capra F 1983 The turning point. Flamingo, London

Carr P, Butterworth CA, Hodges BEL 1980 Community psychiatric nursing. Churchill Livingstone, Edinburgh

Cross F-L, Livingstone E-A 1986 Oxford dictionary of the Christian church, 2nd edn. Oxford University Press, Oxford

Eisenberg L 1986 Mindless and brainless in psychiatry. British Journal of Psychiatry 148: 497–508

Karasu T B 1986 The specificity versus nonspecificity dilemma: toward identifying therapeutic change agents. American Journal of Psychiatry 143(6):687–695

Kenny A 1973 Wittgenstein. Penguin, Harmondsworth

Pirsig R 1976 Zen and the art of motorcycle maintenance. Corgi, London

Scheff T 1975 Being mentally ill. Aldine, Chicago

Smail D 1987 Taking care. JM Dent, London

Szasz T S 1970 The myth of mental illness. Paladin, London

Szasz T S 1987. Insanity: the idea and its consequences. John Wiley, New York

Wittgenstein L 1980 Philosophical investigations (trans GEM Allscombe). Blackwell, Oxford

Commentary

Hugh McKenna

> *With the same cement, ever sure to bind*
> *We bring to one dead level every mind*
> (*Alexander Pope 1713*)

Pope saw the need for having some sort of binding agent to focus our thinking on important issues for the benefit of mankind. He also saw the threat to flexibility and creativity if everyone is bonded to the same ideology. Phil Barker also shares these perceptions. He employs the metaphor of a binding agent to examine a wide range of issues. These include how nurses and people interact, how language distorts reality and how people are inappropriately bound together by diagnostic classification.

He begins by berating the trend in theory shopping that psychiatric nurses engage in from time to time. He realises that borrowing philosophies from other disciplines can bind nurses to beliefs and practices that are inappropriate to their craft. One way to avoid this, especially for an emergent discipline, is to gain a worldview (Fawcett 1989). A worldview is like the view of a country from a satellite. The image is so all-encompassing that it is difficult to begin to describe the detail. Nonetheless, Barker sees the importance of this for psychiatric nursing. A worldview can provide a truly philosophic vantage point, a global perspective which identifies phenomena of interest to the discipline and explains how that discipline deals with those phenomena in an unique manner.

In an effort to gain a worldview of psychiatric nursing, Barker poses questions relating to patients, persons, population and sex. How he attempts to answer these questions makes entertaining and interesting reading. A substantial part of the answers lies in an understanding of language. It is a truism that language affects our understanding, our understanding affects our knowledge, our knowledge affects our attitudes and our attitudes affect our behaviour (Peplau 1987). Therefore language is powerful and power is a theme that Barker returns to again and again in this paper, none more so when he discusses the relationship between patients and people.

The term 'patient' was a relatively innocuous word before becoming hijacked by the medical model. Barker wonders why we do not call recipients of our services people rather than patients – after all, that is what they are! Yet he admits that his use of the term person to describe the recipients of the service may be just a token gesture.

As we enter the third millennium it may not be too late to rediscover the term patient and rescue it from the powerful illness model. The current emphasis on community and primary care means that more people are being treated in their own homes. Therefore, the term patient is no longer merely associated with acute or chronic hospitalisation – now your next door neighbour is a patient of the local primary care practice and you too are a patient. Barker's paper was written in 1990 before the most recent changes in the NHS (DoH 1997). Could his view of the patient be anachronistic?

Rather than bind us, models, holistic or otherwise, can blind us to people and their care. Those who adhere to a medical model of schizophrenia subscribe to a different causation, presentation and treatment than those who adhere to cognitive-behavioural, psychoanalytical or social models. Barker appears to be suggesting that different models create different mirages, and of course the purpose of a mirage is to enchant by fooling us.

Psychiatric nurses should retain a healthy scepticism of all models, for to worship one model's view of the world is inviting enslavement to an ideology. Barker hints at this in his entertaining story of the Psyches family. In 1998, like Damien in the Omen, the Psyche's youngest child 'neuroscience' has grown (if not matured) and has even found fervent disciples among some psychiatric nurses (Gournay 1996).

Psychiatric nurses are good at criticising the medical model of psychiatry. They point to its reductionist approach. However, so-called nursing theories are also reductionist – they reduce people to four adaptation modes, twelve activities of living or eight self-care requisites. One track is one track regardless of philosophy. So, Barker is right to urge readers not to be too enchanted by the 'black hole' of holism – it too is a form of reductionism.

While people are different from plants and soils, nurses consistently adopt the physical science habit of classification and categorisation. Barker argues against the trend of allocating people who have problems of living into taxonomies such as mental illness, mental handicap and psychogeriatrics. His view has much in common with that of the American Nurses Association. It perceives nursing as being concerned with the patient and families' responses to health and illness. I find this view of nursing helpful. Whether a person has a diagnosis of schizophrenia, Down's syndrome or dementia should be a matter for the briefest consideration. Regardless of diagnostic category, nurses should be focusing on how people and their families respond to having these 'disorders' – does it, for example, affect their sleeping, working or communication patterns. This supports Phil's point that, regardless of psychiatric labels, people have needs relating to being human.

The final section on sexuality poses more questions than answers. Nonetheless, it returns the reader to the issue of power. In Ken Kesey's 1992 novel *One Flew Over The Cuckoo's Nest*, McMurphy experiences the disempowerment of the psychiatric system. Barker recognises vestiges of this in the 1990s. There are only so many slices in the power cake, and if one person receives extra, this means there is less for others. To empower patients means a disempowerment of nurses and doctors. Hence the aim of all good psychiatric nurses should be to empower patients by disempowering themselves. This fits in with Barker's view that true nursing involves helping people to need nurses much less. Could it be that true nursing is about ultimately making nursing extinct?

Accepting Barker's distinction between Nightingale and Cuidad, I would contest that psychiatric and general nursing have much to learn from both these individuals. In particular, general nurses would do well to follow Cuidad's humanistic practices. Nightingale also has something to offer psychiatric nurses. She believed that nurses and doctors could not cure illness, rather they placed the patient in the best position for nature to cure him (sic). Similarly, members of the psychiatric team cannot cure mental disorders; their energies should be focused on working with people to remove the barriers to recovery from distress – 'nature' can do the rest.

In nursing, there appears to be a trend where fads and fashions bring with them a plethora of published papers and conference presentations. The authors then move on to other topics and related publications and presentations. An examination of Barker's career to date shows that he has sticking power. Even though he presented the paper on which this chapter is based at a conference in 1990, it is gratifying to note that he is still working diligently on a philosophy of psychiatric nursing and on what people need psychiatric nurses for. A perusal of his recent publications on the development of a psychiatric nursing theory (Barker 1997) shows how he has built well upon the philosophic foundations of this early paper.

REFERENCES

Barker P 1997 Towards a meta theory of psychiatric and mental health nursing. Mental Health Practice 1(4):18–21

Department of Health 1997 The new NHS: modern, dependable. HMSO, London

Fawcett J 1989 Analysis and evaluation of conceptual models of nursing, 2nd edn. F A Davis, Philadelphia

Gourney K 1996 What to do with nursing models. Journal of Psychiatric and Mental Health Nursing 2: 325–327

Kesey K 1962 One flew over the cuckoo's nest. New American Library, New York

Peplau H E 1987 Nursing science: a historical perspective. Conference presentation, Discovery International, Pittsburgh

Pope A 1713 The dying Christian to his soul. In: Harvey P (ed) 1967 The Oxford companion to English literature. Clarendon Press, Oxford

The eye of the needle: research and the proper focus of nursing

Research within nursing is not only in a healthy state, but is far from being a one-dimensional activity. In discussion we discover that research means different things to different people. Research may mean the study of some phenomenon 'within rigorously controlled conditions, for the purpose of prediction or explanation' (Treece & Treece 1986). It may also mean the use of systematic inquiry to 'promote discovery of new facts or relationships between facts' (Clark & Hockey 1989). This may 'lead to generalisable contributions to knowledge' (DoH 1993). When we turn our attention more preciously to *nursing science*, research focuses on what we are really interested in. Woods & Catanzaro (1987) suggest that this is 'the *adaptation* of individuals and groups to actual or potential health problems, the *environments* that influence health in humans, and the *therapeutic interventions* that affect the consequences of illness and promote health' (emphasis added). Research implies, therefore, the systematic *search* for *facts* within any discipline, maybe with the emphasis upon the search.

At least to the layperson, such research implies *scientific* investigation: extending the frontiers of knowledge; trampling ignorance underfoot. Like many journeys, research is more about travelling and exploring than arriving. If there is an after-life for researchers, perhaps they will be likely to assume that it is no more than a way station. Researchers rarely arrive, and certainly not at that place called 'absolute findings'. I find that I am no longer sure what is, or is not, a fact. Day by day, I might add, I become less and less certain of what is science.

I shall adopt a more vernacular definition of research. The *aim* of research is to create new knowledge (Hockey 1996). How it does that is through any *course of critical investigation* (Baker 1932). The downside to the use of such a simple – if not honest – definition of research, is that the layperson may wonder why we make such a fuss about *doing* what appears to come naturally to most animals: *being curious* and, if we are fortunate, *finding out*.

I may, however, be giving myself away too early. My aim is to explore a little of the present, and possible future, territory of nursing research, and to return, for the heart of my reflection, to a consideration of their implications for nursing research as we approach the millenium. Given the changes going on around us – nationally and globally; and within us, as a discipline – I might have called this chapter 'grasping the mercury' or, to take a title from one of my Zen mentors, 'Playing ball on running water' (Reynolds 1984). Instead, I have adopted a biblical metaphor, recognising that many of us would gladly try our hand at passing a camel through the eye of that needle, rather than submit to more of the frustrations of the research life. My own frustration – I gladly confess – is not with *doing* research, but in finding the opportunity to do research *in nursing*, rather than in health care in general, or within psychiatric medicine. However, more of that confession later.

THE PROCESS OF CHANGE

The only constant in our current climate – as the saying goes – is change. This applies both within our academic and clinical cultures. It might be folly, however, to assume that change means progress. Dora Russell left me with that thought when I read her reflections on the alleged progress of 'modern societies'. Progress, in the 20th century, she observed, was little more than the history of – if not the reification of – the 'Great God Machine'; and machines and all things mechanical, including mechanical thinking were, she asserted, yet further examples of the competitiveness which exemplified the men of science and their cohorts. 'Ingenuity and skill, indeed, [she asked] but where are goodness and wisdom?' (Russell 1983:222).

I may be shifting the context of Russell's concern when I compare her concern for the corruption of 'knowledge' – through its association with a male sense of power – to our current concerns for understanding the 'proper focus of nursing' (Barker & Reynolds 1994). The general question I pose is 'to what extent is our knowledge a celebration of our understanding of the human condition?'. Some of us almost worship numbers. Through quantification we believe that we might realise some wisdom. We might care to recall, however, the aged saying that, when fifty thousand voices utter falsehoods it does not become truth. We have learned much *about* people, and health and illness. Many nurses – here and abroad – are beginning to ask, but what do we know of *people*, and *their* health and *their* illness?

I find it difficult to separate Russell's 'power' agenda from the health care agenda. We remain strongly focused on the belligerent metaphors that have characterised the history of medicine: tackling, fighting and struggling, to overcome or control this or that disease or disorder. Often, when we are unable to control the illnesses or disorders, we settle for controlling the people with the disorders. Given the overlap between some recent developments within nursing and some aspects of medical practice, we might consider their significance for nursing science. There appears to be an obvious economic value in developing nurse-surgeons or nurse-anaesthetists. However, what is the fundamental relevance of such developments for nursing science? Many of you will be aware that I am fumbling with that question which has almost become unfashionable: what is the value of *care* within our increasingly pragmatic health markets? One of my doctoral students suggested recently that her study of primary nursing appeared to show that nurses were *either* pragmatic or visionary. The business culture that has enveloped us tries to suggest that pragmatism may be married to vision. My student's experience is telling her – informing her through the research process – that these may well be highly divergent paths in the clinical arena, and perhaps also within the research culture.

THE RE-EMERGENCE OF TENDER, LOVING CARE

I recently commissioned one of my colleagues to write about her experience of being a long-term user of psychiatric services in general and nursing in particular. She wrote about two experiences of nursing that turned out also to be very different (Whitehill 1996). She wrote warmly and with appreciation of the care she received when she had a hysterectomy. Despite the potential trauma associated with a childless woman having a hysterectomy, she felt strangely peaceful and safe in what she could only describe as a 'tender, loving and caring' nursing environment. Only a month or so earlier she had emerged from her 18th admission to a psychiatric unit, where she had been treated for an acute episode of a serious mental illness. One might expect that (all) psychiatric nurses would focus, unequivocally, on the mind, the person and emotional life – if not the inherent spirituality of human life and its distress. However, my colleague felt traumatised (again) by a nursing environment that lacked the fundamental compassion that she found in the surgical unit. Important research questions emerge from her account: not least, what is the value of nursing in the absence of caring? Indeed, in a phenomenological sense, can there *be* nursing in the absence of caring?

I have a favourite hypothesis, which was first framed by Isobel Menzies in 1961 and is therefore hardly original, but remains largely untested. Certain forms of vulnerability, when shown by patients, stimulate hostile defences in nurses. We often avoid talking about death, or we trivialise it, for we fear our own death. We alienate certain kinds of 'patients' – the 'unpopular patient' so vividly described 25 years ago by Felicity Stockwell – because these people reveal, unwittingly, flaws in our own human make up. *We*, rather than *they*, are the difficult patients. My colleague has issued a public call for nurses to fly again the banner of TLC proudly from our ideological masthead (Whitehill 1996). However, in addition to asserting TLC, in the way that we assert many other so-called qualities in nursing, we need also to reveal further the processes which underlie our lack of caring when it all too often occurs.

CULTURE, CUSTOMS AND BELIEFS

My colleague's call for the reinstatement of TLC appears to confirm the importance of establishing what, exactly, are people's needs. There is an apocryphal tale of the young health care executive who was sent by his mentor to find the Ultimate Quality Assurance Manual. He searched and searched but each time he thought that he had found it, returning proudly with a new manual, his old mentor would point out the same deficiency: 'it is too long'. Each time he would find a shorter manual, that too would prove 'too long' for his old mentor. Seeing his young charge so downcast, the old mentor decided to let him off the hook. He pointed to a slim document on his desk and said, 'there it is, that is all you will ever need'. The young CEO picked up the 'manual' which was a cover and three thin pages. On page one, the manual read simply, 'first, *identify the people*'. On the second page, it read, 'then, *ask them what they need*', and on the third page, it read – you've guessed it – 'then, *give it to them*'. Too many nurses appear to be groaning under the weight of some 'manual', which they hope will help them deliver quality care, when a three-page manual might suffice. Small may not necessarily be beautiful, but simple invariably is.

One way to add to our knowledge base is to reveal the essential nature of the needs of individuals, their families and, in principle, whole communities. One hazard of crossing cultural boundaries is that one is brought face to face with one's ignorance, prejudice and narrowness of vision. A couple of years ago I first made contact with colleagues in the USA who offer what is called a 'compassionate approach to recovery from psychosis at home'. I recognised within their approach a complex of caring actions which has all but been submerged by the techno-hype of modern psychiatric treatment. Their approach has been called, quite rightly, 'a genuine nursing of the mind (Podvoll 1991)'. Ironically, only some of those who apply this 'nursing of the mind' are nurses. Their guiding principle is a postmodern update on Nightingale: by providing the necessary conditions for renewal and emotional rescue, patients may be afforded the opportunity to heal themselves – or as Florence would have said, be healed by Nature or by God. The philosophy of this compassionate culture derives from a range of age-old wisdoms – notably that of the Native Americans and Tibetan Buddhism. My vicarious experience of that culture of care brought a sobering set of realisations. In particular, it appeared possible to offer nursing, *par excellence*, when those offering it did not even call themselves nurses. More strikingly, the theoretical basis of this form of nursing was not the wonders of neuroscience or information technology, but shamanism, meditation and the spiritual traditions of ancient societies.

> 'One way to add to our knowledge base is to reveal the essential nature of the needs of individuals, their families and, in principle, whole communities'

In 1995, I went on a lecture tour of Australia where my cultural education was further extended by meeting a range of aboriginal peoples from Australia and New Zealand, who provided a powerful range of alternatives to what we would call psychiatric services. We may look askance at the plethora of 'new age' promises of health care alternatives, which are peddled by the kindred spirits of the modern world, but in the Antipodes I encountered the genuine article and felt curiously humble. Two thousand years ago, Epictetus suggested that difficult circumstances do not so much enoble a person as reveal him. I discovered a strange power of acceptance inherent in what might be called 'primitive' narratives of illness, healing and health. Those accounts begged me to look afresh at some of our assumptions about illness, health and treatment in our multicultural society.

The nursing research literature is beginning now to bulge with accounts of transcultural nursing: from Zambian studies of how families cope with HIV and AIDS on a large scale within urban settings (Nokwane 1993), through the specific role that nursing plays in the lives of Southeast Asian refugee women, unsettled emotionally and psychiatrically by war- (Fox et al 1995), to the identification of expressed needs for health care information in Canadian aboriginals (Shestowsky 1995). As I reflect on my two personal experiences, I feel the ring of fire that is scientific reductionism encircling me. In my own discipline of psychiatry, some nurses assume that it is only a matter of time before we demonstrate that thought, beliefs and emotions are mere manifestations of chemical activity in the brain. It is hardly a research question, but I wonder who would want to know that? Indeed, one might ask how could anyone know that, if 'we' – as distinct from our brains – cease to exist? Alan Watts compared such a question to being in a Chinese box:

> 'Whoever knows *that he knows must be amazed. This is both to wonder and be lost in a maze: to wonder because knowing and being is downright weird, and to be lost in a maze because knowing that one knows generates a confusion of echoes in which the original sound is lost. For when I know that I know, which one is I? The first which knows, the second which knows that I know, or the third which knows that I know that I know?' (Watts 1973:3).*

This is no idle philosophical reflection. When we consider 'what' we study when we study the people in our care, we need to consider what *is* this 'human' experience? Also, *who* is this human who is experiencing this human experience? And, also, *how* does this human come to experience this human experience of the human experience of illness or health?

SPIRITUALITY AND HOLISM

We often act 'as if' we have solved this riddle by simply affirming, repeatedly, that nursing is an holistic activity and that this multidimensional view of the patient will include a consideration of his or her spiritual needs. Although the repetition of such affirmations may be professionally uplifting, as researchers we need to ask to what extent affirmation translates into physical reality. My colleagues and I are currently studying nurses' constructions of terms like 'holism'. The first senior nurse we approached to negotiate access to 'her' nurses asked: 'why would you want to know that?'. My polite answer perhaps gave too much emphasis to the need to dispel ignorance. Had I been more honest I would have said that exploring nurses' ideas about holism and whole people might be vital, if we were not to slide into reductionism.

I also share with other research colleagues an interest in the role of spirituality in health care. One of our recent rejections from a research committee was a project which aimed to study people with a diagnosis of psychosis, inviting them to describe the 'human significance' of their mental distress. The rejection was accompanied by the observation that our study sampling method was flawed, as we would likely only obtain people with religious fixations. We had been at pains to emphasise a secular view of spirituality, using Viktor Frankl's definition: spirituality is the 'meanings which people give to the experiences in their lives'. This appeared to have escaped the committee. This led me to ask if we are not confronted by a curious intellectual paradox. The more we come to 'know' about people – at least in a psychological, sociological and biological sense – the more that we tend to believe that there is nothing 'out there', beyond the demarcation lines of the scientific description of *homo sapiens*. It follows therefore that we should become less keen to explore the unlit corners of human experience.

The discomfort which many researchers – or research committees – feel when invited to look at abstract phenomena, like the spiritual realm of human experience, may have something to do with the secular age in which we now live. Viktor Frankl was himself once challenged forty years ago on his views of spirituality and religion, on the grounds that the concept of God was no more than an archetype. All primitive peoples, he was told, ultimately reach an identical concept of God – which indicated the existence of a 'God-archetype'. Frankl replied by asking rhetorically is there such a thing as a 'Four-archetype', since all people discover independently that two and two make four. 'Perhaps', he said, 'we do not need the concept of the archetype to explain this: perhaps two and two do make four!' (Frankl 1973:18).

Viktor Frankl was a Viennese psychiatrist who found his own 'road to Damascus' in the Nazi concentration camps, where he realised that no matter what was done *to* him – as a biological body – his tormentors could not touch *him*. Although Frankl is almost a forgotten figure, even within psychiatry, we owe him a great debt, if only for alerting us to the importance of 'quality of life'. I fear, however, that even that value is being *MacDonaldised* as we speak. Frankl observed that in addition to the will-to-pleasure, and the will-to-power, shown by people down the ages, there was also the *will-to-meaning*: the desire to give as much meaning as possible to our lives, to actualise our values. When the agnostic scientist challenged him, Frankl had only just begun to feel his newfound freedom from the torments of Auschwitz and Dachau. His concern for spirituality was not, however, a religious fact, so much as a human fact. He saw the rejection of spirituality as part of the dehumanisation process which was characteristic of the 'modern world'. We can only thank fate that he did not have to endure too much of the 'postmodern' world.

Frankl saw man (sic) being reduced to an automaton of reflexes, a mind machine, a bundle of instincts, a pawn of drives and reactions, a mere product of instinct, heredity and environment. Such views, he observed, merely fed the nihilism to which modern man was prone. His experiences at the hands of the Nazis had given him the final warning regarding the ultimate consequences of the theory that man is nothing but the product of heredity and the environment – or, as the Nazis liked to say, 'of Blood and Soil' (Frankl 1973). He saw the horrors of the gas chambers not as a function of some perverse ministry, but as the end point from the lecture halls of nihilistic scientists and philosophers.

'Whether or not nurses can or will address the whole person, encompassing [a] spiritual dimension, is clearly a moral and ethical question... *How* nurses might translate those ambitions into a meaningful practice, caring for *people* rather than *patients*, or *clients* or *consumers*, is undoubtedly a research question well worth asking'

Today we are all confronted by philosophical and scientific challenges that may betray similar nihilistic attitudes toward the human condition. Whether or not nurses can or will address the whole person, encompassing that spiritual dimension, is clearly a moral and ethical question. Of course, as soon as we accept that people are inherently spiritual, everything changes. *How* nurses might translate those ambitions into a meaningful practice, caring for *people* rather than *patients*, or *clients* or *consumers*, is undoubtedly a research question well worth asking.

ENLIGHTENMENT AND UNDERSTANDING

All this talk of human experience, human needs and spiritual dimensions might seem far removed from the necessary concerns of a research conference. There is, of course, a sense of urgency that governs the health care agenda. Nothing lasts! All our systems are provisional and so also is our knowledge base. The ever-changing context of care and the mercurial nature of the management of health care systems, to which I alluded in my opening remarks, demand that researchers become focused: especially in terms of addressing the 'problems' of responding to illness, far less accounting for health. I noted briefly the wealthy divergence of research targets that might be subsumed under that 'health care delivery problem' heading. Some of you are addressing truly vital questions – some literally concerned with life or death. By doing so, you may establish a value for what we do already and also a value for what alternatively might be done.

In Alison Tierney's words, such a research focus recognises that one way in which research may be 'useful' is through its potential for direct use. Tierney reminds us, however, that such a research portfolio is, of necessity, narrow in its focus. The emphasis upon finding a way, or developing a technology of caring, ignores the *value of* – or even the *possibility of* – an 'enlightenment model' for research (Tierney 1996:394). The parallel between 'enlightenment' research and Schon's notion of 'reflective practice' is apposite. Although reflective practice has often been described as a means to bridge the 'theory–practice gap', in how many nursing situations might 'theory' be – as yet – undiscovered. I say 'undiscovered', since one of the processes inherent in reflective practice is to 'bring past experience to bear on current action' (Cervero 1988:44). In the proper sense of the word – as used I think by Tierney – 'enlightenment' means coming to know, perhaps cognitively or literally, what either we already knew intuitively, or which appears to represent a further meaningful dimension of our relationship with the world.

Either I am getting old, or at long last I have brushed against the wise so often that I begin to feel the *sense of life* and also the senseless way that we try to reframe life. Not only do we want to arrest degeneration if not death itself, but also we now believe that if genetic engineering doesn't come soon enough, we can live till we are 120 by eating like mice. These ambitions betray the visually impaired status of the biological sciences. We know that people who find life *meaningful* are more likely to live long or to live full lives, irrespective of what they eat, and irrespective – to some extent – of their genes. As Neitzsche said, 'Whoever has a reason for living endures almost any mode of life'.

'Enlightenment' research changes nurses directly. Those changes – felt within nurses – will resound through the care that they deliver. It is such a philosophical cliche that is worth repeating: there is nothing wrong with nursing since nursing does not exist, other than as an idea in the minds of people called nurses, or in the minds of the people who can observe nursing. If we accept this premise then that is where our search for understanding about nursing begins, in the mental pictures and the word-plays of people called nurses and their patients. Once we know what needs to be done, literally in the *name* of nursing, then – and perhaps only then – shall we begin to find the technology which might enable that idea to take shape.

As a psychiatric nurse it is easy for me to emphasise the importance of the mind and the abstract nature of the nursing relationship. What else is the mind but a word. Yet that single word embraces all the stories which might be told about our world and our relations with it. A casual examination of the nursing research literature suggests that the exploration of the 'whole lived experience' (Parse 1991) has been addressed best by nurses working outside of the psychiatric setting. Indeed, such human inquiry is most often focused on people with the most threatening *physical* problems: those on the edges of life – especially children with cancers, people with AIDS and people served by the hospice movement. The emphasis given by Parse and her colleagues to 'process-oriented theory' provides a framework for interpreting the 'living' knowledge that first concerned William Dilthey a hundred years ago. Indeed, Dilthey was an early manifestation of Frankl's concern: fearing that the natural sciences would strip life of all meaning. As result he called for a human science founded on living knowledge: the subject matter of which would be 'the interrelation of life, expression and understanding'. I have a sense that within such a conception of a human science may lie a key to what my colleague Bill Reynolds and I have called, somewhat improperly, the 'proper focus of nursing' (Barker & Reynolds 1995). Science-as-process rather than science-as-product is rooted in the belief that there are multiple realities and multiple truths about human experience and health. As Gail Mitchell has observed:

> 'Nurses require a knowledge base that explicates the full range of human experience so that new ways of theory-guided practice can be invented and evaluated from the perspectives of those receiving services' (Mitchell 1995).

Although it is over thirty years since Kuhn's famous exposition of the paradigm shift, that shift appears only now to be gaining a wide audience within nursing science. A fine example is Martinson & Liu's (1988) development of a care-planning system for children with cancer which began with those children's stories: their 'three wishes' appeared to have a more profound effect on the care-planning process than any theory of nursing, oncological or otherwise. I often lie awake in the depths of the night, waiting on the formation of research questions. One question that has kept me awake at night for years by its simplicity, if not ineffability, is: 'why do we only take the time to consider the *meaning* of a person's life, when they appear to be nearing the end of it?'. It seems axiomatic that we need to understand something of what life *means*

'It seems axiomatic that we need to understand something of what life *means* for the person, and where they *need* to go next on their journey down the life path, if we are ever to offer them anything remotely resembling *human* care. If nursing is a human science, *how* we do that must be high on our list of research priorities'

for the person, and where they *need* to go next on their journey down the life path, if we are ever to offer them anything remotely resembling *human* care. If nursing is a human science, *how* we do that must be high on our list of research priorities.

There should – in principle – be no obstacle to researching the human processes that might both underpin and explicate an enlightenment model of nursing research and theory. In practice, there are a number of obvious problems. First of all we are encouraged increasingly to take the view that randomised controlled trials (RCTs) offer the only means of realising knowledge. The Chief Nurse's question: 'how can we all ensure our professional practice is based on research evidence?' may, in time, be reframed to read 'based on RCTs'. In the Department of Health's report of the conference on nursing and therapy professions contribution to health services research and development, Adrian Webb observed that the consensus was that:

> 'the field of nursing was far too large and central to be ignored. Nursing practices (and services) need to be subjected to rigorous analysis through research to ensure that the efficacy and also the cost efficacy of nursing interventions can be demonstrated.'

I interpreted Webb's 'can' to mean 'might' be demonstrated. However, the need to subject every inch of nursing to 'rigorous analysis' may not be quite so obvious a research goal. Kendell, the Chief Medical Officer from the Scottish Home and Health Department, has pointed out recently that much medical treatment is not validated by research, for the simple reason that 'nobody doubts for one minute that those treatments are life saving' (Kendell 1995). Do nurses fail to subject 'holistic caring' to 'rigorous analysis through research' because nobody doubts for one minute that it is vital? Or do we take caring so much for granted that we have not thought to study it? Or, do we think it would be impossible to study? What would an RCT of 'holistic caring' look like? A randomised controlled trial of *caring* – far less holistic caring – would present not only methodological problems, but major ethical problems.

'Do nurses fail to subject "holistic caring" to "rigorous analysis through research' because nobody doubts for one minute that it is vital? Or do we take caring so much for granted that we have not thought to study it? Or, do we think it would be impossible to study?… A randomised controlled trial of *caring* – far less holistic caring – would present not only methodological problems, but major ethical problems'.

HEALTH: DREAM, MYTH OR EVERYDAY REALITY

I do not dispute the value of counting some things and measuring others. There is clearly a need, on occasions, to translate people into statistics, to build ever more pigeon holes for human experience, in an attempt to throw a net over the moving target called health and illness. All such activities – which belong to the positivist scientific tradition – assume that life has products. From a constructivist position, however, the same life may only be a process. Life is a journey and it may be understood by using the metaphor of a river as the life route, with time as the constant flow, which often escapes our attention. The fluid nature of life, human behaviour, human actions and interactions – the whole chaotic order of it (Barker 1996) – is not amenable to a form of inquiry which assumes that the target can be rendered stationary. Our snapshots of life in motion are no more than snapshots: the name is not the thing and the map is not the territory (Korzybski 1995)

In a more expansive mood, Robert Pirsig tossed me into the waters of reality twenty years ago:

> 'Forms of reasoning are human inventions. There is no way of measuring whether one entity is more true than another. That which is adopted is generally only more convenient.'

He might have said our adoption of the truth is 'more pragmatic'. However, he went on to observe that:

> 'Traditional scientific method has always been at very best, 20–20 hindsight. It's good for seeing where you've been. It's good for testing the truth of what you think you know, but it can't tell you where you ought to go, unless where you ought to go is a continuation of where you were going in the past. Creativity, originality, inventiveness, intuition, imagination, are completely outside its domain' (Pirsig 1974:279).

As we head for the millenium, that symbolic beacon of renewal and rebirth, we all need to ask, what will help us find our way? What kind of research methodology or ideology might help inform the proper focus of nursing? In 1996, Virginia Henderson, who seemed to have a remarkable capacity to 'envision' nursing, died. I turn to another great nursing visionary to help me reach some kind of a conclusion. Hilda Peplau is not only a great nursing philosopher but possesses the kind of human quality which allows one to feel safe, uplifted and optimistic in her company. I can vouch for that through direct experience. Like my other mentor, Annie Altschul, Dr Peplau finds no difficulty in locating the focus of her attention within the interpersonal domain. For both Hilda and Annie, the personal (and interpersonal) is also political. Recently Dr Peplau returned to one of her enduring interests: the nursing care of people in schizophrenia. Her thoughts are, as usual, topical, given our national (moral) panic about serious mental illness in this country. Dr Peplau suggested that if nursing is ever to become the holistic, person-focused activity which it believes it is already, then it must reject the notion of packaging people and their care according to medical diagnostic criteria. For Peplau – and indeed many North American nurses – the focus of nursing is quite clear: we have no real interest in people's diseases or their health for that matter, nurses are interested in people's relationships with their illness, or with their health. Today I have been begging the question, is such a focus *proper* – is it right and fitting – in our culture at this time? That too may be a research question.

I turn the clock back again to prepare for my conclusion. Over fifty years ago, Thomas Mann published *Dr Faustus*: his re-writing of Marlowe and Goethe's earlier excursions into the myth of Faust, who sold his soul to the devil. Mann's *Dr Faustus* is a novel about the illness of the 20th century and, as such, requires us, as Rollo May observed, to rethink health in a declining civilization and to consider how we might use our great progress in medicine (May 1991). It is, in that sense, a book very much for our time, although not of our time.

The sickness which Mann was talking about – and which Herman Hesse also discussed in *Steppenwolf* – is a spiritual illness. The Devil's lines are the finest example of the devil's advocacy in action.

> *'Have you forgotten what you learned in schools, that God can bring good out of evil?' (and later adds) 'A man must have been always ill and mad in order that others no longer need be so'.*

In Rollo May's view, the passion of modern human beings is to conquer the world of medicine and therefore of health – to arrive at a concept of health which Mann believed was vanity rather than health. Rollo May – an existential psychotherapist in the tradition of Frankl – fears that people who come for therapy might also want a version of a pact with the devil: they want power over whatever ails them and which they cannot achieve. Shall they sell their souls to the devil – who might today be called heroin, cocaine or alcohol – to attain that power? We might consider whether our concerns for our physical health betray a similar unhealthy lust for power, especially power over ourselves.

In May's view much of our self-improvement is Faustian. Even in a conservative society like England, increasingly we see adverts where someone offers to relieve your stress, offers crisis management, offers to help you with goal selection, decision-making, life style, orientation, imaging, premarital strategies, social networking and person evaluation. The new disease of the post-modern world is *wannabe-ism*. Whether we really *want* to be someone, or something, other than who we already are, is unclear. However, it seems remarkably easy to sell the idea that we need to improve ourselves. Today, we have multiple choices for such self-improvement: from the pharmaceutical to the psychotherapeutic to the surgical. George Orwell predicted the National Lottery in *1984*, and Aldous Huxley predicted Prozac Nation in *Brave New World*. However, who would have predicted that in the late 20th century the boys-in-men would lust after women whose assets may be more than 50% silicone implant. More importantly, who would have predicted that women would value either such lusting or such implants?

Although these may appear odd reflections for a research conference, for me our passion for health and our almost obsessive desire to rid ourselves of disease, if not also death, offers at least one context for the research agenda. When we dream of holistic nursing, and then set about researching its existence, we need to ask why we think we are not already whole, even if the whole of *who* and *what* we are becoming is flawed, weak and fickle? When we dream of advancing or enhancing nursing practice, what is it that we wish to advance, to what particular purpose and to fulfil whose particular needs? When we talk of clarifying the status of basic nursing care, how do we approach the notion of what is, or is not, basic to the human condition of health, and where do we go to seek the answers to such ineffable questions?

Once, we, as a people, spent much time reflecting on these kinds of philosophical questions. At some point, recently, in our development we became less interested in 'why' we should do this or that, but became more interested in 'how' we might do it, how well we might do it and how efficiently it might be done. I suppose I am proposing a wider platform for what might be called the moral and ethical underpinnings of research. However, I think it would be unfortunate if we separated off these kinds of questions, labelling them 'ethical issues', and attending to them somehow as a distinct part of the research process. We appear to be growing towards an old understanding of health: that health means whole, and that the possession or loss of health is likely to be linked to the way we live our lives, in the broadest sense. This 'living' includes the social, economic, cultural and spiritual context of our lives. Nursing research *can* avoid dealing with the multidimensional nature of whole/health but it *may* end up rendering a knowledge largely divorced from the life which we set out, first, to study.

'Nursing research *can* avoid dealing with the multidimensional nature of whole/health but it *may* end up rendering a knowledge largely divorced from the life which we set out, first, to study'

These reflections bring me full circle, I hope, and tie up again with Dora Russell's concerns about power and the corruption of knowledge. And I choose to close on another philosophical note. Doing research can be arduous, but attaching a value to research findings may be much harder. Our problem today is not that we do not have enough research, or that we have not implemented enough research. Rather, we have not yet agreed as to how we might place a value on the various forms of knowledge that have emerged from our researches. When we have agreed that, the proper focus of nursing might become clearer.

NOTE

This chapter is based on a paper first given at the Royal College of Nursing, UK Annual Research Conference: Civic Centre, Newcastle upon Tyne, England, Sunday 31 March 1996.

REFERENCES

Baker E A 1932 The new English dictionary. Odhams, London

Baker P 1996 Chaos and the way of Zen: psychiatric nursing and the uncertainty principle. Journal of Psychiatric and Mental Health Nursing 3(1): 75–80

Barker P, Reynolds W 1994 A critique: Watson's caring ideology, the proper focus of psychiatric nursing. Journal of Psychosocial Nursing and Mental Health Services 82(5): 17–22

Clark J M, Hockey L (eds) 1989 Further research for nursing: a new guide for the enquiring nurse. Scutari Press, London

Department of Health 1993 Report of the task force on the strategy for nursing research, midwifery and health visiting. Au, London

Fox P G, Cowell J M, Johnson M M 1995 Effects of family disruption on Southeast Asian refugee women. International Nursing Review 42(1):27–30

Frankl V 1973 *The doctor* and the soul: from psychotherapy to logotherapy. Pelican, Harmondsworth

Hockey L 1996 The nature and purpose of research. In: Cormack D F S (ed) The research process in nursing, 3rd edn. Blackwell Science, Oxford

Hunt J 1984 Why don't we use these findings? Nursing Mirror 158(8):29

Kendell R 1995 From the Chief Medical Officer. Health Bulletin 53(2): 87–88

Korzybski A 1995 Science and sanity: an introduction to non-Aristotelian systems and general semantics, 5th edn. Institute of General Semantics, New York

Martinson I M, Liu B Y 1988 Three wishes of a child with cancer. International Nursing Review 35(5):143–146.

May R 1991 The cry for myth. WW Norton, New York

Mitchell G 1995 The view of freedom in human becoming theory. In: Parse RR (ed) Illuminations: the human becoming theory in practice and research. National League for Nursing, New York

Nkowane AM 1993 Breaking the silence: the need for counselling of HIV/AIDS patients. International Nursing Review 40(1): 17–20

Parse RR 1991 Parse's theory of human becoming. In: Goertzen IE (ed) Differentiating nursing practice in the 21st century. American Nurses Association, New York

Pirsig R 1974 Zen and the art of motorcycle maintenance. Corgi, London

Podvoll E 1991 The seduction of madness: a compassionate approach to recovery from psychosis at home. Century, London

Reynolds D 1984 Playing ball on running water. Sheldon Press, London

Russell D 1983 The religion of the machine age. Routledge and Kegan Paul, London

Shestowsky B 1995 Health related concerns of Canadian aboriginal people residing in urban areas. International Nursing Review 42(1):23–25

Tierney A 1996 Research in nursing practice. In: Cormack DFS (ed) The research process in nursing, 3rd edn. Blackwell Science, Oxford

Treece E W, Treece W 1986 Elements of research in nursing, 4th edn. Mosby, St Louis

Watts A 1973 Beyond theology: the art of Godmanship. Vintage, New York

Whitehill I 1996 General reflection. Nursing Times 92(21): 61–62

Woods N F, Catanzaro M 1988 Nursing research: theory and practice. Mosby, St Louis

Commentary

Dr Colin Holmes

Phil Barker admits that, 'Day by day', he becomes 'less and less certain of what science is'. In recent years, science's underlying philosophy and methodology have been shown to be largely untenable, and since the products of science are as likely to be the cause of human suffering as its relief, it is in danger of failing to justify itself by its fruits. Unfortunately, science is so ubiquitous that it re-fashions our perception of what our needs are, and so, unless we are careful, our own values and identities become indistinguishable from those of science, and the control of our own destiny is secreted away without our even realising. Barker recognises this problem when he refers to 'The importance of establishing what, exactly, are people's needs'. Furthermore, orthodox scientists continue to declare that science is morally and ideologically neutral. From this perspective, technique and ingenuity are what make good science, and they are their own morality. That is why Barker finds sympathy with Dora Russell when she admits that science is awash with 'ingenuity and skill', and asks somewhat plaintively 'where are goodness and wisdom?'

It is not difficult to see how science has been complicit in what Jürgen Habermas calls the 'colonisation of the lifeworld'. The lifeworld – that aspect of human daily life which we have hitherto taken for granted as part of what it means to be human – has been gradually 'colonised' by science, technique, and quantification, and by the associated forms of thinking and feeling. Out of this process arises an obsession with measuring, and with numbers – what Barker here calls 'the worship of numbers'. The reification of such phenomena as 'mental health', 'mental illness' and 'danger-ousness', and the desire to measure these as if they were natural objects 'out there', is one way in which the colonisation of the lifeworld is currently impacting upon psychiatric nursing. In this kind of environment, it is not surprising that the premium placed on obstinately 'lifeworld' phenomena like care and caring has been correspondingly reduced. Care and caring, in such a milieu, only count if we can demonstrate that they work, and we must do this by quantifying them, engaging in some statistical wizardry and thereby 'proving' that they are value for money. Barker protests that caring actions should have a natural authority: they are natural, moral human phenomena, and require sensitive encouragement rather than scientific justification.

Of course, the lifeworld is not immune from our natural tendency to theorisation, systematisation and mastery, but any effort to define, quantify, or technicise it hits at our essential humanity and diminishes us as people. The negative effects of this colonisation of the lifeworld have been extensively described by critical cultural theorists. Most recently, the American psychologist, Tod Sloan, has developed a lucid account of how it undermines our humanity and contributes to individual and social psycho-pathology (Sloan 1996). The impact of this process on psychiatric nurses, whose sensitivity to the lifeworld and ability to operate successfully within its realm are her/his most valuable professional assets, is liable to be destructive of genuine therapeutic engagement.

An obvious postmodernist thread is Barker's allusion to the 'post-disciplinary' attitude. Several factors have created this potential: firstly, the epistemological bases of existing professions have been called into question by postmodernism's attack on foundationalism; secondly, economic imperatives coupled with loosening of the religious anchors around which people once conducted their affairs, have led to an increased concern with 'value for money', and this is leading to creative ways of organising roles in the workplace which are cutting across traditional disciplinary groupings; thirdly, it has long been recognised that multidisciplinary collaboration is a very fruitful approach to research, and in the case of applied research also corresponds more closely to the complex nature of real-world problems. Although the combined effect is a strong move toward postdisciplinarity, the established professions are fearful of losing their identities, and so there are also powerful, solidly entrenched resistances. As Barker notes, at the most basic level, 'individual professionals are fearful of losing their jobs'. Nursing is no different from any other occupation: it is socially constructed and, given sufficiently powerful forces, can be literally deconstructed, and we see evidence of this happening all around us. Barker notes that this does not necessarily entail a reduction in the quality of services; however, it appeared possible, he admits, 'to offer nursing, par excellence, when those offering it did not even call themselves nurses'.

Barker makes, perhaps unconsciously, a postmodern call for the secular rehabilitation of spirituality in nursing. In citing Frankl's definition of spirituality he admits the polysemous nature of human experience and the multiplicity of meanings to which it gives rise. The postmodern age involves a return to esotericism, mysticism, occult religious beliefs and irrationalism, and, for Frankl, these are all strategies people employ in order to construct a meaning for their lives. Significantly, Barker also links Frankl to the contemporary concern for the 'quality of life'. In positing this as a central concern, Barker further justifies the breaking of traditional disciplinary boundaries and role identities, and legitimises a progressive, unbounded concern for human wellbeing which runs counter to regressive efforts to restrict health care to a narrow individualised 'sickness orientation'. Since, as Barker says, 'There are multiple realities and multiple truths about human experience and health', any suggestion that we can actually measure a person's 'quality of life' is simplistic reification. It is another attempt by 'systems' to colonise the 'lifeworld', and, in many senses, we could say that Frankl's 'will-to-meaning' is an inherent form of resistance to that process.

Barker's link with postmodernism becomes more obvious when he suggests that 'value' is 'being McDonaldised as we speak'. When Ritzer (1993) coined the term 'McDonalidization' he wished to refer to a process he considered emblematic of postmodern cultural homogenisation. McDonalds' success, like that of many multinationals, is based on the certainty that the products sold and the style of service are virtually identical anywhere in the world. This strategy crushes the initiative and personal interactive styles of the employees, and reshapes local, traditional tastes so that they fit the standard McDonald product. In referring this process to 'values', Barker invokes the spectre of a world in which there are no differences of opinion over right and wrong, or good and bad, indeed no disagreements of any kind because we have all been socialized into a single 'structure of feeling' (Ang 1985).

Barker notes that the more we study the person, the more we begin to believe that there is nothing out there! This reflects the fragmentation of sense of self which characterises a postmodern society. Traditional anchoring beliefs and role definitions have broken down, and we are bombarded by such a kaleidoscope of images and expectations, that we are no longer sure who we, or others, are supposed to be. My own preference is to think of the self as a 'narrative self', based on the words and images that others use in relation to me, and that I use to describe myself and relate my experiences to myself and others. I know who I am by listening to the stories that my environment, other people, and I myself, tell about me. 'What else is the mind', asks Barker, 'but a word and the story it tells about us and our relations with the world?'. Issues surrounding personal identity, its care, management and redevelopment, constitute the very area in which psychiatric nurses should excel. As Barker says, 'we have no real interest in people's diseases or their health … nurses are interested in people's relationships with their illness, or with their health'.

The final postmodern thread I want to suggest as being immanent in this chapter is that of 'Otherness'. Psychoanalysts, among others, have recognised that it is by contrasting ourselves with 'not-self' that our personal identity is formed in infancy, and that this remains a persistent feature of our adult lifeworld. To define a group of individuals as 'mad', for example, on the basis of their irrationality, emotional disorder or loss of control, allows us to reaffirm our own sense of being rational, emotionally stable and in control. Someone must be defined as 'mad' in order that we may be defined as 'sane'. This is the meaning, I believe, of Barker's quotation from the work of Thomas Mann: 'A man must have been always ill and mad in order that others no longer need to be so'.

REFERENCES

Ang I 1985 Watching Dallas. Methuen, London

Ritzer G 1993 The McDonaldization of society: an investigation into the changing character of contemporary social life. Pine Forge Press, Thousand Oaks, CA

Sloan T 1996 Damaged life: the crisis of the modern psyche. Routledge, New York

Commentary

Ian Beech

As I write, the film 'Titanic' has just won 11 Oscars. We are reminded of the enormity of the disaster in 1912 in which fifteen hundred people lost their lives. The ship that was built as a testament to the ascendancy of science over nature succumbed to the very forces of nature that had supposedly been conquered. The strength of faith in science and technology at the turn of the century and just beyond was momentarily shaken, only to return a few years later with machine guns and mustard gas providing hitherto undreamed of ways of scientifically achieving mankind's objectives.

As we progress towards a new century's turn that brings with it the turn of the millennium, a reflection on the story that says science will give nursing the answer to all of its problems may be apposite. Phil Barker questions whether empirical science will illuminate the path for nursing in the next century. Like Phil, I remain unconvinced by the assumption that nursing's problems equate to the problems of the people in our care (Gournay 1997) and that objective measures of clinical effectiveness should be the single truth adopted in determining how nurses should be with people. Indeed the question of whether we really should define all of 'our' problems as 'their' problems is one that touches on some of the challenging questions Phil Barker has asked us within this chapter. I am reminded of the story of the farmer who meets the Buddha and asks for help in solving numerous problems that he recounts:

> 'After all of the problems had been described the Buddha replied "I can't help you, we all have problems, in fact we each have eighty-three. Even if you work really hard and solve one another one will merely take its place". The farmer was furious at this and asked "what good are your teachings if you cannot help me to solve my problems?"

> The Buddha replied "the teachings might help you with the eighty-fourth problem".

> "What's that?" asked the confused farmer.

> "You don't want to have any problems!"' (Hagan 1997)

A group of mental health service users recently told me of their experiences of being nursed by psychiatric nurses, and their list of complaints was somewhat depressing. They brainstormed a list of where they felt nurses failed to meet their expectations; included in this were issues such as:

- not being treated as individuals
- not being listened to
- not being given time
- being herded around
- being seen as a diagnosis not a person
- being given medication when they wanted to talk
- being fed no information or misinformation
- nurses being separate physically from them.

The experiences described echo those of Irene Whitehill related by Phil in this paper. There is a strong suggestion that mental health service users find that nurses are uncomfortable in their presence, and that the nurses respond to people's problems of living by reaching for the appropriate pro re nata (PRN) medication. This is a response that my colleague Lee Lanciotti and I have (half) jokingly referred to as the 'Star Trek school of nursing' – when faced with a problem the nurse, to paraphrase Captain Kirk, sets the (acu)phaser to stun.[1] I have no doubt that the medications that nurses reach for have been subjected to rigorous RCTs in which they have been shown to be effective. My concern is that those RCTs should not be, and never have been, the true focus of nursing.

In wanting to solve problems in nursing, the nurses described above are, like the farmer, merely replacing one problem with another. They may create quiet, compliant people in their care and they may avoid having to be with someone who is expressing thoughts and emotions that are distressing, but they are moving further and further, both physically and emotionally, from the people on their wards.

In the film 'As Good As It Gets', the character played by Jack Nicholson arrives at his psychiatrist's clinic without an appointment and is refused a session with the psychiatrist. His response is to berate the psychiatrist with the logic that after diagnosing him as suffering from obsessive compulsive disorder, the psychiatrist has no right to then say that he has any control over when he arrives at the clinic demanding to see the psychiatrist. The psychiatrist dismisses the argument and refuses to see him. However, when Ron Coleman (1997) fights against his diagnosis of schizophrenia, he is deemed to be agitated and therefore presenting symptoms of his diagnosis. Here we have one of the paradoxes of the scientific approach. If we solve the problem of mental illness and show it to be anatomically, physiologically or genetically determined, might we not relegate the life experiences of sufferers to mere symptomatology? If we do that, nurses will be able to solve the problem of managing awkward symptoms with an ever-increasing array of smart drugs but will be no nearer to understanding the experience of life for the person whose life is pathologised. R D Laing may have fallen out of favour in the eyes of many psychiatrists, but the sentiment he expressed in *The Divided Self* is a salient point and a warning to researchers in nursing:

> *'It is just possible to have a thorough knowledge of what has been discovered about the hereditary or familial incidence of manic-depressive psychosis or schizophrenia, to have a facility in recognizing schizoid 'ego distortion' and schizophrenic ego defects, plus the various 'disorders' of thought, memory, perceptions, etc., to know, in fact, just about everything that can be known about the psychopathology of schizophrenia or of schizophrenia as a disease without being able to understand one single schizophrenic. Such data are all ways of* not *understanding him' (1960:33).*

Phil is fond of referring to the philosopher Alan Watts in his writing, and I turn to him to end this piece. Watts (1995) believed that the most fascinating problem in the world is 'who am I?'. In much nursing research, nursing is attempting to answer that question and define itself as a scientific profession. Nurses have for many years been described in the popular press as 'Angels'. Watts (1977) reminds us of the words of G K Chesterton that 'The angels fly because they take themselves lightly'. In refocusing the eyes of the nursing profession onto the possibility of the more feminine, lighter, yin areas of nursing research, Phil Barker may just be showing the profession and the people in our care the wonder of flight.

Note

1. Acuphase is a psychotropic medication that has gained favour in acute psychiatric units in recent years.

REFERENCES

Coleman R 1997 The politics of illness. Asylum 10(1):11–15
Gournay K 1997 Clinical effectiveness: what we need to do. Psychiatric Care 4(5):221–224
Hagan S 1997 Buddhism: plain and simple. Tuttle, Boston
Laing R D 1960 The divided self. Penguin, Harmondsworth
Watts A 1977 The essential Alan Watts (ed Mark Watts). Celestial Arts, Berkeley, CA
Watts A 1995 The Tao of philosophy (ed Mark Watts). Eden Grove, London

The last wave? Promoting growth and development in community psychiatric and mental health nursing

4

TAKING A HORSTORY

The American psychotherapist Milton Erickson was a great story teller, as well as an enigmatic therapist. One day, he was in a field with a friend when a horse galloped in, saddle-less but wearing a bridle. Erickson and his friend cornered the horse and Milton, mounting it, said he would take it back to where it came from. 'But you don't know where it came from' protested his friend. 'It could be from anywhere!'

Erickson set off on his mount, keeping to the road. Each time the horse turned in the direction of a field, Erickson gently reined it back in the direction of the road. Mostly, he just let the horse trot 'aimlessly', all the time keeping it 'to the road'. Eventually, the horse turned up a small track leading to a farmyard where a delighted farmer greeted Erickson: 'Well I thought that I had seen the end of him. Where on earth was he? And how did you know where to bring him?'. Erickson replied 'Oh, about five miles from here. *I* had no idea where he was from … *but he did*!'.

I don't remember when I read that story first but it amused me greatly. The mere fact that I recall it now suggests that I found more than humour in the story.

My early training and my practical experience in psychiatry confirmed the importance of always taking a patient's *history*: patently as a means to gaining an understanding of the person and where (s)he came from. Life may be *lived* forwards – to paraphrase Kierkegaard's dictum – but it is *understood* backwards. The taking of such histories – for there are many possibilities depending on one's theoretical persuasion – has long been seen as the starting point of the therapeutic process. As a novice, I accepted the proposition that the *beginning* of care and treatment could only lie in an appreciation of the *past*. Such was my faith in this received wisdom that it took me some years to even begin to dream of alternatives.

When I reflected on the Erickson story I realised that it carried a strong message. Feminism helped us to appreciate some of the problems with *hi*story – and its tendency to reframe or distort the life narrative, through the exercise of a certain (masculine) power. The *her*story might well be a more valid acount of events, as they were witnessed, closer to the lived experience. The Erickson story suggested that I might be better off taking a *horstory*, rather than a traditional *hi*story. I had met many patients who had been unable to tell me their 'history' – at least not in a way that satisfied either them or me. The Erickson story implied that horses – and by implication people – might intuitively know *where* they were *from* and indeed where they needed to be *going*. Call this some kind of 'horse-sense' if you like. Whether or not they could express such knowledge in words is, of course, another story.

Taking a *horstory* seems to involve following the person; giving gentle guidance in a positive direction when (s)he appears to be about to stray from the main path, of the story. For the rest of the time, however, the person leads: this is only right and fitting, it is their story after all. No-one knows their life path better than the person. Of course (s)he is, for the moment, like the Erickson horse, *lost*. We both know that. Once this is agreed – openly or tacitly – we need to agree that the person at least knows, intuitively, the location of the life path. All change is about tramping that path with a purpose. For too long we professionals have assumed that we know the life destination better than the people themselves.

I have been involved in the 'community care' of people with psychiatric problems for twenty years. The opportunity to learn, at first hand, something of what people might need by way of psychiatric nursing services, was the first professional compliment I received. The second compliment came ten years later when the Community Psychiatric Nurses' Association (CPNA) invited me to become a Trustee of the Association. This gained me many new friends and colleagues, and many opportunities to learn from the many CPNs whom I met over the years. My invitation to address the CPNA Annual Conference[1] was the third community psychiatric nursing compliment. This illustrates that good fortune, as well as bad luck, has a habit of coming in threes.

THERAPY AS EDUCATION

I have spent much of my professional career pursuing the notion of the 'nurse as therapist' (Barker 1982, 1985). Yet, I have always experienced great difficulty in distinguishing 'therapy' from the proper meaning of *education*. I believe that people *own* their destiny, but often do not *know* this in any conscious sense. People who ask for – or are referred for – therapy own a wealth of learning, which needs only to be drawn out. I believe this to be true even when people do not ask for help, or may even actively reject the support of the care team. For too long we have maintained the professional myth that people need therapists more than therapists need 'patients'. Reality details a very different relationship: people-in-therapy learn a little from therapists about themselves; and therapists learn a great deal about those *persons*, and often also about themselves. People do not need therapists to change them. Indeed, it is universally acknowledged, but rarely stated, that the therapist *cannot* change a person. Instead, people need help to draw out, *from within*, the personal resources which they use to shape the necessary changes in their lives. This is the proper meaning of education: from the Latin *educere* – to draw out latent potential from within. When therapy achieves this aim it blesses both therapist and patient in the process.

We spend too much time cataloguing the deficits of the person. My father-in-law spent much of his adult life, less that thirty miles from here, a mile underground, mining the valuable black seams of coal that were threaded through this Fifeshire landscape. The miner's trick was to 'draw out from within' the earth that black gold without being crushed beneath the weight of the rock which sometimes supported, and at other times rested on, the coal reserves. This may be a fitting analogy, perhaps for the human mining that might go on within the therapeutic relationship. How do we mine the person's 'valuable reserves', without forgetting that these may lie embedded in their rocky past, traumatic experiences which may, at times, appear to have turned them completely to stone. Such traumas – in a metaphorical sense – may even hold people together, providing the context for the golden (valued) seams of their human development. If our function is to 'draw forth' or facilitate the human education of the person, then the gold must be laid bare and the dark earth and rock of trauma put to one side. There is a world of difference, however, between exploring the weak seams that thread through the individual when we encounter them, and looking out for the factors that keep people going despite their adversity.

Psychotherapy is bedevilled by the assumption that the 'therapist' knows the patient better than the person obscured by the 'patient' label. As community psychiatric nursing increasingly becomes defined as a therapeutic – as well as a caring – activity, this criticism might apply to us also. We obtain this 'knowledge' by generalising, sometimes wildly, from the experience of other people with whom we have worked. What we have found in the case of one person, we attach to the experience of another, to establish some kind of theory of the human condition. However, if we believe – as we so often assert – in the uniqueness of the individual, and in the need for person-centred care, defined by some holistic paradigm, then what can we ever really *know* that can be transferred so readily from me, to you to everyone else?

> 'Psychotherapy is bedevilled by the assumption that the 'therapist' knows the patient better than the person obscured by the 'patient' label. As community psychiatric nursing increasingly becomes defined as a therapeutic – as well as a caring – activity, this criticism might apply to us also'

Every person is, in some respects
like all other people,
like some other people
like no other person!

THE LAST WAVE?

Like most of you, I am fortunate in that I usually work with the person or family alone. Except when I record my sessions for teaching or supervision purposes, I work without a net and without a critical observer. Such a critical observer might encounter some difficulty in accepting much of my description of what I do as 'therapy'. This will be true whether or not they are nurse-psychotherapists, counsellors or generic nurse practitioners. Such is the narrow focus of the work of some therapists that they assume that psychotherapy is – or can be – only one thing: one school, one model or theory of human experience. When I joined the field almost thirty years ago, if it wasn't psychoanalytic, in one form or another, it wasn't worth the candle. Today if it isn't cognitive – or, increasingly, cognitive-behavioural – many believe that it is not state-of-the-art. Long ago I realised that 'not knowing' was a respectable position. Indeed, not knowing allows one to be surprised.

Not knowing maintains one's interest over long periods. Not knowing encourages one to keep a respectable distance from the person's *own* experiences. At the first encounter, how can I not shudder with embarrassment – if not awe – at my woeful ignorance of the human being presented before me? If mental health services are meant to help people to rediscover themselves – or to learn how to live with themselves – is it not obvious that I, the helper, should start from a position of ignorance, not knowing anything of any significance about the person who is the patient? Such reflections on the relative positions of knowledge and ignorance shared by the therapist and the patient, leads me to consider where our various therapeutic journeys might be taking us.

Today, a new wave of therapy appears to be washing over us. This has been called the 'third wave' of psychotherapy (O'Hanlon 1995), and I want to consider the relevance of these ideas to the present and future context of CPNs. The *first* wave began with Freud when he laid the foundation for the field by developing intrapsychic theories. These focused upon the *pathology* of persons: what was 'wrong' with them in some fundamental sense. This focus was of course wholly appropriate given Freud's background as a physician. This *first* wave was important because it provided an alternative explanation of people and their mental ills: they were no longer merely 'morally deficient', but were 'suffering' from disorders of the human psyche which were analogous to physical conditions. That first wave gave us a new language to describe these phenomena. Few people today, however, might be grateful for labels such as 'narcissistic personality disorder' or 'borderline personality', both of which are the descendants of that first wave tradition. Most of us are neurotics but few would thank the diagnostician for advising us, officially, of this fact.

The *second* wave emerged at the end of the Second World War when 'problem-focused therapies' overlapped with the first-wave tradition. Behaviour therapy, cognitive therapy and family therapy did not assume that people were 'sick'. Some of these approaches took the view that people constructed meanings, within their present experience – the 'here and now' of their relationship to self, others and the world at large. Approaches like the cognitive therapies assumed that people influenced themselves through their internal dialogue. In Hilda Peplau's terms, people make themselves up as they talk (H E Peplau, personal communication). And, of course, much talk is 'self-talk'. These therapies appeared to take the view that people were more flexible than the first-wave theories suggested. Personality was something that developed, and changed, as a function of the person's communications with others and with him/herself. The aims of these *second-wave* therapists were to help people repair, or fix, the problems they brought with them, and then to help them back into everyday life. It was as simple as that. Of course, the first-wave therapists took the view that these changes were superficial. Major underlying defects existed, and the person who was 'treated' by the second-wave therapists remained 'faulty'. This did not stop the march of behaviour therapy, and it isn't stopping the march of cognitive therapy, but it is interesting how fashions change and what was here today may be gone tomorrow.

There is no doubt that Freud and his followers released people from the prejudice of moralising judgement, by attributing their problems to a hypothetical set of *intrapsychic* events. People were not innately weak and indecisive, they suffered from a neurosis. Even today, many people are comforted by the observation that their distress is a function of some hypothetical mental illness. I thought I was going crazy – but then I found out it was *only* schizophrenia!

The various second-wave theorists freed people further by suggesting that 'mental distress' was the acceptable face of one 'problem of living' or another. (This of course was another idea borrowed from Tom Szasz who borrowed it from Harry Stack Sullivan.) Like any life problem, pragmatic solutions might be available to resolve such distress. Countless people have been freed from disabling anxiety, or have extended the boundaries of their lives through second-wave psycho-technology. It is interesting to note, however, that the demand for such a service continues unabated, if not increasing.

The *third wave* washing around us at present promises to free people further by assuming that the therapist is not the source of solutions (far less the font of all wisdom). Instead, we assume that the person – and people around the person – already possess the solutions to these life problems. Therapy – in this *third-wave* sense – is all about drawing out the solutions that lie within the individual and her/his interpersonal context.

'we assume that the person – and people around the person – already possess the solutions to [their] life problems. Therapy – in this *third-wave* sense – is all about drawing out the solutions that lie within the individual and her/his interpersonal context'

As we approach the millenium I sense an atmosphere of conviction: too many people claim to *know* the route to humankind's salvation. And such certainty fits all too neatly into a number of *prescriptions*, any one of which, it is proposed, offers individuals, families or even communities and cultures, *release* from human suffering. This story is by definition exclusively a professional story; the people served by professionals appear to have a different agenda.

The rate of technological change is truly staggering. It is estimated that most of the world could be linked to the Internet by 2005. Whereas it was once argued that the meek would inherit the Earth, they now risk being elbowed out by the cyberpunks and technofreaks. Even if this technological brave new world does materialise, it remains likely that vast areas of the world will still not be plumbed in to clean running water. Before we get too excited about the latest psycho-technology, maybe we should ask how many of those in our care are valued as human beings? Technology is exciting, but may not solve some of the more basic problems of the planet. Before we get too carried away by the promise of technology, we might consider the human significance of technological innovation in late 20th century life.

Many of our concerns and anxieties about the promise (or threat) of technology are very pertinent to the future of community psychiatric *and* mental health (CPMH) nursing. Given that we address the person's psychiatric problems while trying to promote mental health it may be appropriate now to refer to ourselves as CPMH nurses rather than CPNs. The massive acceleration in biomedical research – much of it stimulated by the 'decade of the brain' – holds the promise, for some, of definitive answers to our age-old questions about mental illness, its causes and solutions. To what extent, however, is any of this about mental health?

Brain-imaging techniques suggest the possible relationships between anatomical structure, functional changes in brain metabolism, and forms of mental disorder. *Human genome mapping* suggests the genetic contribution to different disorders but, so far, has failed to solve the riddle of schizophrenia or manic-depressive psychosis. Finally, developments in *psychopharmacology*, such as the selective serotonin reuptake inhibitors (SSRIs), most notably Prozac, promise more sophisticated drug treatment, especially for more 'treatment resistant' forms of mental illness. These developments suggest the state of the art in the 'hard science' of psychiatric enquiry. But what is the relevance of these developments for mental health nurses? My answer is: 'not much'. At the risk of sounding like a Luddite I would argue that the main influence of these developments, although important in their own right, would be to prompt us to reconsider the *human* dimensions of mental illness and health. Such human issues are in danger of being subjugated by the over-investment of importance in technology and the control which technology promises.

'Technology may offer intriguing insights into what appears to be "happening" on a biological level but tells us little or nothing about the *human experience* of mental illness, disorder, dysfunction or disability'

Technology may offer intriguing insights into what appears to be 'happening' on a biological level but tells us little or nothing about the *human experience* of mental illness, disorder, dysfunction or disability. Such technology remains within the sphere of the *first wave* of therapeutic innovation: purporting to explain the problem, without appreciating its human significance. Indeed, the only possible source of true information about such 'mental' phenomena, is the person her or himself. If we really wish to know more about what is going on within people described as suffering from mental illness, we need to develop more sophisticated ways of helping them tell us about their experiences.

Such a viewpoint was the basis for most of the recommendations in the Report of the Mental Health Nursing Review Team (DoH 1994). How can we develop our capacity to 'work in partnership' through developing more 'collaborative' forms of care, if we do not pay more attention to the *lived experience* of people with mental illness in our care (Banonis 1994, Cody 1994, Mitchell & Heidt 1993)? If people with mental illness are metaphorically 'lost' then nurses need to establish 'where' they need to go. The answers to questions about the need for nursing can only be established by 'learning from the patient' (Barker 1994). We need to ask *'what do people need CPMH nurses for*, as distinct from doctors, psychologists and social workers?'.

Although technological innovation *may* be important for biological scientists, for CPMH nursing it is a distraction from the proper focus of nursing – the development of appropriate systems of human care (Barker & Reynolds 1994). As *psychiatric* nurses begin to reprofessionalise, growing into *mental health* nurses, we need to remind ourselves of the true goals of *health* care. An illness service may revolve around the identification, measurement and fixing of some assumed deficit in human beings. A health care system must, of necessity, have different goals and processes. But what might they be?

Twenty years ago Illich offered a useful definition of health:

'Health is [the result of] an autonomous yet culturally shaped reaction to socially created reality. [Health] designates the ability to adapt to growing up and ageing, to healing when damaged, to suffering, and to the peaceful expectation of death' (Illich 1976).

Nurses become concerned with the challenge of promoting health when a person presents with some illness, disease, disorder or dysfunction. We should not forget, however, that *what* people present to nurses as 'symptoms' is qualitatively very different from the 'symptoms' they present to doctors or other members of the health care team. 'What patients present to nurses, with the expectation of receiving helpful nursing services from them, are *human* responses' (Peplau 1995). This distinction between the province of medicine and the province of nursing is not semantic. We may only now be beginning to realise the importance of discovering and working with the lived-experiences of the people in our care.

The problems presented by technology are not confined to computerised biomedical assessment and pharmacology. Much concern has been expressed in recent years over the relative lack of emphasis on 'skills' in CPMH nursing. As a result, an expectation has developed that nurses should acquire skills to 'help' people with mental illness more effectively. What these might be is open to question. Since at least the early 1970s, there has been an emphasis on defining discrete 'therapeutic processes'. CPMH nurses who redefined themselves as behavioural or cognitive-behavioural psychothcrapists may be the best examples of nurses who have defined their 'skills' through the use of such psychotechnologies (Barker 1982, 1985). Other innovations in therapeutic technology are emerging, such as Psychosocial Intervention (PSI) with the families of people with schizophrenia (Brooker 1990). These promise to clarify some of the needs in specific care settings and how they might be addressed. This may be an appropriate stage in our professional development to ask, 'to what extent does the introduction of such technologies clarify the business of *nursing*?'. Is this what people *need nurses for* – to offer PSI, cognitive therapy or any other psycho-technology?

- To what extent do such psycho-technologies address the unique lived-experience of mental distress?
- Are these psycho-technologies part of a passing fancy? Are these *second-wave* technologies doomed to fade – like the film-star's good looks?
- Should we be looking for something more substantial?

Users of mental health services are beginning to regain their rightful place at the heart of the care process. More and more user groups in the UK, and worldwide, are commenting on the structure and content of psychiatric services and calling for a 'paradigm shift' in the design and delivery of mental health care. Several studies suggest that fewer people are prepared to identify their problems as an 'illness', viewing the traditional biomedical paradigm as unhelpful and stigmatising. They would rather view their difficulties as 'meaningful in the context of their life experiences in regard to past disappointments, current dilemmas and future concerns' (Rogers et al 1993). These *existential* problems are by definition vague, personal and in a constant state of flux. They are also, by definition, not the same 'thing' as depression, schizophrenia or any of the other *diagnoses* of mental disorder. When I am *in* depression, I do not *have* depression: I have a *human response* to depression. The recognition that such human responses to illness, disease, disability or dysfunction are distinct from the pathological 'things' themselves, is further illustration of Peplau's emphasis on addressing the 'interpersonal relations' dimensions of illness, etc. People *relate* to their illness. We need to find out how they *do* that.

In the same vein, some user surveys advocate strongly the need for more 'personal contact and understanding and [less] specialised treatments and techniques' (Rogers et al 1993). Such expectations conflict with the trend for 'creating increasingly specialised services and modes of intervention … [which] runs counter to the emphasis on *deskilling*, which is implied by what users identify as being beneficial' (Rogers et al 1993). A major conflict is unfolding before our very eyes. On the one hand lie explicit requests by users for a more *humanised* mental health service, emphasising the unique, *personal* dimensions of their mental health problems. Such requests are supported by the Report of the Mental Health Nursing Review Team and reflect the proper focus of nursing, as described by Peplau and numerous others in the USA over the past four decades (Barker and Reynolds 1994). On the other hand, the market culture of the NHS has enhanced our belief in the value of 'fixing' discrete patient groups. At the same time, we have encouraged the development of courses to equip nurses with 'state of the art' psychotherapeutic technologies, appropriate for different populations. Clearly, we need to decide which of these agendas we afford the highest priority.

We may choose to adopt the view that people *have* discrete mental illnesses (like schizophrenia) that can, somehow, be 'fixed' by one psycho-technology or another. This philosophy of care allows a comforting distance between the 'patient' and the 'professional'. Alternatively, if we take the view that people are presenting human responses to complex human situations (which may include some abstract notion of their illness), we acknowledge the common ground between ourselves and those in our care. By acknowledging Harry Stack Sullivan's dictum that 'we are all more alike than different', we may begin building the collaborative approaches to care, which *Working in Partnership* requires of us. Such a beginning might involve the offer of a human, personal, existential service which people in our care appear to need, by developing ourselves, as humans.

The demand for a humanised approach to health care and genuine empowerement is growing across all areas of health care and reflects the new wave of therapy to which I have alluded. It may be that the demand for greater attention to the human factor in care may be a natural reaction to the complex nature of the technologies that threaten to influence, and perhaps control, all our lives. Just as we need to ensure that all people have access to clean drinking water, we need to ensure that the people in our care get the human care and attention which is theirs by right. How we develop a technology of *human care*, which is undeniably about nursing, and which will take us into the 21st century, is the major challenge that faces CPMH nursing.

So far we have talked much of the past, a little of the present but have only alluded to the future, in terms of my 'new wave' theory. In this chapter, I reflect on our professional journey, but mainly with a view to the road ahead.

The changes in mental health care involve more than deinstitutionalisation and the rise and rise of the market culture. All modern societies are experiencing a major epidemic of depression, prompting the view that we are entering a second 'Age of Melancholy' (Barker 1992). The risk of depression in the general population has increased *almost tenfold* since the Second World War. This silent epidemic has not been overlooked, but has been overshadowed by the attention paid to enduring forms of schizophrenia. Although not a proper epidemic, people born within the last thirty years are ten times more likely to experience depression than were their grandparents (Seligman 1990). Although any causal analysis is complex, there are reasons for believing that the social revolution of the past thirty years has contributed greatly. Despite the ebb and flow of economic affluence since the 1960s, one factor has remained constant: the traditional social supports of family, local and religious community have been eroded, to be replaced by a rampant 'individualism'. When people are successful, this individual ethic can enhance self-esteem. However, when people meet with failure, it can contribute greatly to feelings of helplessness and despair.

That focus on 'individual responsibility' shows little sign of abating. It has brought in its wake an escalation in depression, anxiety, substance abuse, addictions and eating disorders. Violent crime and some forms of domestic violence might also be related to the sense of *anomie* engendered by a society where traditional supports and networks are weakening, often to the point of collapse. As the number of psychiatric units in general hospitals increases, the number of admissions tend to rise, due to a reduction in stigma. At the same time, the expansion of community services highlights more cases of mental illness which, in turn, may require hospitalisation. Many of these 'new cases' are part of the rising tide of mental ill-health which is in danger of being declassified as the 'worried well', the 'heart-sink' patient or any one of a number of expressions of frustration. Notably, such frustration is perceived as being wholly professional – or administrative – in character. If the professionals are only too aware of how little they have to offer such people, where does that leave the individual patient?

As the 'goalposts' for mental health care move, this will have an impact on everyone especially on CPMH nurses. Four major factors are likely to influence our future role. These are the discrete, but related demands for

- a wider bandwidth of nursing provision
- more emphasis upon care management
- more involvement of people and their carers in the treatment process
- more cost-efficient provision.

These demands will require, in turn, a reconsideration of the educational preparation necessary to fulfil new roles and the organisational structures necessary to support them in practice.

GENERAL TRENDS AND INFLUENCES

The last twenty years have witnessed the development of a more comprehensive care and treatment 'menu' – comprising various behavioural, cognitive, psychodynamic and family or systems-based psychotherapies. The wider range of research-based options has made multidimensional care a real possibility, and the return to ordinary living more likely. True 'holistic' care may even be just around the corner. These shifts in philosophy have led to greater recognition of the needs of individuals and their families, and has coincided with the growth of the self-advocacy and prosumer movements (Manos 1993, Toffler 1990), promising the return of natural rights to people disempowered by the experience of mental illness.

These trends have highlighted the role differences in CPMH nurses. Some work as generic practitioners, serving the whole gamut of mental health needs, across all populations within one geographical 'patch'. Others have developed more specialist orientations within fields such as child and adolescent psychiatry or the psychiatry of old age (Hughes 1991), some even defining their approach more specifically in terms of a treatment modality – such as family therapy or behavioural psychotherapy (Barker & Fraser 1985, White 1993). The need to define the 'proper focus' of community psychiatric and mental health nursing cannot be disputed. What kind of nurse needs to offer what kind of care, to which particular groups of people, in which specific locations; and what kind of preparation and support do they need to develop such services?

DEMAND FOR A WIDER ROLE BANDWIDTH

In the early 1960s, May and Moore believed that regular home visits by nurses fulfilling 'extra mural duties' relieved the anxiety of relatives and encouraged them to accept responsibility – even if only temporarily (May & Moore, 1963). In the subsequent thirty-five years the needs of patients and their families have diversified, due largely to the changes in family and societal structures. As quickly as we have changed our service, the nature of the problem itself has changed. Such is the chaotic order of life. Natural support structures, such as the extended family, have gone into decline, coinciding with increases in the homeless and itinerant populations. If these changes have not actually influenced rates of mental breakdown, they have reduced the support available to the individual sufferer. We need to ask how best we might organise support for people with mental illness, at risk from social isolation with all the attendant problems this might entail.

Greater recognition is increasingly being paid also to the discrete needs of women, as consumers of mental health services. To what extent should women, long over-represented in the psychiatric population, be viewed as a 'special case'? As I have noted, the international view is that everyone should have some say in determining *who* provides their services. Such a principle is not without its problems given that health care provision is limited by economic factors. We need to ask whether mental health services should be *generic* – serving the widest possible range of populations; or should they be *specific* – focusing upon subpopulations, such as people with enduring mental illness, or addictions. This question can be complicated further by consideration of the extent to which services should be redefined by age – children or the elderly; gender – focusing on women or men; sexual orientation – gay, lesbian, heterosexual, bisexual; or other demographic factors – the unemployed, the homeless or itinerant populations?

What seems clear is that the traditional domiciliary-visiting, quasi-public health role of the CPMH nurses must be consigned to history. Although the provision of mental health services within the home may be appropriate for some patients, *what* kind of service, offered by *whom*, for *how long* and to *what* particular end, are the critical questions which need to be asked. Given the rise to prominence of various voluntary sector organisations, the traditional 'supportive' role of the community nurse may be returned to more natural agencies, such as befriending schemes and mutual-support groups within the natural community. If a comprehensive nursing service is to be offered, we must acknowledge that a range of role-options is required, rather than any single service design.

'What seems clear is that the traditional domiciallary visiting, quasi-public health role of the CPMH nurses must be consigned to history. Although the provision of mental health services within the home may be appropriate for some patients, *what* kind of service, offered by *whom*, for *how long* and to *what* particular end, are the critical questions that need to be asked'

There is a need for a wider bandwidth of role function (Patients' Association 1994). Some people may need the services of an autonomous nurse practitioner, capable of providing a full service with only minimal support from other members of the mental health care team. Many such independent practitioners already exist. We need to ask, however, whether such specialists are the beginning, or the end, of the story. At present, where they function as 'therapists', they may only replicate services that might also be provided by clinical psychologists, psychiatrists or social workers. Further research is required to establish to what extent such psychosocial interventions are a uniquely nursing venture. What do people with mental health problems need CPMH nurses for?

At the other end of the spectrum there is an increasing need for nurses working out of institutional services: offering outreach support to people following discharge from hospital care, based upon careful pre-discharge planning (Waters 1987). There is no logical reason why nurses offering specialised, intensive care in hospital settings should not follow their patients into the community, to provide a bridge to the natural community. This will, naturally, have implications for the structure of community services.

A wide range of other community nursing roles lie between the discharge follow-up and the primary care setting – including the liaison function with accident and emergency departments, providing specific support to people when they return home (Atha 1990). Experimental teams are also looking at alternative ways of responding to psychiatric crises in the natural community. One example is the rapid assessment team, which, having identified the need, offers intensive, but relatively short duration, home treatment services by another specialist team, thereby reducing the likelihood of hospitalisation (Holdsworth & Guy 1994).

The traditional distinction between hospital and community nurses is being blurred. Perhaps the emphasis needs to be on the patient population with, for example, rehabilitation nurses working from the hospital setting out into the community and back again; providing a 'seamless service' of support, care and treatment. We need to ask why the CPN does not continue to be the 'keyworker' for her/his patients when they require to be admitted for acute, or crisis care. Thirty years ago, Altschul identified the 'bonding' which occurred between the vulnerable patient and the first nurse (s)he contacted. Today, most services still appear to allocate 'keyworkers' to patients on a randomised basis. Given Altschul's seminal research, we might ask why we blithely break the relationship which has been established between a CPN and a patient, just because the patient is admitted to hospital? Why cannot the CPN 'seamlessly' carry over the care management into the hospital, facilitating the care and treatment process to allow the patient to be returned to community care, at the earliest opportunity? We might also consider whether the most sophisticated nurses should be based in the community, acting as 'consultants' to the hospital service, or vice versa.

THE DEMAND FOR MANAGED CARE

Health care provision is determined, to a major extent, by its funding base. However, many of the deficiencies of health care services will never be resolved by additional capital. Indeed, there is a need to ensure that health care funds are deployed appropriately. The emphasis upon accountability has shaped new directions in service provision, characterised by clinical audit and continuous quality improvement.

The emphasis upon the quality of service reached its zenith in the USA with the concept of 'managed care', where the 'package' offered to the patient is linked to the availability of funds to pay for the service. Although the North American experience, with its heavy reliance on medical insurance, does not translate easily to the mixed economy of most European countries, the principle of cost-effective care and treatment is generalisable. There is evidence that much traditional psychiatric care and treatment has been poorly coordinated and has often employed inefficient, ineffective or untested methods which, in the final analysis, equate with cost-inefficiency. Increasingly, there is a need to question carefully the validity of both the interventions offered by nurses, and the reliability of the organisational systems that support them. As we focus more attention on the natural community we need to ask again *what* kind of care needs to be offered *to whom*, by *what* specific kind of nurse, at what *level* of proficiency, to *what* particular end?

These are the 'hot' research questions of the day. Already some authorities have argued that the traditional counselling role of CPMH nurses is idiosyncratic and produces highly variable results (Gournay et al 1993) and should be reoriented in the direction of providing psychosocial interventions such as cognitive-behavioural therapy. I suspect that the choice is not between counselling and PSI; indeed both of these models of therapeutic support may be part of a passing wave of psycho-technology. In research terms we need to be asking, 'what do people need from *nurses?*' Then we might progress to studying the many ways such needs might be met. If the expressed views of the user/consumer movement are to be trusted – both here and in the USA – then people want a very different form of care, albeit one that is both effective *and* efficient.

THE DEMAND FOR EMPOWERMENT

The international growth of interest in patient satisfaction and charters for health and 'citizenhood', are part of an increasing 'consumerism' which ties in with the emphasis upon cost-efficiency. The social and technological changes of the last thirty years mean that people are much more discriminating than a generation ago. Those with experience of mental illness have an understanding of the experiences and services received by fellow sufferers, in other parts of the country, if not also from abroad. Mental illness, which once was spoken of only in hushed tones, is now featured regularly in newspaper and magazine features, and on the stage as well as within television and film scripts. The stigma remains, but the image of mental illness and its sufferers has changed dramatically.

Through the advocacy and self-advocacy movement, sufferers of mental illness increasingly define their needs and how best they might be met. Although this development is patchy and fragmented, it is clearly a rising tide. Throughout all democratic societies, it is now taken for granted that the experience of mental illness, even in its most severe forms, does not remove the rights of the individual to involvement in the decision-making process. How the right to self-determination can be accommodated when the individual concerned is suicidally depressed or suffering from an acute psychotic state, is the challenge which faces nurses, given that they are the most constant medium for the provision of care and treatment.

Those nurses who have not yet worked out how to involve people in their care need to begin this important process. Research suggests that any kind of involvement of the patient and/or family, enhances the resultant care, renders it more effective, reduces non-compliance, and increases reports of satisfaction (Wallcraft 1994). All the charters in the world will, however, be of no avail if the relationship between the service provider (nurse) and the service recipient (person and/or family) does not change. Psychiatric care, in all its forms, aims to restore the independent status of the person. Individual autonomy can be restored through careful negotiation of the goals and processes of care. We might consider beginning by:

- learning to talk more effectively in the person's own language
- assuming that the person knows (intuitively) what is good for him or her
- recognising that the person solves problems day in and day out, and might be capable of solving 'this' one

- allowing the person, or the family, to set and 'own' their own goals
- acknowledging – openly – that the person (patient) is the expert on their 'condition'
- giving more emphasis to their assets, as opposed to deficits
- building the whole idea of collaboration and cooperation around a careful recognition of the need to respect – although not necessarily agree with – the person's cultural and familial boundaries.

Perhaps this might lead us closer to some sense of an alliance between nurse and patient where both might learn together what kind of interventions best suit the individual needs, or the specific context, of the person and family. This will not only 'empower' the person but might also further strengthen the role of the nurse as the facilitator of human growth and development.

THE DEMAND FOR NEEDS-LED SERVICES

These three demands – for a more comprehensive 'menu' of community nursing options, using quality systems of care, which promote empowerment – lead us to consider what these developments might mean for nursing. An enduring concern of the past thirty years has involved the 'proper focus of nursing': what do nurses do, which other agencies do not? I see nursing as primarily a developmental activity: nurses provide the conditions under which people can grow and develop – within the limitations of their natures and the restrictions imposed upon them by their illness or their circumstances. If nursing care is not a complex form of 'human nourishment' – if it is not *trephotaxic* – I am not sure it can be properly called nursing (Barker 1989, 1992).

'I see nursing as primarily a development activity: nurses provide the conditions under which people can grow and develop – within the limitations of their natures and the restrictions imposed upon them by their illness or their circumstances. If nursing care is not a complex form of 'human noursihment' ... I am not sure it can be properly called nursing'

How does this philosophy of care relate to the development of community-based psychiatric practice? Nurses are redefining their art by focusing upon what people *need* nurses for. Rather than asking what nurses can borrow from other disciplines to offer patients, they are asking what do patients need from nurses, which they cannot get from psychiatrists, psychologists, social workers or the voluntary sector? This question underpins the notion of the development of a 'needs-led' service. Nurses should not be called upon to treat illnesses – such as schizophrenia or depression – by, for example, collaborating in prescribing medication. Rather, nurses should address the *human problems* which people experience when they are described as 'depressed' or perceived as suffering an acute psychotic disturbance. We risk losing sight of our proper objective by paying too much attention to the classification of mental distress as 'schizophrenia' or 'depression'. When we can address the *human problems* of the people in our care, we shall have begun to define the uniqueness of nursing.

This is not a new challenge. In the USA, theorists such as Hildegard Peplau and her followers have been disentangling the human problems that traverse the boundaries of different diagnoses for fifty years (ANA 1980, Barker &

Reynolds 1994). I have added to this debate by suggesting that the emphasis upon such human problems, rather than the medical diagnoses with which they can be associated, is *the proper focus of nursing* (Barker & Reynolds 1994). The signals are becoming clearer that people need, and are asking for, 'real care' and they want such care to be anchored to the whole of their lives, not simply focused upon some pathological part of themselves. What Capra called 'the turning point' is now past and receding into history. As science falls back into the trap of reductionism, it risks imposing its shrinking view of the human condition on research and teaching. It also threatens to change the way we perceive the world and our place within it (Monbiot 1995). It is time for all of us to learn to be braver, especially in admitting that the world is best seen by the naked eye and not by a sequencing machine. This is especially the case when we return our gaze to notions of the community, mental health and the care that might cement them together. Our ambitions to become 'mental health' nurses might hold the key. Through mental *health* nursing we might begin to develop a personal science of human problems.

There is much talk of mental health, but little agreement on its constituents, its whole shape, far less its function. Newnes has suggested that mental health is

> *'clarity of thought, kindness, calm, intimacy, enjoyment of life, the ability to work, love and co-operate with others, saying what you mean and meaning what you say' (Newnes 1994:46).*

Such sentiments sprang from workshops involving users and providers of mental health services. The same workshops prompted the observation that 'no-one has suggested that cognitive therapy, ECT, medication, hospitalisation, psychoanalysis or the plethora of "therapeutic" interventions on offer should be added to the list of factors which sustain mental health' (Newnes 1994). And what were those factors thought to be?

> *'Privacy, peace, quiet, physical comfort, friendship, love, freedom to participate, support, money, work, information, exercise, a sense of belonging and realistic expectations' (Newnes 1994:46).*

In Newnes' view, it was possible that a person with a diagnosis of severe mental illness, who nevertheless had the capacity to express sensitivity, might be more mentally healthy than a psychologist wedded to rigid empirical views about the nature of reality. (Given that Newnes is a psychologist, this was quite an assertion.) We need to consider carefully the challenges posed by such a notion of mental health: to what extent do we provide the conditions necessary for the promotion of its growth and development?

Such conditions are bound up in notions of true community. Mental illness robs people of much of the meaning of their lives. They become like the horse in Erickson's story – temporarily lost. We have a responsibility to help them find their way back to their life path, by moving forward in their lives. That must involve reconnecting them to a meaningful community. Thirty years ago Klein observed that the community 'may be defined as patterned interactions within a domain of individuals seeking to achieve security and physical safety, to derive support at times of stress, and to gain selfhood and significance throughout the life cycle' (Klein 1968). In that sense, community is not 'man's habitat, community is man *in the* habitat, for the habitat is not meaningful without its inhabitants' (Klein 1968). The extent to which many people with mental health problems are actually *in* their habitat, as opposed to being located somewhere on a map, is open to question. A major emphasis of CPMH nursing must be to help people join the *human* network that defines the community.

And in so doing we need to help people to recognise their own life path, for by following it they may, metaphorically, find their way back home. This may sound like metaphysics or mysticism but it is neither. It merely suggests how a new wave of psychotherapeutic thinking is beginning to wash over us. Perhaps – as a result – we shall begin to develop more ways of genuinely empowering the people in our care, reconnecting them to their natural habitat, from which they will gain, and will in turn give, meaning. Nurses will in turn become ecological practitioners, involved in providing the necessary conditions for the promotion of growth and development. Such ecological activity will of course be defined by the aperiodic and holistic paradigm, which in turn is underpinned by chaos theory. If we thought the last thirty years of the development of CPMH nursing were exciting, to paraphrase Al Jolson, 'we aint seen nothing yet'.

NOTE

1. This paper was given as *The Stanley Moore Memorial Lecture* to the Annual Conference of the Community Psychiatric Nurses' Association of Great Britain, at the University of St Andrews, Scotland on 30 March 1995.

REFERENCES

American Nurses Association 1980 A social policy statement. AMA, Kansas

Atha C 1990 The role of the CPN with clients who deliberately harm themselves. In: Brooker C (ed) Community psychiatric nursing: a research perspective. Chapman and Hall, London

Banonis B C 1994 Metaphors in the practice of human becoming theory. In: Parse R R (ed) Illuminations: the human becoming theory in practice and research. National League for Nursing, New York

Barker P 1982 Behaviour therapy nursing. Croom Helm, London

Barker P, Fraser D 1985 The nurse as therapist: a behavioural model. Croom Helm, London

Barker P 1989 The philosophy of caring in mental health. International Journal of Nursing Studies 26(2): 131–141

Barker P 1992 Severe depression: a practitioner's guide. Chapman and Hall, London

Barker P 1994 A partnership for change. Nursing Times 90(20):62

Barker P, Reynolds W 1994 A critique of Watson's caring ideology: the proper focus of psychiatric nursing. Journal of Psychosocial Nursing and Mental Health Services 32(5):17–22

Brooker C 1990 Expressed emotion and psychosocial intervention: a review.

International Journal of Nursing Studies 27(3):267–276

Cody W K 1994 The lived experience of grieving for families living with AIDS: family centred research using Parse's method. In: Parse R R (ed) Illuminations: the human becoming theory in practice and research. National League for Nursing, New York

Department of Health 1994 Working in partnership: a collaborative approach to care. HMSO, London

Gournay K, Devilly G, Brooker C 1993 The CPN in primary care: a pilot study of the process of assessment. In: Brooker C, White E (eds) Community psychiatric nursing: a research perspective, Volume 2. Chapman and Hall, London

Holdsworth N, Guy W 1994 Research and evaluation relating to a new early intervention community psychiatric nursing service. Journal of Advanced Nursing 19:290–298

Hughes C P 1991 Community psychiatric nursing and the depressed elderly: a case for using cognitive therapy. Journal of Advanced Nursing 16:565–572.

Illich I 1976 Limits to medicine: medical nemesis – the expropriation of health. Marion Boyars, London

Klein D C 1968 Community dynamics and mental health. Harper and Row, New York

Manos E 1993 Speaking out. Psychosocial Rehabilitation Journal 16(4):117–120

May A R, Moore S 1963 The mental nurse in the community. Lancet i:213–214

Mitchell G J, Heidt P 1993 The lived experience of wanting to help another: research with Parse's method. Nursing Science Quarterly 7(3):119–127

Monbiot G 1995 Misappliance of science. The Guardian, March 22, p 22

Newnes C 1994 Defining mental health. Nursing Times 90(19):46

O'Hanlon B 1995 Psychotherapy's third wave? The promise of narrative. The Therapist 2(4):24–31

Patients' Association 1994 Mental health nursing: a spectrum of skills. Mental Health Nursing 14(3):6–8

Peplau H E 1995 Another look at schizophrenia from a nursing standpoint. In: Anderson C A (ed) Psychiatric nursing *1974–1994:* a report on the state of the art. Mosby Year Book, St Louis

Rogers A, Pilgrim D, Lacey R 1993 Experiencing psychiatry: users' views of services. Macmillan in association with MIND publications, London

Seligman M E P 1990 Why is there so much depression today? The waxing of the individual and the waning of the commons. In: Ingram R E (ed) Contemporary psychological approaches to depression: theory, research and treatment. Plenum Press, New York

Sills G M 1995 Future trends for clinicans in systems. In: Anderson C A (ed) Psychiatric nursing *1974–1994:* a report on the state of the art. Mosby Year Book, St Louis

Toffler A 1990 Powershift. Bantam Books, New York

Vicenzi A E 1994 Chaos and social change: metaphysics of the postmodern. The Social Science Journal 28:289–305

Wallcraft J 1994 Empowering empowerment: professionals and self-advocacy projects. Mental Health Nursing 14(2):6–9

Waters K R 1987 Discharge planning – an exploratory study of the process of discharge planning in geriatric wards. Journal of Advanced Nursing 12:71–78

White E 1993 Community psychiatric nursing 1980–1990: a review of organization, education and practice. In: Brooker C, White E (eds) Community psychiatric nursing: a research perspective, Volume 2. Chapman and Hall, London

Commentary

Dr Liam Clarke

The history of psychiatric nursing practice is about evolving patterns of relationships, the slow emancipation of the pauper lunatic with his attendant keeper to the current standing of the person (be this expressed as patient, consumer, client or whatever) in the company of his mental health nurse. There is much to be proud of in this past: there are aspects of shame also. Lest we forget, the relative freedom to debate patient's rights in psychiatric contexts was not easily achieved. In part, it involved developing forms of discourse over and above the medical (psychiatric) discourse, forms derived from myth and/or literature, politics and human rights. For some, such non-medical discussions are a wanton intrusion of sloppy and wishful thinking into what would otherwise be a clear-cut/scientific domain. For others, Barker included, metaphor, alliteration and the philosophical muse are a precious resource: failure to nurture such resources induces a lesser understanding of the meaning of mental illness or, as Barker might put it, 'the prostration of human affairs before the juggernaut of technology and inflexible thinking'. Those who espouse an objective, 'scientific', psychiatry would dismiss this as sheer romanticism, believing instead that the axioms of contemporary psychiatric practice are sufficient protection for anyone.

The 'romanticism' allegation (which is gaining influence) is in need of refutation. To say that something is romantic is to attribute a quality to that something over and above that which it already possesses. On the other hand, when we call something medical, we customarily assume that that is the thing itself, the language of medicine being the starting point to which other dialogues must attend. This is a mistake; for to call something medical is to say as much about it as to call it romantic: both words are adjectives. We have attenuated to medical discourse as an abstract, objective entity. Whereas, here, Barker (resolutely) embraces a dialectic which addresses the nature of psychological illness as an experience, and attributes to that experience which R D Laing used to call 'internal honour'.

Placing the experiencing individual centre-fold, the author asks: 'what can we really *know* [his italics] that can be transferred so readily from me, to you, to everyone else?'.

The reader may wish to examine the extent to which this (unanswerable?) question is answered, or ask if it is a question which nurses should be tackling at all. One's answer to that will certainly give the clue to one's reaction (to this chapter) overall. My hunch is that it will polarise readers into two groups. For the first group, the searching is almost over: i.e. the physical sciences have already answered most of the 'big' mental illness questions and are on the cusp of solving whatever remains. Likewise, behavioural/cognitive sciences are seen as having produced a workable range of cognitive and socially focused interventions. There remains only the task of working out the most economical ways of applying this knowledge to defined target groups.

For the second group, the searching has hardly begun: it's not that they see biological 'discoveries' as unworthy; it is simply that they are inappropriate questions for nurses. This is why, for Barker, understanding schizophrenia must always proceed from the experiencing of it by the person concerned. It is to this sea of doubt which nurses must attend with its endless misgivings as to what is, or is not, true (about schizophrenia). The fact is, engaging people at the level of their experience is wildly at odds with any approach claiming a defined knowledge base. The fact is, psychiatric practice has evolved various schools of expertise but all of which possess the common thread of a knowledge base which propels them beyond experience and often whether the experiencing person likes it or not. Society requires this (for the greater good), and professional groups with their professed knowledge, expertise (and treatment) seek to satisfy the public need by treating affected individuals.

Alternatively, forging a nursing role from the take-off point of existentialism is never going to be easy. We can be sure that Barker is right (at least) when he defines that role as qualitatively different to conventional psychiatric practice. A problem with that, however, is to find a way of communicating one's terms precisely and recognisably. With Professor Barker there occurs an incessant quest for the purity of nursing and, it seems to me, he makes life difficult for himself because, unlike other (mainly US) philosopher nurses, he has saddled himself with the conviction that nursing is something which people 'do': nursing is a practical endeavour. So that although his writing can embrace flights of fancy and, occasionally, unorthodox stances, it is (thankfully) unable to free itself from a need to connect. Of course, there is little import in that: most of us value some point of connection with patients and their worlds. What matters is how we achieve it. Reading this book, some people will say Barker abandons practice, given his alienation from developments in psycho-technology, biological and behavioural sciences, and, no doubt, they will cackle at what they see as his pseudo preoccupation with philosophy and 'the meaning of things'. The fact is, however, he is never on a more sure footing than when playing down current attempts to refocus interest on physical science explanations. Barker's point is not to criticise these *per se* but rather to explore what it is that nurses might contribute to people with an illness (by whatever name). People who find fault with this, aficionados of PET scans and (randomised) trials, are the ones who have jettisoned nursing since what they seek is a kind of mini-medic practitioner, basking in the displaced 'glory' of medical-sounding achievements.

Barker's problem – and that of others like him – is that he employs a dialogue (often taking the form of a duet for one) for which it is hard to find any measurable application to care. An exposed flank if ever there was one. In many ways, what we have here is a kind of 'staying the course', an unabashed refusal to jettison the existential critique of dehumanising psychiatry; an unfashionable attachment to dignity, justice, relationships, freedom and the like. It seems (to me) an essential balance to that wretched scientism which claims to explain all: indeed, in respect of the latter, there is present here a yearning to be as sure of one 'thing' as they appear to be of everything.

Will psychiatric nurses ever offer mental health nursing?

5

THE ENDURING LEGACY

The conventional histories of the care and treatment of people with mental illness, like most histories, invariably features the 'great and the good': the distinguished pioneers, the theorists, the reformers and, occasionally, even the famous patients (cf. Porter 1989). There is of course a subtext to that history, wherein can be found the histories of those whose only distinction was to deliver the care, or to implement the treatments. Among their ranks we find the foot-soldiers: those who were at the 'care-face', whoever they were, and whatever was their rank, title or location in the pecking order. Many different kinds of people have placed their stamp on our cultural appreciation of those twin concepts, mental illness and health. However, the enduring legacy of the social history of the modern discipline of psychiatry is to be found in the close relationship between the alienist and the attendant; or between nurses and doctors, as we know them today.

Dr Eric Cunningham Dax came to Melbourne in 1951, to find huge, overcrowded asylums, which were as inhospitable towards staff as they were towards patients. Nurses were expected to clean wards, as well as care for patients, but were largely denied the means to do either. One of Dr Dax's first initiatives was to release cleaning materials and to persuade the government to hire cleaners. He also engaged the support of the Country Women's Association to make curtains and bedspreads and to raise funds for other essential developments. He then began his formal contribution to nursing, by having separate nurses' homes built, and after developing a curriculum, persuaded the Victorian Nurses' College to accept psychiatric nursing as a legitimate 'nursing course'. The rest, one might say, is history. More than forty years later, he was asked to join the Board of the Institute for Psychiatric Nursing Research,[1] on which he served for over two years. Perhaps, better than anyone else, Dr Dax has witnessed the emergence of psychiatric nursing as a discrete aspect of the care and treatment of the mentally ill. He has also witnessed its emergence as an academic discipline, eager to see its discrete contribution, formalised, clarified and evaluated. I hope that that eagerness will prove a fitting compliment to his own eagerness to see nursing released from its servile status of yesteryear.

As we approach the threshold of the millennium, it remains unclear whether or not nursing is a profession, a semi-profession or even the discrete discipline of which I speak. Shaw's wry observation that all professions are a conspiracy against the laity may seem harsh, but it serves to remind us to question what 'professionalism' in nursing might mean and, more importantly, whom it would best serve. We might also recall Thoreau's observation that: 'As for Doing-good, *that* is one of the professions which are full'. Could we but be certain that we always wish to do the 'good' which is meaningful for the person in our care, rather than merely to make ourselves 'feel' that we are doing good and therefore we *are* good. Currently, in all developed countries, significant steps are being taken towards making mental health care more accessible. We might care to ponder what the formal creation of a 'proper' profession of nursing, or even of 'good-doers', would contribute to the widening of that access. If we are to learn anything from the history of the true professions, we might conclude that the formal creation of a profession of nursing is the least of our ambitions.

THE MAP OF CARING

However, even if the discipline of psychiatric nursing remains ill-defined, or even half-formed, there is no doubt that the activity undertaken by people called psychiatric nurses lies at the heart of all our mental health services, and has been established there for a very long time. I feel a certain thread running through me, extending far back in time to the earliest recorded carers of the people whom we now call the mentally ill or mentally disordered. That those earliest recorded carers were monks stimulates a sense of male bonding. That they, like me, were of Celtic origin promotes a sense of kinship. Those monks practised their care in the old kingdom of Northumbria that extended from Tayside in Scotland, where I first trained, through Fife, where I was born, to Newcastle on the river Tyne where I have worked for the past four years. That historical fact makes me feel that my current work is only the most recent page in my book of destiny. I am conscious that I am making a small scratch in the margins of history.[2]

As we stand on the threshold of a new millennium, we all might sense something of the rhythms of the caring relationship which has pulsed through humanity, down the past one thousand years (Nolan 1993, Barker & Davidson 1997). Caring *is* part of the human condition. Indeed, as Pat Deegan, the American psychologist and psychiatric survivor has said, it is a vital part:

> 'although it's possible to quit, to sever ties, and to give up trying, it is not possible to completely stop caring. To be human means to care. In a sense to be human means to be condemned to caring' (Deegan 1994:19).

'Irrespective of the gender of the carer, we should not forget that true caring speaks always in a feminine voice. It is characterised by gentleness, by creativity, by flexibility and by understanding. Caring, in that sense, may be distinguished from treatment – which speaks perhaps in a masculine voice, characterised by rigour, by reason, by provocation and by control. These two voices, I shall argue, are complementary'.

Any map of caring which I might draw would be an extensive one, at least in terms of its lineage. I shall return to this historical map in my conclusion. Florence Nightingale's success in establishing the modern concept of nursing has largely overshadowed that history. Not insignificantly, the towering presence of Nightingale also overshadowed the role played by men as carers: men working alongside women as carers, first in the religious orders, and later in the asylum tradition. Irrespective of the gender of the carer, we should not forget that true caring speaks always in a feminine voice. It is characterised by gentleness, by creativity, by flexibility and by understanding. Caring, in that sense, may be distinguished from treatment – which speaks perhaps in a masculine voice, characterised by rigour, by reason, by provocation and by control. These two voices, I shall argue, are complementary. Although polar opposites, like the poles of our planet, they are what makes the world of mental health care go round. In their distinctive forms and functions they define the balance which we hold as a desirable human ambition – desirable as much for us as for those whom we are charged to serve.

TOWARDS A HUMAN SCIENCE OF CARING

That said, it is beyond dispute that the loudest voice in psychiatric history has been the masculine voice of treatment. Yet even this is a young voice which, as I have indicated, stands in the shadow of an aged tradition of caring; a tradition that straddles cultures and contexts as easily as it straddles the millennia. Only within the past fifty years, however, has any significant effort been made to understand and represent what that psychiatric caring might involve. In that sense the study of the art of caring, in pursuit of something resembling a human science of caring (Barker et al 1997) is a mere infant.

Having devoted so much time to introducing psychiatric nursing, I appreciate the irony in the title of this chapter. What exactly has *psychiatric* nursing to do with *mental health* nursing? In the USA, the term psychiatric/ mental health nursing tends to suggest its hybrid nature (cf. ANA 1994, Lego 1996). In the UK, nurses originally were called 'mental' – rather than psychiatric – nurses. Today, all *mental* nurses have been redefined by fiat as mental *health* nurses, although what this change means in practice remains unclear. Perhaps because I am a Celt and, like many Celts, enjoy playing with the English language, the meaning of words is important to me. By the end of this paper I hope that I shall have put Tweedledum and Tweedledee back where they belong, in the pages of a book which emphasised a play on language as much as it involved conjuring with reality. I hope to convince you that there is a *real* distinction between the experience of psychiatric, as opposed to mental health, nursing; and that these are not simply terms that mean whatever we want them to mean.

To explore that distinction, we need to return to the root of nursing practice, and the caring which is central to the nurse–patient relationship. And we could not even begin to discuss this relationship without acknowledging the contribution made to our understanding of interpersonal relations by Hildegard Peplau.

Peplau has been dubbed, rightly, the 'mother of psychiatric nursing' (Lego 1996). She has been recognised by her colleagues as a:

> 'wise, caring and gentle person [who] is one of the finest and best scholars the profession has known … for over sixty years her scholarship has been evocative, informative, and provocative' (Sills 1989:viii).

Although not specifically concerned with consciousness *per se*, Peplau's interpretation of the theory of interpersonal relations encouraged nurses like me to look beyond the delimiting parameters of the patient label, and to begin to consider what it might mean to *be* the person. In that sense, her work, over six decades, has consistently emphasised the need to focus on *human* issues (Peplau 1952, 1990, 1995), reminding us of the need, perhaps, to cure the patient as well as the illness.

Although it would be an impertinence to summarise Peplau's life work in a few sentences, at its heart lies a gentle curiosity; a willingness to relate *and* to understand; and a concern to provide people with the support they need to free themselves from their distress. Peplau clearly felt little inclination just to be a 'good-doer'. Echoes of Peplau were found in the work of Annie T Altschul in Britain in the 1950s and early 1960s. Altschul developed the interpersonal paradigm to include a consideration of systems theory and the idea that groups and communities might be, in one sense, more whole (even) than the individuals who peopled them.

These two women are obvious choices as models of virtue in psychiatric nursing. These were women who practised what they preached, so to speak, although both are more concerned with facilitating than telling. Both are women who are as comfortable sharpening their analytical skills, as they are in laughing at their own failings. I choose them as exemplars for their own radiant humanity. As I have known both as mentors and as friends, my choice is perhaps flawed by that most human of characteristics: *affection*.

THE INTERPERSONAL LEGACY

Altschul might well have found her own way to explore the 'personal' and 'human' context of the expression of mental distress, but she tended to acknowledge the guiding influence of Peplau and others from the fields of psychology and psychotherapy. Peplau, in turn, tended to attribute a generous degree of influence to the work of Harry Stack Sullivan, with whom she worked at Chestnut Lodge in the late 1940s. Sullivan had observed that even the 'most peculiar behaviour' of the acutely psychotic patient, was intelligible, since it comprised interpersonal processes with which each one of us is, or has historically been, familiar. This led him to conclude that we (staff), and our patients, are all more alike than different. This was a provocative view fifty years ago and, potentially, is even more provocative today. Despite her advancing years, Peplau maintains her allegiance to the radical humanism that she sees as the proper focus of psychiatric nursing. In that sense, she echoes the quality attributed to Sullivan by a long-time colleague Clara Thompson, who said that Sullivan's principal contribution was a very simple idea:

> *'ever present awareness of the need to convey respect for the patient and to maintain the patient's own self-esteem'* (Hausdorff 1985).

A similar sense of the simple, yet grand, idea underpins Peplau and Altschul's work. For that very reason I hope that they will never be forgotten by future generations of psychiatric nurses: they symbolised *what* needed to be done; and they opened the door into establishing *how* it might be done.

THE PHENOMENOLOGICAL FOCUS OF NURSING

My hope may, however, be a vain one. Already, some eminent nurses are consigning Peplau to a position as a mere footnote to history (cf. Gournay 1995). The late 20th century is manifesting an infatuation in health care with quantification, experimentation and replication. This emotionalism, disguised in the language of reason, risks losing sight of the point of all such analytic strivings. Increasingly it is asserted that all mental health disciplines must group together behind a single ideal, or perhaps ideology, of treatment; and must acquire and sharpen a similar armamentarium of skills and knowledge. To my ear, this argument sounds analogous to every member of an orchestra playing the same notes, or (worse) the same notes on the same instruments. However, a critique of interdisciplinary teamwork is not appropriate here. Teamwork does, however, prompt us to reconsider what nurses might be doing with, for or to the patient, family or community, that is not being done by other disciplines. What is the phenomenological focus of psychiatric nursing?

In her keynote address to the second 'State of the Art in Psychiatric Nursing' Conference, in Ohio in 1994, Peplau returned to one of her prevailing interests – people in schizophrenia. She reminded her audience that nurses needed to address the *human responses* associated with schizophrenia (cf. ANA 1980), rather than with schizophrenia as a disease process. More importantly, she recognised that nurses were regularly asserting that they advocated for, and considered, the personal interests and needs of patients. Given such assertions, Peplau noted that: 'it would behove nurses to … think exclusively of patients as persons' (Peplau 1995:2).

This simple assertion summarises, in my view, the proper focus of nursing: identifying the needs of individuals, and their families, which may be unique, given the influence of a unique life experience. This assertion appears to conflict with Sullivan's dictum about the commonality of human experience. However, there is no conflict in recognising that all of us breathe – and therefore share the breath experience. What that experience means to us, its importance and our attachment to it, will of course vary greatly, even within individuals, across changing life contexts. We know, for instance, that even when forms of mental illness are common to different cultural groups, the sense organs involved can vary from one culture to the next, and even within subcultures belonging to the same racial group (A1-Issa 1978). This suggests something of the complexity of human experience. All people are, in some respects *like all other people, like some other people* and *like no other person*.

At this time, when they are embracing a commitment to *holistic* care, involving the *whole person*, nurses might care to consider whether they have any option *but* to focus on the uniquely defined experience of the person *qua* patient. The proper focus of nursing is to help reveal what that meaning is now, and to establish what – if anything – needs to be done, now or shortly, to address such needs.

THE MEDICAL-EXPRESSIVE TRADITION

Traditionally, nurses assumed that their proper focus was to act as a support for doctors. They remain so at present and, one hopes, will continue to do so in the future. John Connolly complained that his attendants would not do *exactly* what he wanted. Connolly's complaint is echoed in many a hospital ward or community team today, often rightfully so. Doctors and nurses have not always seen eye to eye, and that creative tension has often been of benefit to the patient. The pain of discord has often been the prelude to growth.

Psychiatric medicine was once described by the British psychiatrist Albert Kushlick as a 'hit and run' activity. Using a related metaphor, doctors were like DC 10s, offering only direct care for 10 minutes before 'flying off' somewhere else. Given this status, doctors had to rely on nurses to express their treatment, especially the administration of drugs and the maintenance of the therapeutic milieu (Cormack 1983). Perhaps, however, patients might have nursing needs which extend far beyond nurses acting as the long arm of medicine – or more recently, psychology, social work or other disciplines also characterised by their 'hit and run' status. We might care to ask what these needs might be.

FINDING A ROLE – BUT LOSING OUR WAY?

Nurses in the USA have found a new security by extending the boundaries of their traditional role to include processes previously the preserve of psychiatrists or physicians. This is hardly a new phenomenon: it began when nurses were given permission to take over medical procedures of which doctors had long since tired, such as taking blood pressure readings. Given the nature of current economic pressures, the so-called extension of the nurse's role is unlikely to rest here, with physical examination and prescribing privileges. The issue which needs to more fully explored is, are these the kind of developments which people (and occasionally their families) *need*; or are we meeting the needs of another agenda, which may ultimately be to the disadvantage of the people served by nursing?

CONTEMPORARY AMBITIONS

What we claim to 'know', is our *knowledge*; and that knowledge determines our view of the world and our place within it. Even a nodding acquaintance ship with the philosophy of science shows how tenuous is the state of our knowledge at any point in time. This is most obvious today, living in a postmodern society where almost everything goes and there is a worldview for almost every occasion. However, Kuhn noted that this had always been the case: there always was more than one theoretical interpretation for any event. More importantly, we have always been fickle about our allegiances to particular scientific worldviews. Often theoretical allegiances have been shifted – or paradigms have been swapped – in the same way as people have shifted their political allegiances. As Kuhn pointed out thirty-five years ago:

'The act of judgement that leads scientists to reject a previously accepted theory is always based upon more than a comparison of that theory with the world. The decision to reject one paradigm is always simultaneously the decision to accept another, and the judgement leading to that decision involves the comparison of both paradigms with nature and with each other' (Kuhn 1962).

Since psychiatric nursing is not a science, it is – in a Kuhnian sense – pre-paradigmatic. Yet it has always been underpinned by a kind of paradigm: a set of practice-based principles and assumptions – some of which were hypotheses about human conduct if not quite theories in a proper sense. Psychiatric nursing has also felt the influence of paradigm shifts, not least the shift from the construction of illness to the construction of health.

THE CONCEPT OF MENTAL HEALTH

One dimension of the paradigm shift is the generalised acceptance of the concept of 'mental health'. Increasingly, psychiatric services are described as *mental health* services, despite maintaining their focus on dealing with manifest illness, using traditional forms of psychiatric intervention. As I have noted, in my own country, nurses who were once defined as *mental* nurses are now called mental *health* nurses. One does not need to be a pedant to argue that simply changing titles is not good enough. In what way might a mental *health* nursing service differ from that which was previously offered by *mental* nurses?

Our current ambitions to acquire 'mental health' represents, in some important senses, an echo of the ambitions for the pursuit of happiness and the good life, embraced by the Greeks. In Plato's view, the 'good life' was something which was both an art to be practised and an ideal to be contemplated. Plato's emphasis on the need to 'labor (sic) toward that goal,' (Arnett 1955) echoed Freud's well-known characterisation of mental health as being represented by the capacity to both love *and* work. The importance of love, as one essence of mental health, seems obvious, but what is love and how do we acquire a proper appreciation for it?

Lucretius (55 BC) recognised that the vigour with which a man pursues happiness might, paradoxically, reveal how fast he might be running away from it.

The man who is tired of staying at home, often goes out abroad from his great mansion, and of a sudden returns home, for indeed abroad he feels no better. He races to his country home, furiously driving his ponies, as though he were hurrying to bring help to a burning house; he yawns at once, when he has set foot on the threshold of the villa, or sinks into a heavy sleep and seeks forgetfulness, or even in hot haste makes for town, eager to be back. In this way each man struggles to escape himself: yet despite his will he clings to the self' (1924:141–142).

By recognising the importance of the relationship to the self, the person may reveal the essence of happiness and the good life: the exchange of love with oneself and other persons. That interpersonal dimension of *loving* and *giving*, was defined specifically by Sullivan:

'[when] the satisfactions and security which are being experienced by someone else, some particular other person, begin to be as significant to a person as his own satisfactions and security, (Sullivan 1947).

'People who are receiving mental health care want mental *health* care, not something which people define so, only to be politically correct, or to make them feel more positive about their work. We might care to consider how nursing rebuilds an appreciation of the importance of love and work within its mental health service provision'

People who are receiving mental health care want mental *health* care, not something which people define so, only to be politically correct, or to make them feel more positive about their work. We might care to consider how nursing rebuilds an appreciation of the importance of love and work within its mental health service provision.

THE SPIRIT OF COLLABORATION

However, the mere fact that we are even considering what people in mental distress might *want*, takes us closer to the heart of this issue, if not lifts us on to the horns of the dilemma. The past two decades has witnessed an emerging spirit of collaboration. Arguably, this has been greatest among the various sub-groups of dispossessed people defined by psychiatry: those who redefined themselves, provocatively, as psychiatric survivors,[3] among other things; and those who said they were oppressed because they were women, or defined by some other sexual, racial or cultural 'minority status' (Campbell 1997). Now we are learning that the people in our care might wish to define the parameters of their 'selfhood', or their own notions of 'empowerment', or the boundaries and limits of 'choice'. Now we realise that the political correctness which underpins many of our so-called improvements, may not be sufficient to support us in doing what *really* needs to be done.

SHAPED AND RESTRAINED BY COMPLEXITY

History will show that the 1990s were characterised by an attempt to redefine the parameters of mental health services, by deploying the suspect concept of 'serious mental illness'. The alien anthropologist who has stepped out of the X-Files might be forgiven for assuming that mental illness is, by definition, a serious business; and that we were wasting words again, or perhaps not really meaning what we say, or not really saying what we mean. Several psychiatric survivor groups in Britain have drawn to my attention the obvious corollary that, if they are not 'serious', then their mental illness must be 'trivial'; a damning indictment of our play on administrative language.[4]

The concept of schizophrenia is perhaps the best index of our current difficulties in working out where we should go within psychiatric nursing. Some of my nursing colleagues accept uncritically the notion that schizophrenia is a biologically based disorder, albeit aggravated by social factors. In this country, Dawson has illustrated the gross oversimplification of this viewpoint. We are almost knee-deep in hypotheses about the causes of schizophrenia, many of them swallowed readily by nurses and the lay public as 'new facts' (Gournay 1995). If nursing is to become a discipline, far less a profession, it might care to ask what is the relevance of such developments for our work? I am often asked, is it not important for me to be able to tell patients and their families what they are suffering from? The answer is, for me, a clear 'No'. People tell me what they are 'suffering' from! My responsibility is to be able to help them express themselves to the best of their abilities. Hopefully, that extends – as Peplau observed forty years ago – to their naming their distress and coming to understand its human significance.

The idea of 'giving' patients information about their 'condition' and treatment has become increasingly popular. As a libertarian I have long been an advocate of sharing information. However, much of what passes today as information-exchange is little more than ideological territoriality. I could never approve of nurses giving patients or families information about any condition involving mental distress, since the issue is so complex. This does not mean that I do not think that nurses should help people understand better what is 'going on' within their experience – to develop, if you like, a 'personal epistemology', or a local knowledge of mental distress. A woman with whom I recently worked complained of voices and presences. She also talked about selling up her home, becoming a traveller and also claimed to be able to read my thoughts. We addressed each of these phenomena as and when they arose, focusing on what these experiences meant for her, and sometimes – at her urging – what they meant for me. Her doctor said she was moving into mania. When she 'came down' again, she acknowledged that she had sensed that intuitively – but that knowledge did not dispel her need to address those specific experiences as they flowed through her and over her life, day in and day out.

That woman's experience reminded me of the experience of one of my colleagues, from Northumberland in England, who wrote recently about a woman whom he had met who observed that:

> 'Two snow-white cats crossed my path yesterday and I knew at once that God protects me. I wonder [he asked] what it is in her life that she trusts God to protect her from, and she replies with nice circularity, that she trusts God to protect her from people who persecute her because of her trust in God' (Holdsworth 1993).

I have spent almost thirty years trying to establish what such elliptical forms of reasoning *mean*. I may have been slightly unusual in trying to understand such people, rather than *explain away* such phenomena as this or that kind of psychotic presentation. Such explanations echo the comedian's aside: 'Gee, I thought I was going crazy, then I found out it was *only* schizophrenia'. By virtue of their linguistic development, people are labelling animals. People *can* and *do* describe. Perhaps there is still a place for awe and wonder; for being surprised by the reports of patients and their families; for working out *with* people what needs to be done, and how it might be accomplished; rather than always working from an established, standardised template of human experience.

The idea that anyone might understand madness disturbed Wittgenstein, who commented that:

> 'You must always be puzzled by mental illness. The thing I would dread most, if I became mentally ill would be your adopting a common sense attitude; that you could take it for granted that I was deluded'.

If I had the power to teach *all* nurses *one* thing, it would be that the line between impeccable logic and incorrigible lunacy is a very fine line indeed.

THE TYNESIDE VIEW

By 1994 I had become frustrated with the empty rhetoric of much nursing theorising. I had tired of the arcane language we often used to express our understanding of care and caring (see Barker & Reynolds 1995, Barker et al 1995). I had also grown weary of the promiscuous borrowing from other disciplines, which nurses engaged in, in an effort to shore up the weak theoretical basis of nursing practice. A little late in the day, I realised that I had been doing all of these things for much of my career.

I found echoes of my frustration around the world but none which resonated more closely with both my feelings and my thinking than Dawson in Melbourne who argued that:

> 'the language of nursing, of meaning, of care, of subjectivity and of spirituality has been suborned by the one-dimensional language of the technocratic society which purchases a spurious exactness at the cost of meaning' (Dawson 1997:40).

As I noted earlier, some nurses had tried to validate themselves by learning the lines of dominant narrative; by translating nursing into the healthcare-speak of the disciplines with the power to move mountains. Usually, that meant learning to objectify the person as a patient, and learning how to speak of psycho-technologies (at least), if not implement them. However, even those nurses who opted for alternative paradigms often get entrapped:

> 'revealed in the tortured vocabulary that attempts to reconstitute the whole from the pieces left strewn on the battlefield of rational investigation: "biopsychosociocultral", "psychosocial" mantras that are repeated ad nauseam in psychiatric nursing texts. The words themselves indicate the essentially divided and atomistic nature of the constructed reality that their enforced unity parodies; the mode of reasoning being employed is still, in essence, analytic rather than holistic; and the praxis is instrumental and objectifying' (Dawson 1997:70).

So, with some trepidation, I brought together a group of colleagues in Newcastle and undertook to study the 'collective consciousness' of psychiatric nursing. We asked – what did we do? Why did we do this rather than anything else? And we asked – what did we think this was for? Our aim was to develop a framework for practice which was grounded in practice, in practitioner's language, and practitioner's direct experience of caring for people.

The study, which employed the cooperative inquiry research methodology described first by Rowan and Reason, and more recently by John Heron (1996), focused on an established, heterogeneous group of nurses, including nurse specialists, managers, practitioners and educationalists and researchers, with a wide range of experience. Twelve months of inquiry was distilled in the following four premises.

Firstly, psychiatric nursing is an interactive, developmental human activity, more concerned with the future development of the person than with the origins or causes of his/her present mental distress. Psychiatric nursing is concerned, therefore, to establish the conditions necessary for the promotion of the person's unique growth and development (Barker 1989, Barker 1995). Such growth and development will, of necessity, involve the person's adjustment to, or overcoming of, the life problems associated with psychiatric disorder. Such conditions will, by definition, be determined by individual norms and by the interpersonal structure of family and cultural mores and are virtually infinite. Nurses manipulate such complex variables in an effort to establish what is an appropriate form of care. This represents the *process of caring*.

> 'psychiatric nursing is an interactive, developmental human activity, more concerned with the future development of the person than with the origins or causes of his/her present mental distress'

This first assumption is more radical than it might appear. It returns to the root of the caring issue. It assumes that, contrary to received wisdom, the establishment of *common* patterns of managing or caring for groups of patients, with, for example, common diagnoses, is not an appropriate ambition for nursing. At least, such an ambition appears at odds with nurses' expressed concern for the uniqueness of the individual, expressed through person-centred, holistic care (cf. Peplau 1995).

Secondly, the experience of mental distress, associated with psychiatric disorder, is represented through public behavioural disturbance, or reports of private events that are known only to the individual concerned. These represent the phenomena that are the *proper focus of caring* (Barker & Reynolds 1994, Barker et al 1997). Psychiatric nursing involves the provision of the necessary conditions under which people may access and review such experiences. Such collaborative re-authoring of the person's life might result in the healing of past distress, the alleviation of present distress, and the opening of ways to further human development.

> 'the experience of mental distress, associated with psychiatric disorder, is represented through public behavioural disturbance, or reports of private events that are known only to the individual concerned. These represent the phenomena that are the *proper focus of caring*'

If nurses are ever to develop true working alliances with the people in their care, they must begin with the person's experience of themselves, working with that experience, rather than with their experience of them as 'patients'. *Thirdly*, the nurse and the person are involved in a relationship based on mutual influence. This is the *interpersonal context of caring*. It is assumed that the reflexive nature of the caring experience will produce changes for the nurse, the person and significant others. In that sense, nursing involves caring *with* rather than caring *for* people, irrespective of the context of care.

How nurses adapt themselves to meet the needs of the person is the challenge; not how the person adapts to the nurse's construction of them as a patient.

The idea that nurses might be influenced by patients receives little attention today. Instead much of our focus on the nurse–patient relationship assumes a kind of one-way traffic: nurses influencing (for the good) their patients. This third assumption also adopts a radical position, asuming that nurses adapt to the needs of their patients, expressed through the relationship. It also assumes, of course, that nurses are open to change, by this process of relating. The patient is not the only one who might be affected (for good or ill) by this relationship.

Finally, the experience of psychiatric disorder is translated into a variety of problems of everyday living (Szasz 1961). The practice of psychiatric nursing is located uniquely within the context of the everyday life of the person, even when they are located in extraordinary care settings. This is the *social context of caring*. As a result, nursing is invariably an *in vivo* activity, focused on the person's relationship with self and with others, enacted within their everyday experience. Nursing is focused on helping people (cf. ANA 1980) rather than the disorders themselves, which are – by definition – professional, rather than human, constructs.

This last assumption echoes some of the history of psychiatric nursing, especially the idea of the nurse sharing the 'lifespace' of the patient. In the asylum era, this extended even to nurses sharing the accommodation of the hospital. Although nurses increasingly engage with the patient in formal therapeutic settings, much benefit still may be accrued in the more ordinary space of the patient's real world. Indeed, one of the most *extra*ordinary features of psychiatric nursing may be that the patient might gain so much from such extraordinarily 'ordinary' relationships.

These quasi-philosophical premises are currently the subject of an extensive validation project, involving an even wider range of practitioners and those in their care, seeking to clarify the extent to which these assumptions do represent what people *need* psychiatric nurses for.

CLOSING THE LOOP: SEARCHING FOR RAPPROCHEMENT

At the risk of sounding old-fashioned, I would suggest that it might be time to resurrect an interest in the mind. Although the mind is clearly dependent on brain cells and related biological structures for its existence, knowledge of individual brain cells or related biological structures, cannot explain the mind (Gregory 1987). Our minds may be 'of' the brain, but are not 'in' the brain and certainly are not synonymous 'with' the brain. Indeed, one might argue that the mind is 'non-biological'; the mind is spiritual; the mind is the 'soul'. Even the functioning of machines is now recognised to involve more than the activity of their individual parts (Pirsig 1974). Peplau observed recently that nursing needed to be promoted as a form of human inquiry: helping 'patients [who] are embarked on a search for truth about themselves and their life experiences' (Peplau 1990:9).

I have no hesitation in suggesting that such a search for truth is a spiritual endeavour, although not necessarily a religious one. Spirituality is – as Frankl (1964) observed – no more, or less, than the meanings which people attach to the experiences in their lives. When nurses respond to people's distress by helping to contain it, delimit it, or otherwise 'fix' it, they may well be practising *psychiatric* nursing. This may be a very important activity, even a life-saving activity. That dimension of care is firmly rooted in the present: both nurse and patient are, metaphorically, stationary – attempting to stem the flow of distress, or keeping a watching (and passive) eye out for signs of exacerbation or remission.

Alternatively, when nurses can join with people in their distress, metaphorically accompanying them, they may help them to appreciate the meaning of Epictetus' dictum that: 'difficult circumstances do not so much enable a person, as reveal him'. Such an alliance may provide the security needed to embark on that 'search for truth'; faltering steps down the life path; the journey we all must take but often would postpone indefinitely. We need to recognise that this involves an alliance, for surely – given the power differential – such a relationship can never properly be called a partnership. Such an alliance may be the basis of mental *health* nursing.

> 'when nurses can join with people in their distress, metaphorically accompanying them, they may help them to appreciate the meaning of Epictetus' dictum that: "difficult circumstances do not so much enable a person, as reveal him". Such an alliance may provide the security needed to embark on that "search for truth", faltering steps down the life path; the journey we all must take but often would postpone indefinitely. … Such an alliance may be the basis of mental *health* nursing'

I am aware that the voice I use here to describe mental *health* nursing may make some nurses uncomfortable. It may well be an echo of the voice of those Celtic monks who learned how to *be* with people in mental distress a thousand years ago in my homeland. Maybe my thinking about caring and nursing seeks, unconsciously, to close a loop in time.

I may also be seeking to close a loop in our relations with the people in our care. Both may have occurred by chance, and may be all the more significant for that fact. In Celtic art, knotwork symbolises the spiritual progress of all humanity on a journey in search of the divine source: the sacred centre. The endless riddle of life is expressed through successive rebirths, expressed graphically by the endless knots. Perhaps those knots are the threads running through me to which I alluded in my opening remarks. My colleague, the British survivor Peter Campbell, has written recently that:

> *'It is no longer acceptable that we should be presumed to have so little of value to say about madness or about living with madness. The crucial debate is about social understandings not service systems. Mental health workers, including nurses, should put aside their notes and badges and work alongside us' (Campbell 1997).*

Having entered nursing almost thirty years ago, keen to understand – on a human level – the experience of madness, Peter's words are a great comfort to me today. A senior manager told me recently that one of his colleagues had said that 'Phil Barker was a great therapist and then he started to go all mystical'. I assumed that this was an expression of disappointment. In reality the only significant change in my thinking over the past fifteen years has been to 'get real' rather than 'get mystical'. The failure to acknowledge the spiritual distress of mental illness is the most damning indictment of our current 'mental health services'. All too often we discover that we have successfully treated the illness but have either damaged or lost the person in the process.

We stand on the threshold of a new millennium. The year 2000 increasingly assumes a symbolic presence: highlighting the need for positive action coupled with the need for vision. As I survey this threshold, I often feel that in health care terms, we may not have come far in the last thousand years. One of the wonders of our 'New Age' health care philosophy is the holistic focus. We appear to have learned – again – that health means whole. As nurses, we may be beginning to learn that psychiatric and mental health nursing are carefully balanced reflections of what those in our care need to be whole. In that sense we may be trying to define what our Celtic forbears practised, perhaps intuitively. This reminds me of Plato's recognition that 'true knowledge is remembering what the soul has always known'. Or as TS Eliot so eloquently put it:

> We shall not cease from exploration
> And the end of all our exploring
> Will be to arrive where we started
> And to know the place for the first time
> ('Little Gidding' – the Four Quartets, 1942).

When I was a boy, my parents had a candle which we kept for emergencies – when the lighting failed. It was a stubby little candle and, for many years, I thought that this was the only *kind* of candle there was, and that this was the only function that a candle might serve. The *meaning* I attached to the word candle was sorely limited indeed. My childlike ignorance might serve as a metaphor for much of our understanding of the meaning of care and caring. I offer these thoughts in the spirit of lighting a candle, to commemorate this most enduring of symbols: a symbol of hope, a symbol of meaning, a symbol of enlightenment. It is my earnest hope that these thoughts will mark a renaissance of nursing interest in the diverse human meanings of mental illness, and an interest in the diverse practices of care and caring. I hope that, for your part, you will confer your own, special meanings, on this symbolic candle, and on all that I have said. In so doing, you will make your own distinctive contribution to what I hope will be a new age of enlightenment in psychiatric and mental health nursing.

NOTES

This paper was given as the Inaugural Eric Cunningham Dax Lecture at the University of Melbourne, on 31 July 1997.

1. The Institute for Psychiatric Nursing Research, Melbourne, Australia.
2. *See* Món C 1996 Scratches in the margin. Random House, Milson's Point, NSW.

3. I have learned a great deal from many of my 'survivor' colleagues, most notably: Ed Manos, Judi Chamberlin and Sally Clay from the USA, and Irene Whitehill, Louise Pembroke and Peter Campbell from England.
4. This gem was given to me by Louise Pembroke, Secretary of the Self-Harm Network, of Survivors Speak Out, UK.

REFERENCES

Al-Issa L 1978 Sociocultural factors in hallucinations. International Journal of Social Psychiatry 167:24–27

American Nurses Association 1980 Nursing: a social policy statement ANA, Kansas

American Nurses Association 1994 A statement on psychiatric-mental health clinical nursing practice and standards of psychiatric-mental health clinical nursing practice. American Nurses Publishing, Washington DC

Arnett W 1955 Santayana and the sense of beauty. Indiana University Press, Bloomington

Barker P 1989 Reflections on the philosophy of caring in mental health. International Journal of Nursing Studies 26:131–141

Barker P 1992 Severe depression: a practitioner's guide. Chapman and Hall, London

Barker P 1995 Promoting growth through mental health nursing. Mental Health Nursing 15:12–15

Barker P, Reynolds B 1994 A critique: Watson's caring ideology: the proper focus of nursing. Journal of Psychosocial Nursing and Mental Health Services 32(5):17–22

Barker P, Reynolds B, Stevenson C 1997 The human science basis of psychiatric nursing: theory and practice. Journal of Advanced Nursing 25:660–667

Barker P, Reynolds B, Ward T 1995 The proper focus of nursing: a critique of the 'caring' ideology. International Journal of Nursing Studies 32:386–397

Barker P, Davidson B (eds) 1997 Psychiatric nursing: ethical strife. Arnold, London

Campbell P 1997 Listening to patients. In: Barker P, Davidson B (eds) Psychiatric nursing: ethical strife. Arnold, London

Cormack D F S 1983 Psychiatric nursing described. Churchill Livingstone, Edinburgh

Dawson P J 1997 Thoughts of a wet mind in a dry season: the rhetoric and ideology of psychiatric nursing. Nursing Inquiry 4:69–71

Deegan P 1994 A letter to my friend who is giving up. The Journal of the California Alliance for the Mentally Ill 5(3):69–71

Frankl V 1964 Man's search for meaning. Hodder and Stoughton, London

Gournay K 1995 New facts on schizophrenia. Nursing Times 91(25):32–33

Gregory R 1987 The Oxford companion to the mind. Oxford University Press, Oxford

Hausdorff D 1985 In: Sullivan H S, Devine E, Held M, Vinson J, Walsh G, (eds), Thinkers of the twentieth century: a biographical, bibliographical and critical dictionary. Firethorn Press, London

Heron J 1996 Cooperative inquiry: research into the human condition. Sage, London

Holdsworth N 1993 Philosophy, wisdom and psychotherapy. Changes 11(2):139–144

Kuhn T 1962 The structure of scientific revolutions. University of Chicago Press, Chicago

Lego S 1996 Psychiatric nursing: a comprehensive reference. Lippincott, New York

Lucretius 1924 On the nature of things (trans C Bailey). Clarendon Press, Oxford

Nolan P 1993 The history of mental health nursing. Chapman and Hall, London

Peplau H E 1952 Interpersonal relations in nursing. Putnam, New York

Peplau H E 1990 Interpersonal relations: theoretical constructs and applications in psychiatric nursing practice. In: Reynolds W E, Cormack D (eds), Psychiatric and mental health nursing: theory and practice. Chapman and Hall, London

Peplau H E 1995 Another look at schizophrenia from a nursing standpoint. In: Anderson CA (ed), Psychiatric nursing 1946–94: the state of the art. Mosby Year Book, St Louis

Pirsig R 1974 Zen and the art of motorcycle maintenance. Corgi, London

Porter R 1989 A social history of madness: stories of the insane. Tavistock, London

Sills G 1989 Foreword. In: O'Toole A W, Welt S R (eds), Hildegard E Peplau: selected works – interpersonal theory in nursing. Springer, New York

Sullivan H S 1947 Conceptions of modern psychiatry. William Alonson White Foundation, Washington, DC

Szasz T S 1961 The myth of mental illness. Hoeber-Harper, New York

Commentary

Ann Benson RPN, BA(Hons)

This chapter is based on a lecture given to honour Dr Eric Cunningham Dax, a psychiatrist who was the director of the Mental Hygiene Authority in Victoria, Australia from 1951 to 1968. Dr Dax then took over as head of mental health services in Tasmania until returning to Melbourne in the late 1970s to concentrate on the Eric Cunningham Dax Collection of Psychiatric Art.

The title – 'Will psychiatric nursing ever offer mental health nursing' – fitted well within the context of this lecture, for before there was mental health nursing there was, and is, psychiatric nursing, and no individual has contributed more to the development of psychiatric nursing in Australia than Dr Eric Dax. During the 1950s he became a foundation member of the Nurses Council and supervised the new curriculum for psychiatric nurses that would culminate in the Council's finally acknowledging psychiatric nursing as a legitimate nursing endeavour in the state of Victoria.

A rose by any other name

In order to set the context for the question mooted in the title, this chapter endeavours to give an historical perspective to the psychiatric nurse, to define mental health nursing and psychiatric nursing. The chapter first examines nursing for evidence of whether or not it is a profession or a semi-profession or even a discipline. While acknowledging the brief existence (and weaknesses) of nursing theory, the author endeavours to trace back psychiatric nursing to a thousand year tradition emanating from Celtic monks, a process he describes as tracing a 'map of caring'. He speaks of the earliest carers as monks of Celtic origin practising in the 'old Kingdom of Northumbria'.

While allowing for a little Celtic bias I believe the chapter would benefit by acknowledging other 'maps of caring', maps from beyond the borders of the Judaeo-Christian tradition. We could have our understanding broadened by a reference to the response in Ancient Greece to madness or the contribution of the Arab peoples, who as early as 1500 AD built an asylum for the insane in Adrianopolis under direction from the sultan and impressed travellers during the seventh and eighth centuries with their enlightened and humane response to madness (Mora 1980).

Professor Barker rightly reminds us of the role of men as carers, of men and women working together to care for society's misfits both in the religious orders and, during the last two centuries, in the asylums. Whatever title these people were given, attendants, nurses, they are rightly, we are reminded, the foundation members of our profession, our forebears, the men and women who, over the ages, have offered care to the mentally ill, the insane, the lunatics, or, in the author's own terminology, those suffering from mental distress.

As the chapter acknowledges, the theory of nursing is still in its infancy, only able to boast of half a century of development. Homage was justly given, however, to Hildegard Peplau and Annie T Altschul, the founders of psychiatric nursing theory, and it says much of the short life of psychiatric nursing as a recognisable entity that both these founders are still with us today. We are reminded, rightly, of Peplau's exhortation for nurses to give up the notion of disease, epitomised in the term schizophrenia, rather to think exclusively of patients as people – wise advise often ignored still.

The chapter invites us to contemplate the change of nomenclature of recent times as the word 'psychiatric' is often replaced with 'mental health' in describing services, despite the emphasis remaining on treatment for what is described as 'serious mental illness', a term Professor Barker finds incongruous.

I can not agree with the argument that if a mental illness is not defined as serious then it must be 'trivial'; can we not accept a continuum of mental illness and distress that ranges from personally 'manageable' to 'unmanageable', to needing the extent of help only available in intensive treatment and care? Cannot the illness/distress range from mild through to serious without mild needing to be correlated with trivial?

In the section 'Mapping the territory', Barker articulates an issue of great concern to many nurses who work with mental health services: the weak theoretical base of nursing coupled with the empty rhetoric of much of the published theory. There is a lack of foundation in nursing theory that leaves us either mute when asked to articulate our philosophy or finds us borrowing theory from our relatives in the mental health profession.

In my view, a major achievement of this chapter is that it offers a definition of psychiatric nursing as an interactive developmental human activity that includes the process of caring, the focus of nursing and the interpersonal content of caring, and that it reminds us of the need to concentrate on helping people, not in treating a disorder.

The question 'will psychiatric nurses ever do mental health nursing' was answered in the following passage: 'when nurses respond to people's distress by helping to contain it, delimit it, otherwise "fix" it, they may well be practising psychiatric nursing, and a very important – often life-saving – activity that can be. When nurses can join with people in their distress, metaphorically accompanying them, … Such an alliance may be the basis of mental health nursing'.

Phil Barker has penned a thought-provoking chapter that describes and defines psychiatric nursing practice and suggests that the further step on the hierarchy of the caring profession might be to form an alliance that provides the necessary security for the person suffering mental distress to embark on the search for the truth; this he sees as the basis for mental health nursing. Whether or not psychiatric nurses will be willing and able to join in such an alliance, or prefer to remain as psychiatric nurses, only time will tell.

As long as the focus of our profession remains caring for people suffering from mental distress and matching that care to the individual's needs, I would argue that both psychiatric nursing and mental health nursing will be needed but that mental health nursing, as envisaged in this chapter, will be a spiritual alliance that will take our profession that step further.

REFERENCE

Mora G 1980 Historical and theoretical trends in psychiatry. In: Kaplan H I, Freedman A M, Sadock B J (eds) Comprehensive textbook of psychiatry. 3rd edn, Vol. 1, Ch 1

Part 2
The Proper Focus of Nursing

It seems trite to even suggest that nursing is about caring for people – or, as they are often called, patients or clients. The naming of *people* and the naming of the human dimensions of people's lived experience, has been an enduring feature of psychiatric history. In pursuit of a psychic version of the Linnaean tradition, we hope that by naming human phenomena, we might grow to understand such phenomena.

People who have the kind of experiences which we have variously called 'madness', 'mental illness' or 'mental health problems', have tried, down the ages, to tell others something of their experience. For various reasons, the audiences have heard only the version of events, which fitted their purpose. In more recent times, especially since the social turbulence of the mid-1960s, people in various walks of life have begun to develop their own 'voice'. The people traditionally referred to as the 'mentally ill' have, at long last, found their voice among that throng of powered-up self- and citizen advocates. Or at least, a tiny proportion of those people has begun to make their voices heard, at least in some quarters.

Having witnessed the counterculture of the 1960s at first hand, I have wondered about the legacy of the spirit of empowerment, which sparked into life all those years ago. The implications for nursing, of the voice of the people, should be enormous. Indeed, in Britain, predictions have been made for almost a decade that nurses will work *in partnership* with the people in their care. How far we have journeyed down that ambitious road remains unclear. However, at least the spirit appears willing. In the next three chapters, I offer some of my reflections on our need, as a discipline, to encounter the people in our care.

It might seem woefully obvious that any effective mental health service must take the fullest account of the *who*, as well as the *what* and *how*, of the people it serves. We have long since claimed to be interested in the people behind the towering patient labels, and have emphasised the whole and person-focused nature of our efforts to assess them, and their needs. We may, all too-often, have emerged from our transactions with little more than a stereotype, or worse, an awareness of just one of the masks which most of us wear in our daily lives.

We might find in the personal history of Leonardo Da Vinci, a fine example of the paradox which challenges all who seek to understand and reveal themselves or others. Despite his status as an icon for the universality of Man (sic) we know virtually nothing of *who* Leonardo was. Indeed, despite his fame for studying the world and the people around him, he penned virtually nothing about himself in his thousands of pages of notes, even in writing intended for his eyes only. Just once he wrote, 'do not reveal if liberty is precious'. Leonardo also turned his back on the methods which were emerging for printing and copying his work. He may have been indifferent but, more likely, he feared public disclosure of his work, and of himself. Richard Turner has argued that: 'Leonardo was vulnerable to being misinterpreted – indeed to being wilfully invented anew'. It seems ironic that the drawing of his aging face should be so well known, centuries after his death, but the man should remain an enigma.

But are not all people destined to remain enigmas, should they decide to follow Leonardo's dictum, and attempt to preserve their liberty through privacy? Although that may once have been true, today society has a rampant culture of interpretation which, in the case of the psychiatric culture, invents people 'willfully anew' whether they like it our not. With the emergence of the user and survivor movements, at home and abroad, the era of the psychiatric 'invention' of patients/clients (etc.) may soon be coming to an end. Perhaps even within my lifetime, we shall witness people defining in their own voice the phenomena associated with their psychic distress and voicing their concerns as to how we, their carers, might respond to such distress. The opportunity to *encounter* people, in their full complexity, rather than to *address* patients, in that limited sense of the word, has always attracted me. I hope that I might get a chance to witness that revolution at first hand.

REFERENCE

Turner A R 1995 Inventing Leonardo: the anatomy of a legend. Papermac, London

Patient participation and the multiple realities of empowerment

THE REIFICATION OF THE TECHNOLOGY OF CARE

We live in an era of rapid change. The technology of information exchange shrinks our view of the outside world, and biotechnology threatens to shrink further our constructions of our inner worlds of health and disorder (McLuhan 1962). The massive acceleration in biomedical research, especially within neuroscience, promises definitive answers to age-old questions about illness, its causes and solutions. In psychiatry, brain-imaging techniques suggest relationships between brain structure and metabolism and forms of mental disorder (or illness); human genome mapping suggests the genetic contribution to different disorders; and psychopharmacology promises treatment for more resistant forms of mental illness. These biomedical developments are reflected in virtually every area of health care provision and have major implications for nursing across all areas of practice.

This suggests the state of the art in the hard science of medical inquiry. But to what extent is any of this about health? Technology may offer us intriguing insights into what appears to be happening at a biological level, but tells us nothing of the human experience of distress, whether mental or physical. Technological models may contribute towards an explanation of the problem, but fail to address the human significance of such problems. Indeed, there is no reason why they should – technology has no ethical basis. However, as nurses who allegedly are involved in an earnest *human* activity, we should be questioning seriously how we respond to such technological developments.

In this chapter, I shall make some observations on nursing, drawn largely from my own experience – both personal and professional. I hope that what I have to say will prove thoughtful and stimulating. I believe that psychiatric nursing may serve as a useful focus for considering empowerment in nursing. Whereas some forms of physical illness or disability are perceived often as affecting only a part of the person, *mental* illness or disability is invariably perceived as affecting the whole person. As such, mental health care may serve as a useful setting to explore the viability of our present interests in being or becoming an holistic discipline.

Some of my colleagues believe that educational curricula should contain more 'up-to-date information on … contemporary neuroanatomy and biochemistry' (Gournay 1995). I disagree strongly. I would go further and suggest that no matter how important these developments may be within the biomedical field, they hold no *direct* implications for nursing. If our aim is to make a contribution toward improving the health of those in our care, such developments may be a major irrelevance. They may represent a distraction from what might be called our proper focus – the development of appropriate systems of *human* care (Barker & Reynolds 1994, Barker et al 1995). More importantly, these developments emphasise the ethical challenge that faces us in trying to develop appropriate systems of human care. Nursing is a craft (Barker 1995) whose product needs to be assured by contextual relevance: i.e. what we offer needs to fit the person and the person's unique context. Those who want to transform nursing into a science, risk sacrificing contextual relevance on the altar of traditional scientific rigour. Adopting a similar view, Glenister (1994) has suggested that psychiatric nursing has failed to take up the challenge of human rights issues for the mentally ill in Britain. In a related vein, Peplau – in the USA – believes that there are great threats inherent in the 'promise of the bio-technological utopia' (Peplau 1995). She quotes Callahan who claimed that:

> *'the marriage of science and business [in the USA], the joining of a mechanistic view of the body with an unrelenting profit motive, has created that most treacherous of American progeny: commerce masquerading as human liberation' (Callahan 1993).*

We might ask: to what extent our services 'free' the people in our care from their distress, or represent only further restraints on their human identities?

HOLISM AND NURSING PRACTICE

It is accepted widely that people are greater than the sum of their parts. By adopting a 'holistic' perspective, we recognise what Martha Rogers called the unitary nature of human beings (Rogers 1989). However, nursing exists within a medical community which – to a great extent – still favours reductionist explanations of illness. Indeed, our western way of thinking about the world and our place within it, still owes a great debt to Plato, who first distinguished 'matter' from 'ideas' and, by consequence, *soma* from *psyche*. The debates that continue to rage concerning the mind–body split may indeed suggest that current notions of the mind are no more than footnotes to Plato's philosophy (Flew 1964). The idea that people might be *unitary* or whole is borrowed largely from eastern philosophy, in particular from Chinese Taoism and Zen Buddhism. Holism not only implies a wholly different way of viewing people, but leads to a wholly different range of possible ways of responding to people who might be viewed as ill, especially mentally ill. Reductionist approaches – both within medicine and psychology – have, by contrast, collapsed the wealth of human behaviour into a range of associations of separate elementary events. Our approach to describing and measuring specific patterns of behaviour (or symptoms) which – when added together – are taken as evidence of the presence or absence of any disorder, might be representative of this approach. A recent CPN research report noted how:

> *'nurses undergoing psychosocial intervention training are now being* taught how to assess symptoms *using the Manchester or K-G-V scale. This scale rates nine areas based on observation and interview and examines both positive and negative symptoms' (Baguely 1995: emphasis added).*

The author suggested, quite appropriately, that by the use of such a scale, a common language would be established within the team. Nurses might care to ask to what extent our use of reductionist measures of the human condition is consonant with the fulfilment of 'holistic care'? What has the measurement of 'medically defined symptoms' to do with the nursing of the whole person?

THE PARADIGM SHIFT?

Nurses' use of the term 'holism' may mean several things. It may mean *only* that they are trying not to care for the person in too reductionist a manner. It might mean that they acknowledge, and try to manipulate, the possible interaction between the psychological, the biological and the social *selves* which make up the person (commonly referred to as the biopsychosocial model). *Or* they may mean that they believe (like Martha Rogers and others) that the elements which go to make up the person are not separate from the elements which make up the universe and, as such, *we* – and all those in our care – are not separate from the universe. Rogers' view – seen by some as science-fiction, by others as mysticism – is consonant with the Taoist view that mind and universe are one, and that to separate them is folly. We need to consider to what extent these trends may exemplify our inherent discomfort with holism, which may be national or cultural in character. We might also consider the inherent power of our ideas about illness and health, since they are so heavily value-laden. Over twenty years ago, Illich (1976) offered a definition of health that remains useful, if not fundamental:

> 'Health is [the result of] an autonomous yet culturally shaped reaction to socially-created reality. [Health] designates the ability to adapt to growing up and aging, to healing when damaged, to suffering, and to the peaceful expectation of death'.

This definition suggested that there is unlikely to be any widespread consensus about how people *should* promote and maintain the state of health. It is, however, certain that they (the people themselves) will have clear ideas as to what health means within their own worldview. It is the task of nursing to establish what is their worldview.

Illich's definition presents us with our first major dilemma. If we believe that people define their experience of growing up, illness, aging and death, *we* should be learning from those in our care rather than *them* learning from us. Yet, much scientific theory of illness comes from the opposite end of the spectrum: scientific paradigms are no more, or less, than the characteristic beliefs and preconceptions of the scientific community that first established the paradigm. Kuhn (1970) argued that paradigm-based science becomes a strenuous and devoted attempt to force nature into the conceptual boxes supplied by a professional education. In the context of psychiatry, various people have argued, for at least the last thirty years, that people do not so much *have* schizophrenia (or indeed any disorder) as are forced into a conceptual box marked 'schizophrenia' by people wedded to a biomedical paradigm (Boyle 1990).

What has all of this to do with nursing and empowerment? Given that we believe that we are committed to 'user-empowerment' and collaborative styles of working in partnership (Department of Health 1994), we need to ask ourselves to what extent do the theories and models of medicine help or hinder us from translating such concepts into action? The community psychiatric nursing research noted earlier included the assumption that:

'If clients and families are to understand their experiences, they need to be given information about the illness' (Falloon et al 1993 – cited by Baguely 1995).

This illustrates two problems concerning the biomedical paradigm. Firstly, the assumption that we know what people *need*. More importantly, it suggests that we know how people might come to an understanding of *their experience* of illness. This simple scenario provokes a complex set of ethical dilemmas for nurses.

Compare Falloon's view with the following:

'A requirement of a nursing model is that nurses become innovative and reframe information about schizophrenia, using their own observations and interview data from patients. The general tendency, in all too many psychiatric-mental health nursing textbooks, is to reiterate or paraphrase what has already been published in journals and books, usually by psychiatrists'.

In a more assertive mood, the same author goes on to say that:

'Nurses claim that advocacy for patients, and consideration of their needs and interests as persons having dignity and worth, are primary values inherent in the design and execution of nursing services. These values should be implicit in a nursing approach for the care of patients having a diagnosis of schizophrenia. In keeping with these claims, it would behoove nurses to give up the the notion of a disease, such as schizophrenia, and to think exclusively of patients as persons' (Peplau 1995: 2).

This insight is not restricted in its application to psychiatric nursing, far less schizophrenia. Not surprisingly, this call for a paradigm shift comes from Hildegard Peplau, who recognised what many nurses have so far chosen to ignore. Whereas physicians see the atypical, socially unacceptable behaviours, which they call symptoms, and view them as indicators of disease, nurses *ought* to recognise such behaviours as problem-solving actions, emblematic of difficulties arising within interpersonal relations, which, of course, includes relationships with oneself. Peplau notes that nursing interactions should be used to help the person retrieve and understand the 'highly personal meaning and purpose' of the phenomena we call illness.

Peplau takes an unashamedly moral position on this: this is what nurses *ought* to be doing. I cannot dodge the issue: I also believe that this is what we ought to be doing. We cannot claim to be *holistic* practitioners, focused upon the *uniqueness* of the individual, promoting *advocacy* and *empowerment*, through *collaborative* styles of *working in partnership*, whilst at the same time asserting that we can 'give people information which they need to understand their illness'. At present most, if not all, our working relationships are predicated on an 'expert' and 'subordinate' relationship: we know and they don't. Partnerships of any kind cannot be based upon such an unequal power relationship. Consideration of this power relationship offers us an opportunity to review the nature of our relationships with the people in our care, if not to review also the nature of nursing.

METAPHORS OLD AND NEW

The term *nursing* fulfilled a significant function in defining interpersonal behaviour, long before it acquired the restricted definition associated with the *practice* and discipline of nursing (Colliere 1979, Barker 1989). Nursing, as an enduring human, interpersonal, activity, involved a focus on the promotion of growth and development, deriving from the Old French and Latin 'to nourish'.

- When people are 'nursing a beer' it is implied that they are drinking *'carefully'* in an effort to prolong a significant activity.
- Athletes are 'nursing an injury' when they adopt a restrained (or careful) style of movement, to prevent the exacerbation of the injury. By 'taking care', they help restore the injured part to its former function.
- The forester 'nurses a sapling' by planting it in the shade of an established tree thereby allowing the 'infant' tree to gain the shelter it needs to promote its chances of growing and developing.
- Finally, in table billiards the player uses a particularly careful stroke (characterised by gentle actions) which increases his chances of achieving a high score. Where the billiard player is 'nursing the balls' his stroke play is characterised by care, attention and the minimum of force needed to move the billiard balls around the table. This can be distinguished from the more forceful 'potting' and power play exhibited often by the snooker or pool player.

These definitions offer metaphorical anchors for the clarification of the meaning of nursing in contemporary health care (*cf.* Szasz 1987: 135–169). They are also important given the central position taken by metaphor in our everyday discourse: people talk of being at the 'end of their tether', 'unable to see the light at the end of the tunnel', 'at the end of the road', 'all washed up', 'not taking it lying down', 'eaten up by jealousy (or any emotion)', or a 'shadow of their former selves'. It is difficult to make any meaningful statement about oneself or life in general without recourse to metaphor. As one of the modern masters of the critical appraisal of metaphor in relation to concepts of illness has noted:

> 'A man dies and his young son is told that he went to heaven. However, when a man dies and goes to heaven, his going is not the same sort of action as that entailed in his widow going to Italy, nor is heaven the same sort of place as

Rome. A man comes home and as he walks through the front door calls to his wife 'Honey, I am home'. Like jokes, which they so closely resemble, metaphors like these cannot be explained. If one tries to do so, in the process – to use another metaphor – one succeeds only in killing *them (Szasz 1987:137).*

Thomas Hobbes saw clearly the benefits and risks associated with being a language-using species: 'For words are wise men's counters, they do but reckon by them; but they are the money of fools' (Hobbes 1651). I have noted already that there has always been a strong professional urge to deconstruct the person's metaphors, transforming their richness into the base language of pathology. This seems to suggest that we take the metaphorical for the actual in some sense. Instead, of accepting the 'as if' proposition made in metaphor, we interpret the metaphor as saying that this 'is' the case. This is particularly so where people are re-presenting their lived-experience. I have never been at the end of my tether: I could not begin to say how long it might be, where it stretches to and of what it is composed. But, my lived-experience has often been 'as if' I were in that strangely undefined place or state.

Even where manifest pathology is present – as in carcinoma – the patient's metaphorical descriptions of pain, fatigue or the perceived ebbing of the life force, do not represent a mirror image of cancerous cells. It is likely that such metaphors *are* – rather than *reflect* – the whole lived-experience of illness (Heidegger 1961).

Some nursing theorists have recognised for some time the importance of metaphor for all areas of nursing practice. Arguably, Parse has given this aspect of human experience the most prominent focus through her 'human becoming theory' (Parse 1981). More recently, Kelly has offered a complex *house–garden–wilderness* metaphor as a means of exploring ways in which Parse's theory might shed light on nursing as a philosophy of caring (Kelly 1995).

All people are, metaphorically, in search of a home – which represents the feeling of 'being in one's own place in the world' (Mayeroff 1971). People find a home through a journeying process, which is the arch metaphor for the life path itself. The *house* is the starting point and end point of all human journeys: the place which is full of familiar and neglected treasures, trophies and souvenirs; and which affords the person a sense of rootedness, security and belonging. Although others may visit or intrude, no one can know the *house* like its owner.

The *garden* is an extension of the *house* whilst being a separate place: a place of growth, renewal, cultivation, work and rest. The *garden* affords an opportunity to grow in discipline and confidence: somewhere that may be viewed by visitors and passers-by, but only known to the gardener for its history and meaning.

The *wilderness* is boundless and unknown and stretches from the garden wall to beyond the horizon. The *wilderness* offers possibilities and threats for the person: opportunities for exploration and new knowledge; an opportunity to balance 'safety and risk, known and unknown, custom and exception, self and others' (Kelly 1995).

In that powerful metaphor Kelly offers a vision of the substantive domain of nursing as co-participating with persons in co-creating quality of life in a universe of open possibilities (Kelly 1995). My colleagues and I have tried to translate such a philosophy of care through use of the following four propositions:

- Nursing is a developmental human activity, more concerned with how people live through or overcome distress, than the causes or origins of their distress.
- The nurse–patient relationship is focused upon helping the person to re-author their lives, healing past distress, alleviating present distress and opening ways to further development.
- Nursing is focused upon everyday life – the person's relationship with themselves, and others within the context of their interpersonal world.
- Nursing involves a process of mutual influence – patients influence nurses who in turn influence patients, and so on. Nursing is, therefore, done with people, not to them.

Embedded within these nursing and health metaphors is the promise held by the interpersonal relationship. Whatever else might be involved, nursing is rooted firmly in the interaction of a *person*-called-patient and a *person*-called-nurse. There have been many attempts to reclassify the interpersonal activity of nursing within a quasi-scientific paradigm. Some commentators have discussed the art *and* science of nursing, and others have suggested that there might even be a 'science of caring' (Watson 1989). Empowerment offers an opportunity to explore a related, but distinctive, set of assumptions about nursing, which invokes yet another metaphor. Nursing is neither a science nor art but is a craft: an activity that requires the exercise of the mind to produce what is generally deemed to be a skill. Craft is neither art nor science but possesses elements of both. More importantly, the process of craftwork is based upon a contractual relationship between the craftsperson and the consumer. Artists make creative statements that are complete and independent. Those who appreciate art rarely influence its production, short of commissioning it. Similarly, scientists either explain phenomena, or, in a technological context, apply scientific theories to some problem. As with art, people use the products of science; they do not change or modify them.

> 'Nursing is neither a science nor art but is a craft: an activity that requires the exercise of the mind to produce what is generally deemed to be a skill. Craft is neither art nor science but possesses elements of both'

Craft belongs to a wholly different context, where a product is made which has a function, but no meaning. The meaning is attributed by the user of the craft-work. A jeweller makes a ring which the wearer transforms into an heirloom, a symbol of attachment, something of sentimental value, or a vehicle for expressing personality. All these characteristics were unknown when the ring was first made. Similarly, potters make pots for which people define uses and attribute meaning; as do the wearers of crafted clothing. The nursing intervention that we craft – in a metaphorical sense – is essentially meaningless. Its meaning, significance and human value is assigned by the person, family or community who are the recipients of the caring intervention. However, for this process to be effective, it needs to be made manifest.

INHERENT POWER AND INHERENT VALUES

The idea that we might 'value' the people in our care or otherwise 'empower' them has become part of late-20th-century healthcarespeak. This raises the question: 'why do we not assume that such people already possess their own value – why should we need to give them value through the creation of a nursing art form or the calculations of a nursing science?'. We also appear to have lost sight of the obvious fact that people *own* the illness, and the related symptoms, although – for obvious reasons – often they might wish that they did not. When we embark on the sophisticated business of measuring, labelling the phenomena associated with illness and disorder, perhaps we are – metaphorically – trying to capture the phenomena as our own 'prize specimen' – or by defining the phenomenon we are staking some claim for territorial rights, albeit of an intellectual nature.

Such medical imperialism is no longer acceptable. All health care providers work *for* the person – learn *from* the person. Given the subservient (if not ignorant) nature of our status, we need to be committed to discovering what the person believes needs to be done. Once that has been established, the nurse may decide whether or not (s)he has the skills and knowledge to meet such needs. In effect, is (s)he the most appropriate person to meet such needs? Moreover, the nurse needs to decide whether or not it would be appropriate – in an ethical as well as practical sense – to attempt to meet such needs.

These developments suggest that we have reached a watershed in our professional developments, where two related but antithetical choices face us. In aiming to extend the boundaries of our practice, should we accommodate more technological information about pathology, anatomy, biochemistry and pharmacology? Clearly, such knowledge would enhance our status as the expert commentator on the patient's illness, disorder or dysfunction, whether these represented actual or metaphorical plights. Or, should we be attempting to enhance the skills needed to appreciate the unique experiences of mental distress, which coexist with what is called mental illness? Arguably, the most common of such illness experiences is the construction of loss: loss of function, loss of life expectancy or – specifically in the case of mental illness – the loss of the sense of self, however that is defined.

> 'Arguably, the most common of ... illness experiences is the construction of loss; loss of function, loss of life expectancy or – specifically in the case of mental illness – the loss of the sense of self, however that is defined'

Some might argue – why 'either/or'? Why not 'both/and'? In some situations, 'both/and' might well be possible. In other situations 'either/or' might be a necessary nettle that requires to be grasped. Let us consider what the poles of these practices might look like.

FIXING ILLNESS OR GROWING WELLNESS?

Helping to *diagnose* problems, believing that we know what *caused* them, and helping to *fix* them, seems a laudable ambition for nursing, especially when it is consonant with medical practice, biomedical research and government health care ideology. It might be seen, however, as akin to the situation where we entrust our car to the garage mechanic, expecting that he will diagnose and fix the fault without any unnecessary recourse to us. Helping people to examine or re-examine their lives is a qualitatively different process. Working *with* people, helping them to identify the nature and function of the problems they meet in their lives, helping them appreciate what those problems *mean* in their terms, in their own language, is a fuzzy process. Helping people to devise *their* own perspectives on *their* lives and *their* human development – as opposed to helping them to 'buy' our perspectives – is a much less secure undertaking. Helping people to devise their own route maps, for their life path, which might lead them out of their current predicaments, perhaps even heal their own lives, is a potentially risky adventure, for both nurse and patient. We might also consider to what extent we might be able to sell such human, person-centred, empowering forms of health-care provision to our health care purchasers as interventions that might deliver 'nursing outcomes'.

'Helping people to devise their own route maps, for their life path, which might lead then out of their current predicaments, perhaps even heal their own lives, is a potentially risky adventure, for both nurse and patient'

Ironically, addressing these human *responses* to illness, dysfunction or disability appears to be what many people want. Various studies of users of mental health services suggest that people want more 'personal contact and understanding and less specialised treatments and techniques' (Rogers et al 1993). Such expectations conflict with the trend for 'creating increasingly specialised services and modes of intervention … [that] runs counter to the emphasis on de-skilling which is implied by what users identify as beneficial' (Rogers et al 1993). To what extent does this prevail across other areas of health care provision?

A major conflict seems to be unfolding before our very eyes. On the one hand there exist explicit requests by users of mental health services for a more humanised service that acknowledges the unique, personal dimensions of their problems, acknowledged by the users who reported to the Mental Health Nursing Review Group (DoH 1994). The emphasis of the conference at which the paper, on which this chapter is based, was presented – on empowerment through patient-centred care – suggests that we may, at last, be sharpening our focus on the *proper focus of nursing*, which Peplau and others have been describing in the USA for the past four decades. However, at the same time, the market culture of the NHS has sensitised us to notions of 'fixing' discrete patient groups – especially through brief 'packages' of interventions. Now it has been proposed that psychiatric nurses might even 'police' patients in the community to ensure that necessary treatment is given. Of course, these are not examples of nursing developments, but are service developments which are likely to become (perhaps a central) part of the nursing role. On a professional level we need to ask, to what extent do such approaches to treatment and care provision clarify the business of nursing, or represent a dangerous blurring of our role boundaries?

To some extent our current predicament – if indeed it is such – derives from our failure to clarify what nursing is *about*: what is its 'proper focus'. Whereas medicine, and perhaps psychology and sociology, are interested in the explanations of how people reached this point in their lives – i.e. to explain the genesis of their present difficulties – I believe that nursing is primarily interested in how people move on from this point. This is the nourishing, or nurturing, root function of nursing.

Almost forty years ago, Hilda Peplau described nursing as 'a developmental activity' which acted as an 'educative instrument'. That definition reminds us, should we require it, that part of the experience of growth involves an acknowledgement that we are lost, stuck or metaphorically grounded. When you are lost in a strange town late at night you need to *know* that you are lost to *find* the good sense to ask for direction. Moreover, your potential guide will have no interest in where you *came from* (origins) or at *what point* you got lost (critical episode), or *how* you got lost (process), but will only be interested to find out *where* you want to go (destination). Here, the help which is offered is a 'developmental activity' – helping you to journey towards a goal the significance of which you define. This activity will also incorporate some aspects of the 'educative instrument', since it will presumably also involve an assessment of your available means to reach that goal. Such means will likely lie somewhere within you – your personal resources. Of course, this assumes that you possess the knowledge of loss. Should you be unaware that you are lost, some kind person might help you towards such a realisation. However, having clarified that you are indeed lost, at least within a true democracy, you remain at liberty to continue to journey on aimlessly, should you so desire. Either way, your potential guide looks to you for guidance to frame the offer of help.

As it is in the metaphor, so it may be in life. The proper focus of nursing appears to resemble what I called *trephotaxis*: providing the necessary conditions for the promotion of growth and development (Barker 1989, 1992). The person and the person's particular context, of course, determine the necessary constituents of growth and development – where the person is on the life path.

Although growth may build on the experience of loss or pain, it is not dependent on the origins of distress for its realisation. I became aware of this, and began to clarify for myself this notion of 'focus' within my role as a psychiatric nurse, when caring for my terminally-ill father over a six month period more than a decade ago. We rarely discussed his carcinoma – indeed I knew little then, on a technical level, and know little more now. What became the focus for our relationship was his life review, his management of himself (in the here-and-now) and his need to prepare – as he saw it – for the final stages of his life path. In truth, father and son met, almost as strangers, but finally could not be parted by death. Over those months his dying became the great, and final gift which continues to sustain me. With his passing came the realisation of what my journeying with countless other patients meant.

In Russian folklore, there is a character called the *yurodivy* – a holy fool – who joins people, mysteriously, on their journeys, asks all sorts of stupid questions and then disappears as suddenly as he arrived.[1] The *yurodivy* is seen as a spiritual guide, serving as a necessary and sufficient means of helping the traveller take the difficult steps, resume the journey, return to the proper focus of the life path. The *yurodivy* is yet another metaphorical slant on the process of caring on life's journey from the cradle to the grave. The caring process may help the person gain a new perspective on his/her illness or disability. This may even help reveal new meanings for his/her life, and may stimulate an awareness of his/her natural power – the power over oneself. This is the power which, Frankl suggested, is beyond the reach of any torment – whether in human form as torturer or abstract as in disease, disability or impending death (Frankl 1971). Our ambitions to promote a vibrant life and a peaceful death must surely involve the development of the person's awareness of his/her power and how it might be used to reach such vibrant and peaceful destinations. In my father's case, it was he who determined what were his needs on those final stages of his life journey. Although he was frail, and failing day by day, my responsibility was to sit – metaphorically – at his feet as he taught me what needed to be done to meet his human needs. I have no doubt that, by abdicating the power which a son usually acquires as his father weakens, I unwittingly fostered something close to a therapeutic relationship: one which healed both our old emotional wounds and opened the way to a closeness of human spirit, until then denied us. Through my own uncertainty, my own clumsiness and my own lack of confidence in knowing what needed to be done, I became my father's *yurodivy*.

We need to ask whether or not nursing needs to include a dimension of 'not knowing'. We might also consider whether it is possible to help nurses learn how to identify what people-in-care need – determining what responses might be appropriate – without invoking powerful ethical principles. Some eminent psychiatric nurses have argued that all models or theories of nursing are hopelessly out of date and should be replaced, in the psychiatric nurse's canon, by the biomedical and pharmacological models of madness. Some have even argued (Gournay 1995) specifically that Peplau's theory cannot fit a disorder such as schizophrenia, because it 'fails to recognise the biological basis of hallucinations'. Such criticisms suggest a failure to appreciate Peplau's work. Such criticisms also suggest a faith in the biomedical explanation of certain human phenomena which, even if relevant, is premature. The argument could be made that because I had a limited knowledge of oncology I was hardly a fit person to address my father's needs in his dying days. Such views suggest a belief in an overarching, single, 'grand theory' which might explain *all* that we need to know. Should such a theoretical 'holy grail' ever be found, what would it tell us of what it *means* to be ill or, more specifically, what we – personally or interpersonally – *need* to do about it?

I believe that we face a major ethical dilemma in choosing between our faith in biomedical explanations of ill-health, on the

'I believe that we face a major ethical dilemma in choosing between our faith in biomedical explanations of ill-health, on the one hand, and listening to, and learning from, the people in our care … on the other'

one hand, and listening to, and learning from, the people in our care in the manner suggested by various nursing theorists – from Peplau to Parse – on the other. As these theorists have so clearly illustrated, one can know much about the disorder or dysfunction but fail to be able to address the meaning which this has for the person and the person's life.

OH BRAVE NEW AGE!

We live in a world where the only constant is change and with it perhaps a loss of traditional meaning. Down the ages, and across all cultures, evangelists have looked for or proclaimed a 'golden age', and we are now firmly embedded somewhere at the beginning of the Aquarian age. This 'new age' is characterised by a regeneration of interest in all things 'touchy and feely' and the many alternatives of the holistic movement. It also features a radical paradigm shift which looks set to influence our sociocultural and scientific views of self and what it means to be human (Capra 1973, 1981). Commentators on the 'crisis of the human spirit' have ranged from the physicist Fritjof Capra in the USA to the Prince of Wales in the UK. It seems folly to refer to this as a 'new age' phenomenon, since the likes of George Bernard Shaw and H G Wells were hoping for a similar kind of apocalyptic redemption at the start of this century. It would be a greater folly, however, to ignore the implications of this paradigm shift for nursing education and practice.

Our yearning for a new or 'golden age' has meaning; we are not yearning in a vacuum. It seems likely that as the millennium draws nearer we shall see an escalation of spiritual angst – as we wonder aloud about the significance of time and life. This will correspond with an even greater proliferation of gurus and forecasters, all determined to explain this significance on our behalf. The millennial scenario echoes similar scenes of reflection and wonder that occur daily as people's lives are disrupted by serious illness. After they have gone beyond the 'why me' stage, a life-review may be stimulated, even for those – like my father – who have rarely reflected before in such a fashion. People who are preparing to become nurses are likely to be involved in addressing similar doubts concerning life and the self: 'Have I got what it takes?'; 'What exactly is the *it* that I need to become a good nurse?'. At that vulnerable stage of their professional development, nurses might come to appreciate something of the spiritual vulnerability that their patients encounter on the journey through illness toward wellness. Maybe we need to develop a philosophy of nursing practice that attempts to maintain such a useful form of insecurity within the professional *persona* of nursing.

HEALTH AND WELLNESS

Increasingly it is recognised that health is an experience, rather than a state, and that even people who are 'seriously ill' – such as those with cancers – may possess an abundance of 'wellness', and that some may even heal themselves through processes of which we, as yet, have little understanding. This suggests the growing of an oncological 'new age' (Simonton et al 1978). There appears to be no ceiling for growth in human terms. Indeed, the concept of growth is a hopeless question for scientific enquiry. All organisms have an urge toward health, wholeness and competency. We need to ask to what extent does the structure of our nursing practice accommodate the person's urge towards wellness or militate against it.

The notion that we might 'empower' those in our care suggests that they do not own such power naturally. Taken literally, empowerment means to delegate legal power, to authorise or to enable. In psychiatric nursing in particular, there exists often an explicit requirement to *restrict* the person through the exercise of legal mechanisms. Nurses in other branches are faced with similar temptations toward beneficence or paternalism, if not autocracy. Indeed, many of the examples of 'knowledgeable doing' in psychiatry which I cited earlier emphasise the development of a nanny-state for people in mental distress. The state often empowers nurses to disempower patients. Such contexts generate significant professional conflict. The other two definitions of empowerment appear more innocuous but may be even more provocative. We might ask, for example, what might lead us to think that people need our *authorisation* to make choices in their lives? People may discuss their options with me – until the proverbial cows come home. However, ultimately, their choice can only be *their* choice if it is to be a choice at all.[2] Perhaps nurses should not be so keen to suggest that they help people to make choices. Rather, nurses might provide the conditions necessary for people to come to realise that they already *possess* such choices, and are free to make them or not.

In some instances, nurses may remove such power from the person. In that sense would we be 'empowering' if we returned such freedoms to the person? We might be engaged in some form of recompense or even justice, but 'empowerment' in such a context seems quite the wrong term. Increasingly, however, empowerment has come to be understood as giving something to people that, previously, they did not possess. If by empowerment we mean to 'enable' – providing the conditions under which the person is able to do (freely) something that previously they appeared unable or unwilling to do – then such a definition would fit squarely with the notion of nursing as a developmental activity. If, by enable, however, we mean *allowing* people to do something, we might care to ask who prevented them in the first place and why?

Professionalism has always been linked to the exercise of power. As nursing aims for greater professionalism, it risks extending its power base – with the potential for disempowering those who fall within its ambit. The establishment of a private language within medicine was the first step taken to control the people in our care. By discussing their experience of illness or disability in an arcane terminology we ensured that they would know little of what we were talking about, and would be – quite literally – *enthralled*: held in bondage.

What might be the alternatives to extending the power-based, false authority of professionalised nursing? One alternative has at least the following four features. We might emphasise the need to:

- show genuine respect for people's experience of themselves
- value those experiences and the unique strengths and capacities of the person
- listen and take full account of what people have to say,

- discuss what has been talked about, offering our views in a manner which is neither patronisingly simple, nor overly complex
- recognise that the above values need to be part of the system of health care, rather than enshrined in the peculiar activities of one individual (nurse).

At the risk of sounding like a Jeremiah, I conclude by suggesting that all our romantic aspirations – from the growing reality of the reflective practitioner to our dreams of empowerment – must accommodate the harsh realities of a social world in turmoil. In the words of the famous *haiku*:

The evening cool
Knowing the bell
Is tolling our life away

Down the ages many people who have experienced illness, and a few of those who have cared for them, have recognised that illness – whether ostensibly mental or physical – can be a curious reflection of that fearful knowledge, that the bell is tolling our life away. The metaphor of the life path, where mental and physical ill health meet, is where we all hear the tolling of that bell. The stories told by the people in our care are distressing variants on age-old themes concerning birth, death and the often-complex life path in between. That troublesome buzzword *empowerment* may well reflect a growing recognition that such stories are not the incoherent ramblings of a diseased brain, nor the meaningless reflection of a body in crisis. At last we may recognise what the German artist Josef Beuys saw as the fundamental nature of all illness:

'Illness are almost always spiritual crises in which older experiences, and phases of thought, are cast off in order to permit positive changes' (Gotz et al 1979).

The adoption of such a view of illness would present many challenges for us as human beings, and many more as professional carers. However, the challenge of such a philosophy would be greatest for the health care market, which often tries not only to mould or fashion the construction of the illness experience but, in so doing, may also unwittingly end up trying to mould our view of our human selves.

NOTE

This chapter is based on a paper presented to the conference 'Empowerment through patient-centred care' at the University of Ulster, Jordanstown Campus, 7 September 1995

1. I am indebted to Eileen Inglesby for helping me appreciate the mythic significance of the *yurodivy*.
2. This does not preclude me from offering my view on the person's situation, but they must remain free to accept or reject my view.

REFERENCES

Baguely I 1995 Evaluation of the Tameside Nursing Development Unit for psychosocial interventions. In: Brooker C, White E (eds) Community psychiatric nursing: a research perspective, Vol 3. Chapman and Hall, London

Barker P 1989 Reflections on caring in mental health. International Journal of Nursing Studies 26(2): 131–141

Barker P 1992 Severe depression: a practitioner's guide. Chapman and Hall, London

Barker P, Reynolds W 1994 A critique of Watson's caring ideology: the proper focus of psychiatric nursing. Journal of Psychosocial Nursing 32:17–22

Barker P, Reynolds W, Ward T 1995 The proper focus of nursing: a critique of the 'caring' ideology. International Journal of Nursing Studies 32:386–397

Boyle M 1990 Schizophrenia: a scientific delusion? Routledge, London

Callahan D 1993 They dream of genes. The New York Times Book Review, September 12, p 26

Capra F 1973 The Tao of physics. Flamingo, London

Capra F 1981 The turning point: science, society and the rising culture. Flamingo Fontana, London

Colliere F 1986 Invisible care and invisible women as health care providers. International Journal of Nursing Studies 23(2): 95–112

Department of Health 1994 Working in partnership: report of the Working Party on Mental Health Nursing. HMSO, London

Falloon I, Lapporta M, Fadden G, Graham Hole V 1993 Managing stress in families: cognitive behavioural strategies for enhancing coping skills. Routledge, London

Flew AGN 1964 Body, mind and death. Collier-Macmillan, London

Frankl V 1971 Man's search for meaning. Penguin, Harmondsworth

Glenister D 1994 Patient participation in psychiatric services. Journal of Advanced Nursing 19:802–811

Gotz A, Konnertz W, Thomas K 1979 Joseph Beuys: life and works. Barran's Educational Series, London

Gournay K 1995 New facts about schizophrenia. Nursing Times 91(25): 32–33

Heidegger M 1961 Being and time. SCM Press, London

Hobbes T 1651 Leviathan. Penguin, Harmondsworth

Illich I 1976 Limits to medicine: medical nemesis – the expropriation of health. Marion Boyars, London

Kelly G 1995 The garden-wilderness metaphor. In: Parse RR (ed) Illuminations – the human becoming theory in practice and research. National League for Nursing, New York

Kuhn T 1970 The structure of scientific revolutions. University of Chicago Press, Chicago

Mayeroff M 1971 On caring. Harper and Row, Perennial Library, New York

McLuhan M 1962 The Gutenberg galaxy: the making of typographic man. University of Toronto Press, Toronto

Parse RR 1981 Man-living-health: a theory of nursing. Wiley, New York

Peplau H E 1995 Another look at schizophrenia from a nursing standpoint. In: Anderson C A (ed) Psychiatric nursing – 1946–1994: a report on the state of the art. Mosby Year Book, St Louis

Rogers ME 1989 Nursing: a science of unitary human beings. In: Reihl-Sisca JP (ed) Conceptual models for nursing practice. Appleton & Lange, Norwalk, CT

Rogers A, Pilgrim D, Lacey R 1993 Experiencing psychiatry: users' views of services. Macmillan/MIND, London

Simonton C, Mathews-Simonton S, Creighton J 1978 Getting well again. Tarcher, Los Angeles

Szasz T S 1987 Insanity: the idea and its consequences. Wiley, New York

Watson J 1989 Watson's philosophy and theory of human caring in nursing. In: Riehl-Sisca J (ed) Conceptual models for nursing practice. Appleton and Lange, Norwalk, CT

Commentary

Dr Cheryl Waters

This chapter raises issues that have disturbed me for some time. It is not possible to address all the issues that have been discussed even though all demand a response if mental health (MH) nursing is to claim its future and help to create a 'brave new age' for itself and the people it serves. Many of the concerns raised by the author signify the dilemmas facing nursing today – there are no easy answers, only hard questions.

The principal dilemma for me is about how to 'grow' MH nurses who are equipped morally and spiritually to help a person make meaning of alienating and distressing events, all in an environment that is increasingly technological and interventionist. How do we design curricula and promote learning about a discipline or occupation about which there is little agreement or cohesion? How do we work with the vulnerability inherent in the self-doubt of nurse/learners in ways that promote their self-awareness and appreciation of the circumstances of the people in their care?

Medicine has fixed the limits of its practice within mental health care to include the diagnosis and treatment of what it defines as mental illness. Most people come into nursing care as a result of coming under the 'care' of medicine and having their life experience 'forced ... into the conceptual box' of a psychiatric diagnosis. Nursing has historically defined itself and its horizon with respect to medicine. This can be explained from several perspectives. An historical analysis that focuses on the legacy of Nightingale offers some explanation for this. Another and less attractive explanation comes from the literature on oppressed group behaviour (Roberts 1983).

I am reminded of a course in graduate MH nursing with which I was involved. In this course was a subject that dealt in depth with neurophysiology and psychopharmacology. The subject was led by an RPN with a BSc (Hons) in neurophysiology, who was enrolled in a PhD, and still practising part-time. The registered nurses who struggled with this subject matter, which they found challenging because of its scientific content, were amazingly positive about its impact on their professional lives (in a way that they were not positive about other more 'nursing' focused subjects in the curriculum). This raised questions about the benefit of such a subject. Who was the true beneficiary of the resulting knowledge and power?

Many of the doctor – nurse skirmishes I have witnessed in practice revolve around issues of medications and the side effects of somatic therapies in general. The students claimed that the subject gave them the confidence and the knowledge to articulately challenge treatment regimes – they claimed to feel 'empowered'. The most innocent interpretation could take the claim at face value, that they had sufficient information to intervene on the patient's behalf to alter treatment and hence its impact on their lives.

The other interpretation acknowledges the power of the language and discourse of the dominant group. There is a seductiveness to power and the language of the powerful that makes it difficult to forego the opportunity to interact as apparent equals. To what extent do we collude with medicine in maintaining its dominance over the lives of the people in our care and over our practice?

One of the quandaries of teaching is that MH nurses do need to understand the language, skills and knowledges of the other disciplines – but the risk is that this knowledge leads to distancing and mystification. We risk co-creating a situation that disempowers and devalues and marginalises the already dispossessed. An arcane knowledge base is acquired that bears little relationship to the everyday experience of living with 'mental distress'.

Although nurses have found it desirable to understand the focus of other disciplines, they appear, on the other hand, to be sublimely unconcerned with the focus of nursing. A fairly cynical view is that MH nurses are probably perceived as the eyes and ears and hands of other MH professional groups. These are the ones who can in fact 'fix' the problem – nurses are not really distinguished as having an autonomous helping and enabling role but as extenders and monitors of the treatments of others – this in spite of the rhetoric (ours and theirs) to the contrary. Nurses are considered useful and caring but I am not sure if they are considered to take an active therapeutic role or to undertake a therapy that is of any real value according to the prevailing and powerful medical model. Who decides on the focus of nursing services within the context of a whole coordinated service for those experiencing the life-altering effects of a mental illness? I agree with Barker that we must define for ourselves the proper focus of nursing, or continue to have it defined for us by the other mental health disciplines who have the power to dictate the agenda of the funding bodies and planners of MH services.

One of the principal puzzles that this paper highlights for me relates to the exercise of power and the endeavours of nursing to advance itself as a discipline and a profession. The strategies of professionalisation may be alien to views of nursing that value co-participation and the co-creation of meaning from lived lives. Professionalism is linked to the exercise of power, as noted by Barker. The recent concern with staking a claim to the phenomena of concern to nursing is a twofold concern – on the one hand it is about the care we give people, on the other, it is a political manoeuvre. The science-versus-art debate and the medicine-versus-nursing debate are both politically motivated. At the roots of these debates is the ongoing turf war between medicine and any occupational group unfortunate enough to fall within the reach of medicine and the territory it perceives as its responsibility and to which it has staked a claim.

An interesting proposition raised by one of my students was that patients and nurses are very much in it together – one can't be emancipated or empowered without the other: that our fates are tied (Linda Duffell 1995, personal communication). Where will that sense of power come from? Probably not from engaging in or winning turf wars, but, as proposed by Barker, through collaborative partnerships with the people in our care and a confident belief in the benefits and congruity of caring ideals implicit in this new age.

REFERENCE AND FURTHER READING

Bishop A, Scudder J Jr 1997 Nursing as practice rather than art or a science. Nursing Outlook 45(2):82–85

Capra F 1982 The turning point: science, society and the rising culture. Flamingo, London

Holmes C 1992 The drama of nursing. Journal of Advanced Nursing 17:941–950

Nightingale F 1980 Notes on nursing: what it is and what it is not. Churchill Livingstone, Edinburgh

Roberts S 1983 Oppressed group behavior. Advances in Nursing Science 5(7): 21–30

The logic of experience: developing appropriate care through effective collaboration

7

Gregory Bateson told the story of the man who wanted to know about the mind, what it was and whether computers would ever be as intelligent as humans. The man asked only one question, which he typed into the most powerful computer he could find: 'Do you compute that you will ever think like a human being?'. The computer rumbled and stuttered as it analysed its own computational habits. Eventually it printed out a single reply which the man grabbed excitedly. On it he found six words which responded without answering the question. The computer had replied 'That reminds me of a story…'.

Our libraries are full of books and papers which purport to explain the concept of mind. Those enquiries and explications are no more than stories themselves. The mind itself may be no more than a meta-story which explores, but fails to explain, the business of being and living. It was once taken for granted that mental illness involved an affliction of the mind. Nowadays some of us are a lot smarter: now we're not so sure.

Although psychiatric nurses complement the care offered by doctors and other health care professions, arguably, however, their unique role has always been to facilitate the *psychosocial*, if not *spiritual*, 'healing' of the person with mental illness. How they exercise this 'psychic healing' function distinguishes them from all other nurses. Nursing may differ from other disciplines in the sense that it has no foundation in explaining how people reached this point in their lives; such hypotheses regarding the origins of mental distress are the preserve of medicine, psychology and sociology. Nursing is concerned more with how people move on from this point: how people change. To establish how people move on from this point on their life path, we need to know something of 'where' they are, and 'where' they might need, personally, to be going. Arguably, we need no real appreciation of where they have come from (Barker 1995).

'Nursing may differ from other disciplines in the sense that it has no foundation in explaining how people reached this point in their lives; such hypotheses regarding the origins of mental distress are the preserve of medicine, psychology and sociology. Nursing is concerned more with how people move on from this point: how people change'

It has become fashionable to assert that nursing is 'holistic': in some way addressing the totality of the person. Given the nature of mental illness, involving in every case some damage or insult to the 'self', care must be focused on the personal, the psychosocial and the spiritual identities of the patient.

My view of the history of psychiatric nursing is uncontroversial, and has been confirmed by archival research. What may be controversial is my belief that psychiatric nursing is a spiritual activity; that nurses participate in the 'psychic healing' of the person with mental illness. The German artist Josef Beuys suggested that: 'Illnesses are almost always spiritual crises in life in which older experiences, and phases of thought, are cast off in order to permit positive changes'. Let this provocative belief serve as the anchor for this chapter.

Whatever nurses do, of necessity, it involves a complex of interpersonal relations. Given the form of care – human meeting human – and the content of those meetings – interaction, exchange and mutual influence – we could not discuss caring without interpersonal relations. If 'psychic healing' is one of the goals of nursing, interpersonal relations must be the process by which it is realised.

Something significant takes place in those relationships. Their ordinary nature often disguises their significance: people telling or enacting the stories of their lives. Often these stories make grim and harrowing telling, as well as hearing; but they remain no more than stories. The significance of *true* psychiatric nursing lies in recognising how such relationships *heal* everyday lives, and that by 'healing our lives' we all might make a contribution to 'mending our minds'. By being party to this process, nurses might also heal their own lives. Before I discuss the relationship between 'healing lives' and 'mending minds', perhaps I should illustrate what I mean by life and the mind.

Two and half thousand years ago Plato warned that 'the unexamined life is not worth living'. Bateson's computer story may be only a witty update on that age-old moral. People are natural philosophers: devoting much of their lives to establishing the meaning and value of their experience; and to constructing explanatory models of the world and their place within it. What we see – when we take a look at ourselves – may, however, not always be what we expected.

People with mental illness spend more time than most reflecting on their experience of self. Sufferers are often only too aware *either* that they are not the person they once were, or that they are, in some way, different from the rest of humanity. The New Zealand writer Janet Frame defined this difference concisely: 'I shall write about the season of peril. I was put in hospital because a great gap opened in the ice floe between myself and the other people whom I watched, with their world, drifting away through a violet-coloured sea where hammer-head sharks in tropical ease swam side by side with the seals and polar bears. I was alone on the ice' (Frame 1980). This state of dis-ease connotes the *illness* of the mind: a human problem with social, psychological and medical relations. These add up to a spiritual, or whole-life, crisis – where the person is trapped in the search for meaning which we all undertake as we journey, metaphorically, from the cradle to the grave.

We remind ourselves of the metaphorical nature of mental illness to emphasise that mental illness often *has* no location: it is everywhere and nowhere, apparently at the same time. Mental illness often reflects the *whole* of a person's lived experience, without emphasising any particular part. It is this 'lived experience', rather than mental illness itself, which nurses manage in the name of care.

Much of our limited understanding of how nurses help people comes from the mutual examination which goes on within the nurse–patient relationship. It is popular today to talk about the 'empowerment' of people with mental illness. *We* do not empower our patients; the person with mental illness empowers the professionals. The only way we can be of real service is to *learn from the patient*. Having learned what to do *for* the patient, *from* the patient, nurses often gain some understanding or insight, which changes them – however imperceptibly. This small change in their professional demeanour influences the next interaction, and so on

> 'We do not empower our patients; the person with mental illness empowers the professionals. The only way we can be of real service is to *learn from the patient*. Having learned what to do *for* the patient, *from* the patient, nurses often gain some understanding or insight, which changes them … This small change in their professional demeanour influences the next interaction, and so on…'

ad infinitum. This limitless process of mutual influence might be an example of what we call co-participation.

If nurses *do* anything of note within those interactions, it is to offer hope. They hold out a *hopeline* to people who are often devoid of hope. One of the key tenets of nursing must be that people *are not* the problem – *the problem is the problem*. Adopting this view allows patients to distance themselves from their problems. The person who has a problem with schizophrenia, or depression, or obsessional thoughts, is neither morally responsible for the problem, nor possessed of some fundamental flaw. They *have problems with* schizophrenia, or whatever.

Effective nurses recognise that we can have relationships even with things which might be seen as parts of ourselves; they assume that people and their problems are not one and the same thing. By adopting this view, nurses facilitate the hope that such problems can be overcome, or otherwise left behind on the life path.

To do so one must first believe that people *can* change and grow. This is more than a philosophy. This is the treasure map of the territory of care. Where patients do not make progress, some of this must be a function of the carer's pessimism. We need to foster a fierce belief in people's possibilities for change. When I became a nurse almost thirty years ago I was entertained to a litany of theories as to how patients became mentally ill. I learned how to recognise deterioration or exacerbation, but we paid little attention to how positive change might be facilitated. We spent a lot of time observing patients, but spent little time *with* them, sharing their lifespace, sharing their life stories. Nurses *looked after* people, which often meant helping them remain stationary. When I reflect on the changes which have occurred in my own beliefs and behaviour, many seem to occur as a consequence of conversations with people. I may only be reading their words in a book, or they may only be talking to me on a telephone line, but my sense of change derives from the stories we tell one another. Today, there exists greater recognition that nurses need to help people change. There has also been a resurgence of interest in the psychopathology of serious mental illness, and some some nurses advocate that the people in their care, or their families, should be 'taught' about the nature of their illness. Such views seem wholly antithetical to the spirit of empowerment.

'People own the experience of distress. We should not forget that we have only translated these experiences into the symptomatology of psychiatric disorder'

People own the experience of distress. We should not forget that we have only translated these experiences into the symptomatology of psychiatric disorder.

Effective nursing helps people develop their natural reflective processes. In that sense, psychiatric nursing is a most ordinary pursuit. Although a few nurses are beginning to work with patients out of consulting rooms, much psychiatric nursing takes place in the most mundane of settings: from the day rooms of hospital wards to the living rooms of the person's own home. What nurses *do* there can all too easily be mistaken for mundane interaction and mundane conversation.

Psychiatric nursing is one semi-public context within which people reaffirm their need for self-examination as a core element in the life process. Almost twenty years ago, I began to work with women with severe depression who had been hospitalised over many years, many of whom had made repeated attempts on their lives (Barker 1992). As I began to explore their experiences – individually, sometimes with their husbands and families, and in groups – I began to feel like an intruder, as I listened in to these stories from the edges of life. Viktor Frankl suggested that the anxiety which people with melancholia experience is what Kierkegaard called 'the giddiness which overcomes us on the peaks of freedom'. For those women, that giddiness involved perception of the gap between what life was and what they thought it ought to be. That gap was experienced as an abyss – over the edge of which they felt themselves falling, along with the rest of the world and its meaning. It was within those experiences that I began to appreciate the edge of my own professional abyss, the gap between what I felt able to do and what I thought I ought to be able to do. In time I realised that the women and I shared the same problem. We both needed to act within our lives *now*, with all our perceived limitations, in the face of all our living nightmares. As Harry Stack Sullivan observed, we were more alike than different (Sullivan 1953).

The 'caring' function of nursing is often misrepresented as doing something 'active' like easing distress through reassurance. I would rather emphasise the way in which nurses influence the *conditions* which allow change to occur, in a way appropriate to the individual, and their individual situation. In this context, an unusual definition of nursing is to be found in table billiards. The term 'to nurse the balls' means the stroke 'used to keep the balls in the best position for the scoring of cannons'. By nursing the balls, rather than employing more vigorous strokes, the billiard player increases the likelihood of achieving a high score; of realising optimum performance. The value, perhaps, of taking care with all due attention.

Hildegard Peplau said that, among other things, nursing was a maturing force and an educative instrument (O'Toole & Welt 1994). By means of effective nursing, individuals and communities can be aided to use their capacities to bring about changes that influence living in desirable ways. Nursing, in Peplau's terms is very much about such a firm, controlled yet gentle facilitation of optimum performance. Nurses do not change people, but help people use their own capacities to bring about their own desirable changes in living.

When people are helped to appraise their life, its problems, the meanings they attach to these events, and the myriad possible actions open to them, they gain a new perspective. That awareness of 'something different' is one of the critical signposts on the human life path. Maybe that is the difference which makes a difference.

The development of such alternative perspectives might be seen as part of a 'personal science of human problems'. Although, people may make discoveries which are similar to those of others, in the final analysis, such discoveries always possess a unique meaning. Take the example of depression. Irrespective of the putative causes of the depression, most people share the experience of fear of what is ailing them, will feel powerless to respond constructively to the depressive event, and with the passage of time, may descend into the 'slough of despond' which Bunyan described in *Pilgrim's Progress* – where hopelessness and desolation become one. These 'sensations' are common to severe depressive states and are reported by most sufferers, although the language and the metaphors may differ. We are all more alike than different. And yet people draw their own meaning out of the experience of illness: a meaning which is, by definition, beyond my ken.

My knowledge of myself and others is bounded by the language which defines my experience. As Peplau wisely remarked, 'language influences thought; thought then influences action; thought and action together evoke feelings in relation to a situation or context' (Peplau 1969). Indeed, how language operates, and how we might help the person reframe their emotions and behaviour, remain highly fertile research territories.

Language is used also to redefine nursing, by the creation of models of nursing practice. I have lost track of how many such models are now in existence, each claiming to be the evocation or distillation of the 'business of care'. Believing that we were getting lost in the many definitions of what is, or is not nursing, I decided to proffer a solution called *trephotaxis:* a neologism I cobbled together from the Greek, meaning 'the provision of the necessary conditions for the promotion of growth and development'. We deploy 'trephotaxis', or we become 'trephotarcs', when we facilitate the conditions under which people discover the experience of growth and development (Barker 1989).

Growth is a possibility for all patients, even for those facing death. I have written elsewhere of my experience in caring for my father who lived with cancer for five years and who, when he had had enough of the struggle, asked me to help him prepare for his death. He did this very explicitly by asking me to bury him: to 'say a few words', since he was not in any sense religious. This was a brave request since, within his culture, everyone was buried by a priest or minister – whether believers or not. His choice was doubly difficult since my mother was, and remains, a strong believer. That invitation began a change in my relationship with my father, which indirectly changed my life. My father had always been a background figure – quiet, supportive, but largely unknown to me. In the last few months of his life he talked for the first time of the joys and the suffering of his life. Barefoot days in the slums of the North East of England were the beginning of joy, and his part in the allied forces' relief of Belsen, which was part of the suffering. These were not the stories of which soap operas are made, far less film scripts. Simple yet profound story telling on the last stages of his life path. Stories which healed his life and began the healing of my own. These stories were to be the final gift from an almost absent father: a gift which helped me understand the true meaning of my metaphorical journeys with the people called patients.

When people fail to realise such growth, they may well be suffering more from professional pessimism than psychopathology. Whatever the presumed 'condition' from which the person suffers, true nursing addresses the potential for growth: how the person can grow in human terms, with the result that the disorder – whatever it might be – presents as less of a problem, or may no longer be manifest. Nursing addresses the person's relationship with the disorder. We have a responsibility to help the person nurture the hope that (s)he might leave the disorder behind. This experience will illustrate Hilda Peplau's dictum that 'people make themselves up as they talk' (Peplau 1986, personal communication). This is, however, no ordinary talk, although to the outsider it might appear so. Nursing, which has always dealt in the currency of language, is illustrating how the careful use of language can aid and abet the growth process. I say 'aid and abet', for clearly we facilitate rather than make this happen.

The history of psychiatric nursing is replete with examples of 'trephotaxis', the most significant being within the territory of interpersonal relationships. Consider the following proposal: 'the nurse has to become an acute observer, who maintains an active curiosity and a habit of asking questions about her own and the patient's feelings and behaviour and an interest in developing insight into her own and other person's stereotyped ways of thinking about and behaving with patients'. The same authors suggested that 'the careful observation of small changes in a patient that could be built upon and expanded is a significant part of this process'. That quote illustrates the value of curiosity: through inquiring into the nature of relationships, both nurse and patient may grow more knowledgeable about what, exactly, is going on between them; and with knowledge might come the understanding which both seek. The authors, Morris Schwartz and Emmy Lanning Shockley, published those American views forty years ago.

A common misconception about psychiatric nursing is that nurses simply encourage patients to talk about how they feel, thereby 'working through' their difficulties. Thirty years ago, Hilda Peplau said 'I am not at all convinced that mere catharsis is useful'. Rather, she went on to say, nurses should allow patients to express negative feelings, whilst encouraging discussion, allowing the nurse an opportunity to observe the behaviour, catalogue it as a pattern, and perhaps get some data to help him/her understand the pattern. Peplau was illustrating the importance of formulating hypotheses: in order, in my words, 'to begin to find out, more exactly, what is going on here' with a view to 'finding out what needs to be done' to facilitate growth and development.

What do I mean when I say that nurses address the whole, lived-experience of the person? The context, illustrated here, is an intimidating example of the complexity of the human situation. At the organic level we need physics, molecular biology, cellular biology, pathology, biochemistry and physiology – in ascending order – to appreciate how the body of any person works. When we move beyond the individual, we need – again in ascending order – psychology, sociology, ecology, political science and finally anthroplogy, to appreciate the psychosocial boundaries of the individual. The person is, metaphorically, the pivot for this human see-saw, at the opposite ends of which lie the atomic self and membership of the human race. The person has various relationships up and down these hierarchies – although, without reflection, most of us are unaware of these relationships. How the person-who-is-patient relates to these various organic and psychosocial selves is the content of the nursing enquiry.

When nursing acts as the educative instrument which Hiledegard Peplau defined, it will draw forth the person's knowledge of her relationship to these distant atomic and racial selves. The inquisitive process of nursing – through which the person is educated – aims not for any final answers to the human predicament, but merely to establish where (s)he is at this point on her/his life path; what sense does the person make of experience at this point in time; and how can such sense-making help the person to make progress? If you think this sounds rather philosophical, you would be right. However, such philosophical uncertainty has great value in practice. In Bertrand Russell's view, philosophy was to be:

'studied, not for the sake of any definite answers to its questions, since no definite answers can, as a rule, be known to be true, but rather for the sake of the questions themselves; because these questions enlarge our conception of what is possible, enrich our intellectual imagination, and diminish the dogmatic assurance which closes the mind against speculation' (Russell 1912).

The most elegant nursing interventions involve asking questions: the most central of which is 'what, exactly, is going on here?'. The extensive repertoire of questions which we might use to facilitate the person's voyage of discovery has only one proper objective: to further her/his relationship with her/him self, her/his world, and all those within it, and to extend her/his appreciation of the meanings (s)he constructs around and about these interacting relationships.

Such 'discovery-based' caring is to be distinguished from the kind of care which is built around the forcible insertion of 'therapy' into the nursing context, which often results in losing sight of the true meaning of care. Too much therapy, and not enough care, can unsettle the person further. The American survivor, Rae Unzicker, described her recent experience thus:

'To be a mental patient is to participate in stupid groups that call themselves therapy. Music isn't music, it's therapy; volleyball isn't a sport, it's therapy; sewing is therapy; washing dishes is therapy. Even the air you breathe is therapy, and that's called the milieu' (Unzicker 1992).

I have a hunch that there is no need to 'change' people, or to 'lessen their distress', through one form of magic or another. People will change only when the conditions are right, but they will be the prime mover in the change process. I recall working with a 72-year-old woman, with a history of manic depressive psychosis extending back to her early 20s. She was

'I have a hunch that there is no need to 'change' people, or to 'lessen their distress', through one form of magic or another. People will change only when the conditions are right, but they will be the prime mover in the change process'

recognised by family, friends and staff as a shy, yet eager to please woman, who had a difficulty acknowledging any success openly – indeed she shrank back physically when success was even suggested. My intervention involved little more than asking her questions, persistently yet carefully, over several weeks. My curiosity helped her to construct a picture of herself haunted by her mother, whose voice and ghostly presence, she translated into auditory hallucinations and apparently delusional beliefs. Ultimately, she used some of the experiences she had gained in 'letting go' her dying husband – which she had told me about in great detail – to release the restrictive ghost of her mother. She used experiences gained – painfully – in one part of her life, to heal another part. I had no idea whether what she reported was 'true' in any absolute sense. That she changed suggested that she had constructed a personal truth which was valid at least at that point in time. I have often asked myself, what more is there?

I have an abiding interest in people who might be called intractably depressed or suffering from psychotic disorder. The proper focus of nursing such people is to help the person clarify the experience: how their experience 'works'; so that they might 'draw forth from within' new perspectives – a definition, I think, of real education; something which we all need. We can facilitate such education even when the person is reluctant to name the problem. I have had several experiences of working with women who had been sexually abused in childhood. I would begin by acknowledging, openly, that the woman *knew* the problem, but that there was no need for *me* to know, unless she explicitly wished this. This exchange would mark the starting point for an exploration of this unidentified problem, an experience which belonged to her, but which she knew she need not necessarily share directly with me.

The Australian writer Pearlie McNeill offers a disturbing but apposite metaphor. She described how her grandmother told a story about a child greatly bothered by a large tapeworm. The child's mother took her to a healer who asked the mother to leave but relented when the mother begged to stay, but sternly instructed her to say nothing. The healer prepared a hot meal and set it before the child, bidding her to lean over and open her mouth. The child did as she was told and in a moment or two the tapeworm emerged past the child's lips, drawn forth by the tantalising smell. But then the mother screamed. A fatal mistake. The tapeworm recoiled suddenly, killing the child, probably by choking her. McNeill noted that although the story was grim she was never frightened by it. Instead she came to accept the inherent wisdom of the story: that the tapeworm symbolised all the hurt that had somehow taken up residence inside her; the mother is the conscious part of her reasoning that wants what is best, but cannot always deal with the pain of the stories as they begin to come out; and the healer is the driving force that motivates her to prod memory, often coaxing forth more than she might like. And the food – the food might be therapy, but therapy might also be writing. I am presently writing a book with a woman who was in the therapy with me and who, like Pearlie McNeill, found that rewriting her stories was a most potent form of re-authoring her life. Like McNeill, she too learned that she was the child, the mother *and* the healer of her own hurt. Therapists of many persuasions often expect that the person *must* openly address the problem if any progress is to be made. This does not match my experience. Indeed, such a requirement may, of itself, be taken as no more than a further form of abuse. I have listened to and collaborated in the re-authoring process of Bobbie Kerr, my co-author. I remain largely in the dark as to what was her root problem, although the therapy was judged to be a success. Sometimes light can appear mysteriously from out of the darkness.

People always own experience, whether or not they can communicate it; or even when their capacity to label and communicate such experiences has deserted them. Wittgenstein suggested that 'language is the only reality'. Recently, I read Alan Bennet's diaries, in which he talked of his dementing mother's difficulty in finding words for ordinary situations. When riding in a car she asked her son 'do you have one of these?'. 'What?' 'One of these … what we're in just now?' 'What … a car?' 'Yes, that's it, do you have a car?' Bennet wisely observed that she knew what she was experiencing but had lost the language to communicate what she knew she wanted to say. He added that he wished Wittgenstein could have been in the back seat.

Many nurses working with people with dementia will have reached similar conclusions. The challenge appears to be not to concern ourselves with the decaying of the physical self – the pathology of dementia – but to focus upon the experiences of confusion and agitation, anger and resentment, which are but some of the human dimensions of this disorder. As Dylan Thomas observed, 'old age *should* burn and rave at close of day; rage, rage against the dying of the light'. At least part of our caring for people with dementia should acknowledge that the disorder may, in human terms, be raging against the dying of the light. How we respond to such rage is one challenge for nursing.

My realisation of what might be the 'proper focus of nursing' has, as I have illustrated, been recognised by other nurses for generations. The renaissance of interest in the compassionate dimension of caring has also been described by people who are not nurses. Twenty-five years ago, the American writer Robert Pirsig wrote in *Zen and the Art of Motor Cycle Maintenance*:

> 'When one isn't dominated by feelings of separateness from what he's working on, then one can be said to "care" about what he is doing. That is what caring really is, a feeling of identification with what one's doing' (Pirsig 1974).

More recently the American psychiatrist Edward Podvoll (1990) has described the importance of a compassionate environment for people suffering from more severe mental illness, like psychosis. Podvoll has defined the ability of staff to 'be fully' with their charges, offering the kind of human support they sorely need. Podvoll suggests that what he called basic attendance 'requires more than just what one knows; it requires that one use everything of who one is and how one relates to the world. It involves a genuine nursing of the mind'.

Mental illness affects the whole person. Recovery must, therefore, address the whole person. True care of the person with mental illness must involve careful attention to bodily needs: in general we remain too fixated on medication, which doubtless has an important place. But what of attention to diet, exercise, physical contact, massage – all of which might promote growth? To what extent are these elemental dimensions of human life part of the everyday care plan?

The psychological dimension requires similar care: through effective interpersonal relations, the sense of alienation, stigma and isolation may be reduced; and the person may uncover hidden psychological resources which may overcome the fears and self-abasement which characterise serious mental illness.

These lead naturally into the social domain, where relationships with nurses under ordinary life circumstances take prominence, and the business of 'healing lives' can begin. These relationships can be powerful, and a sense of kinship and bonding brings rewards as well as challenges for the nurses themselves.

Finally, this excursion into 'therapy *in* life … therapy *through* living' makes an impact on the spiritual identity of the person – and by implication, the nurse also. The patient may begin to develop an awareness of who (s)he is and to appreciate the meaning of distress, which goes far beyond mere personal issues. The American nurse, Rosemary Parse (1995), has suggested that nursing can deal, in this sense, with the art of 'becoming'; treading the path which Maslow charted to the further reaches of human nature.

I am often accused of holding what might be described as an overly optimistic view of the human condition, and of the potential for genuine recovery from mental illness. Such a position seems appropriate to me, given that people with mental illness already know too much of pessimism. Without the compassion, mutual discovery and optimism I have sketched here today, I fear that people may well cope with mental illness, may apparently recover, but will acquire no real human lessons from the experience. I have met many people who changed dramatically following serious physical illness. The confrontation with death encourages many people to become aware of the need to live life, minute by minute; to *live fully* right up to the moment of death. These are lives which have been healed through the challenge of illness. These examples suggest the possibilities also for people 'healing their minds' by becoming aware, in the words of Sheldon Kopp (1974), that: 'This is it; there is nothing else'. This also reminds me of Alan Watts' rephrasing of the Zen addage: 'One is more likely to achieve enlightenment by peeling potatoes than by meditating on the Bhudda'. Our lives – embracing relationships, work, challenges, disasters, hustle and bustle, activity and rest – have the capacity to wound us, but also a capacity for repair. Often the recipe for spiritual repair is under our very noses, if not in the kitchen sink. Some extraordinary life problems may well have ordinary solutions.

'I am often accused of holding what might be described as an overly optimistic view of the human condition, and of the potential for genuine recovery from mental illness. Such a position seems appropriate to me, given that people with mental illness already know too much of pessimism'

Through interpersonal relations with effective nurses, some patients may experience the true meaning of 'taking care'. This experience may be like their original experience of mental illness: something of which they have true knowledge; but which often can be beyond words. True care might begin the development of their true selves – a process which they will continue in their own everyday lives, through their own version of taking care.

People with mental illness have taught me that 'we cannot turn the clock back; there is no going back. The aim of all our strivings may be to help the person express what (s)he experiences and then to learn how to find her/his own faith, through doing what needs to be done'.

And now I am back where I started: the story of our reflection on ourselves and how, through the power of stories, we might learn how to live life fully. Searching for an explanation of what nursing is and how it is done, by deconstructing it, is like analysing the paint in a picture. In art we fumble for an understanding of the idea which the painting conveys. We shall never know the essence of art or life, or indeed of nursing, as long as we observe it like viewer and object. The essential value of life, and indeed of nursing, can only be comprehended by merging fully into the flow of life so that one can become fully a part of it. By losing ourselves in our relationships with our patients and in the stories they tell us, we may come to appreciate the point of the illness, if not also of their lives. The stories of nurses and of nursing will, by implication, become enriched in the process.

NOTE

This chapter is based on a paper presented to the 21st Annual Conference, ANZCMHN – 'Celebrating a new era', Canberra, Australia, 29 September 1995.

REFERENCES

Barker P 1989 Reflections on the philosophy of caring in mental health. International Journal of Nursing Studies 26:131–141
Barker P 1992 Severe depression: a practitioner's guide. Chapman and Hall, London
Barker P 1995 Promoting growth through community mental health nursing. Mental Health Nursing 15:12–15
Barker P, Reynolds W, Ward T 1995 The proper focus of nursing: a critique of the 'caring' ideology. International Journal of Nursing Studies 32:386–397
Dao D M 1992 365 Tao: daily meditations. Harper, San Francisco
Frame J 1980 Faces in the water. The Women's Press, London
Frankl V 1963 Man's search for meaning. Washington Square Press, New York
Gotz A, Konnertz W, Thomas K 1979 Joseph Beuys: life and works. Barron's Educational Series, London
Kopp S 1974 If you meet the Buddha on the road – kill him! Sheldon Press, London
McNeill P 1989 One of the family: an Australian autobiography. The Women's Press, London
O'Toole A W, Welt S R (eds) 1994 H E Peplau – selected works: interpersonal theory in nursing. Macmillan, London
Parse R R 1987 Nursing science: major paradigms, theories and critiques. Saunders, Philadelphia

Parse R R 1995 Illuminations: the human becoming theory in practice and research. National League for Nursing, New York

Partington A (ed) 1992 Oxford dictionary of quotations. Oxford University Press, Oxford

Peplau H E 1969 Psychotherapeutic strategies. Perspectives in Psychiatric Care 6:264–270

Peplau H E 1994 General applications of theory and techniques of psychotherapy in nursing situations. In: O'Toole A W, Welt S R (eds) H E Peplau: selected works. Macmillan, London

Pirsig R 1974 Zen and the art of motorcycle maintenance. Corgi, London

Podvoll E 1990 The seduction of madness: a compassionate approach to recovery at home. Century, London

Russell B 1912 The problems of philosophy. Williams and Norgate, London

Schwartz M S, Shockley E L 1956 The nurse and the mental patient: a study in interpersonal relations. Russell Sage Foundation, New York

Sullivan H S 1953 The interpersonal theory of psychiatry. Norton, New York

Thomas D 1970 Miscellany one: poems, stories and broadcasts. Dent, London

Unzicker R 1992 'To be a mental patient' in Psychopoetry II. Changes 10:226–227

Watts A 1957 The way of Zen. Thames and Hudson, London

Wittgenstein L 1963 Philosophical investigations (trans G E M Anscombe). Basil Blackwell, Oxford

Commentary

Jon Chesterson

'The logic of experience' was a keynote address presented in Canberra in 1995 at the 21st annual conference of the Australian and New Zealand College of Mental Health Nurses. The title of the conference, as it suggests, 'Celebrating a new era' was concerned with acknowledging and sharing the valuable contribution mental health/psychiatric nurses make to mental health within society. This address focused on one of the key themes, 'consumer perspectives and effective collaboration'. Clinton (1996) states, 'scholarly sources can be used to inform the way we think about nursing, but … it is not these sources in themselves that contribute to our insights but our intuitive grasp of them in the light of the most personal of our experiences'. Reflection helps 'us to integrate the concepts we read about with our experience of life to better inform our thoughts about nursing'. Such reflection is also a process within the patient, with which nurses can engage through listening and helping the patient make sense of their illness and their stories and restore or bring meaning to their lives. This reminded me of something I had read, which was written 360 years ago:

> *'I was brought up on letters from my childhood; and since it was urged on me that by means of them one could acquire clear and assured knowledge of all that is useful in life, I was extremely eager to learn them. But as soon as I had finished the whole course of studies at the end of which one is normally admitted among the ranks of the learned, I completely altered my opinion. For I found myself embarassed by so many doubts and errors, that it seemed to me that the only profit I had had from my efforts to acquire knowledge was the progressive discovery of my own ignorance' (Descartes 1637).*

We are reminded of Gregory Bateson's story of the man who wanted to know about the mind. Phil Barker observes that, 'our libraries are full of books and papers that purport to explain the concept of the mind', whilst, 'the mind itself may be no more than a meta-story that explores, but fails to explain, the business of being and living'. The logic of experience, as the title suggests, opens up a new path that invites us to explore our world and our practice from a different perspective: the personal experience of the sufferer. By listening to another's story, the nurse together with the patient have an opportunity to re-affirm their need for self-examination as a core element of the life process. Simon Champ (1997) whilst describing his personal experience of being and living with schizophrenia reflects on this very point: 'I would try not to absorb the negative messages about people who lived with schizophrenia that I was reading and would try instead to find out for myself what this diagnosis would mean for me in my own life. It was the beginning of a mental turn about, trying to re-establish my life and find a more acurate sense of self'. This logic of experience, described by both nurse and patient as a 'defining characteristic of a new era' or 'mental turn about' underpins Descartes' own personal discovery and plan when, in 1618, he abandoned the traditional sciences and predominant schools of thought for what he might find within himself and the 'great book of the world'. He travelled, frequenting courts and armies, mixed with people of various dispositions and ranks, collecting a variety of experiences, wherever fortune placed him, reflecting always on things as they came up that enabled him to derive profit (meaning) from them.

Phil Barker asserts that the unique role of the mental health/psychiatric nurse 'has always been to facilitate the psychosocial, if not spiritual "healing" of the person with mental illness'. Whilst the evidence for this 'always' having been the case is not clearly substantiated in the literature, the epistemology of psychiatric nursing or indeed the observable or documented practices of mental health/psychiatric nurses, it may well be a unique vision for the future which is already emerging. Such a view is controversial since it represents a departure from the predominant neuro-scientific paradigm of the late 20th century, which thrives along with the cognitive-behavioural school, which have articulated well the evidence and research base for health outcomes within the economic-rationalist world in which we live and with good reason and gains.

The empiricist may argue and others concede the scholarly value and humanistic forte of the philosophical arguments but take issue with the lack of evidence presented, particularly that which is research based. Gournay (1996), for instance, claims that Barker does not offer an alternative to research-based interventions and holds very much a minority view. Clinton's (1996) response cautions us about the perils of one orthodoxy being in too high an ascendance over another. Theories or reflections on existence, being and meaning are of no less value than that which is scientific; both are, after all, constructs by which we interpret our experiences within the world and validate or affirm what we know – constructs that provide an instrument to explain different phenomena, just as much as chalk is different from cheese – and they serve different functions, but probably the same master. Arguably, therefore, we most certainly need both. It would be most erroneous to shelve the so-called 'minority view', as this would subjugate not only the potential development of mental health/ psychiatric nursing in the new millenium, the already emerging reality of a new era of collaboration with consumers and potential new and deeper insights about health and recovery, but most importantly the reality and lived experiences of sufferers. It is not correct either to say that Barker presents no alternative, nor is it entirely correct to say that there is no evidence. The logic of experience here is replete with interventions and strategies, and whilst the evidence is less clearly presented, it may be readily validated by talking to consumers and just listening to the many stories they have to tell about their experiences of illness, the ravages, the disconnection and how health professionals, armed with the power of language, status and science, may unwittingly add to this disempowering discourse.

Farrell (1997) reminds us that evidence-based practice in nursing is concerned with clinical expertise, best available research, and individual patient predicaments, which together assist nurses and patients to make informed choices about what might be the optimum care in a given situation. It is interesting to note that there are many significant arguments presented in the logic of experience that parallel what sufferers or consumers are saying, and one such milestone work is that of Simon Champ (1997) and his independent and equally inspiring reflective account, 'A most precious thread', an account of one person's struggle with schizophrenia and the search for meaning over the past 23 years. When talking about the impact of nursing interventions, often in his most vulnerable moments, he has three things to say:

'The nurses I most valued at that time were those who rather than impose their reality on me helped me to explore where reality and well being might exist for me. The best staff allowed me to go over my psychotic experiences gradually diffusing the power they held over me.

I think the best professionals involved in my care have opened themselves to the mystery that is schizophrenia along side me. They have gained my trust, sharing and supporting my inner search for meaning and understanding of self in relation to illness'.

Barker says:

'Effective nursing helps people develop their natural reflective processes. When people are helped to appraise their life, its problems, the meanings that they attach to these events, and the myriad of possible actions open to them, they gain new perspective. That awareness of something different is one of the critical signposts on the human life path. Maybe that is the difference which makes the difference'.

Here in Australia, certain resources are scarce. Within the the health care system, time, human resources and money have become scarce economic commodities. This may be due to the power we give up to the dollar as much as our priorities and attitudes towards helping people with a mental illness. One of the big challenges for mental health/psychiatric nursing will be how to deliver the care that meets the growing and complex needs of sufferers in an effective way, not merely to dress the wounds and take away the symptoms of suffering, but to help people heal their broken lives, to make sense of who they are and where they want to go, to live and to have meaningful lives. These are in part, the elements of mental health which all of us are striving for and consumers are asking us to address. 'The logic of experience' is a landmark work to provide us with both hope and direction, whilst on the other hand, a challenge given the scarce resources required. Perhaps it challenges us all to look within ourselves, reflect upon the resources we have within us and share it with others. That would be part of a new era. When we disover this, we might become more effective in a meaningful way to those entrusted in our care … and that would be grand.

It's grand to be a lot of things
In this fair southern land,
But if the Lord would send us rain
That would, indeed, be grand
(A B 'Banjo' Paterson).

REFERENCES

Champ S 1997 A most precious thread. In: Proceedings of the 23rd annual conference of the Australian & New Zealand College of Mental Health Nurses – 'communication in practice', an international conference hosted by the South Australia branch, Adelaide

Clinton M 1996 Response: letter to the editor. Australian & New Zealand Journal of Mental Health Nursing 5(4):152

Descartes 1970 Philosophical writings: a selection translated and edited by Anscombe E, Geach P T. From: Discourse on the method (French text first published in 1637). Nelson's University Paperbacks for the Open University, London, Part 1, p 9, p 12, p 13

Farrell G A 1997 Getting up to speed with evidence-based practice [monograph]. Australian & New Zealand College of Mental Health Nurses, PO Box 126, Greenacres, South Australia, p 1

Gournay K 1996 Letter to the editor: a response from Britain. Australian & New Zealand Journal of Mental Health Nursing 5(4):149–152

Paterson A B It's grand. From: The collected verse of A B Paterson. In: Along the western road: bush stories and ballads. Angus and Robertson Publishers, Sydney, p 14

Rungs on the ladder: creativity and psychic distress

Leonardo is reputed to have said:

> 'I understand the art of my science and the science of my art. I don't just think in words, but also in pictures, in sounds, smells and tastes. I look for the hidden meaning in every event in life'.

Although not renowned for his literary skill, Leonardo's notebooks provide sketches of a man in almost constant reflection with his experience. For him, there was little repetition; he moved, day by day, progressively forward, seeking new experiences, seeking to solve new problems, celebrating the gift of life and honouring it by acting as a conduit for the very essence of creation (Taylor 1960).

The occasion for the presentation of the paper on which this chapter is based, was an exposition of work of the artist Aidan Shingler, at which he reflected on the creative processes involved in the production of some of his recent works. The state of the visual arts in contemporary society is an uncertain one. Many of the well-known 'young contemporaries' appear to be shocking us with little more than the rewarmed memories of Dada or Pop Art. The dividing line between theatre and performance art began to be blurred, intentionally, more than a half century ago. Something of a zenith, or nadir, was reached by the sociopolitical work of the Fluxus group and by Josef Beuys, who affirmed that everyone was an artist and – by implication – all human experience might be represented as 'art'. Beuys, you will recall, 'exhibited' his memory of being shot down during the war over Russia and, suffering from exposure, being rescued by peasants who wrapped him in felt and animal fat. Beuys, who went on to make numerous constructions and sculptures from felt and fat, identified that experience as his first 'work'.

The parallel between Beuys and Aidan Shingler may be apposite. Some of Shingler's constructions and installations are funny, some tragic, yet all possess an illumination which distinguishes them from the often vacuous displays of outrage or cleverness of some of his 'young contemporaries'. His work is grounded in his experience of himself: in experiences which many of us might all too readily call bizarre, psychotic or delusional, and which has been described, officially, as schizophrenia. Shingler has acquired an enviable understanding of his own experience. In that sense he is both the observer and the observed, and joins a number of other notables from the visual and literary arts, who have journeyed to the farthest reaches of human nature.

Several links may be drawn, between Da Vinci and latter-day celebrants of the creative process. Here, I shall focus, mainly, on the visual arts, emphasising Pablo Picasso – who may have been the conduit, for some of his life, for the heightened consciousness often called mania or psychosis – and Juan Miro, who was an artistic archetype of the depressive experience. I shall refer, briefly, in passing to writers and scientists who might also have been stimulated by an as-yet poorly understood creative process. I propose that the relationship between creativity and so-called madness can involve a 'transcendence' of everyday reality. Such transcendence may be viewed as actual or metaphorical. It is, nonetheless, an essential part of the great works of creation. It would be folly to suggest that all people described as mentally ill are frustrated Da Vincis. However, we should remind ourselves that the nature of the 'experience' called mental illness, remains unclear. Some people defined as mentally ill may experience a transcendence of reality. This may be a good time to reflect on the relationship between creativity and 'madness'. Increasingly, neuroscience encourages us to believe that we know how the brain creates the mind, if not also the person. These assumptions carry the implication that human experience is an epiphenomenon which, ultimately, is meaningless – no more than the waste products of the brain constantly inventing and re-inventing itself (*cf.* Gournay 1995a, 1995b). Personally, I have to admit to grave misgivings about such a view. What brings me to write on this specific topic, may be expressed through my complex neurophysiology, but is infinitely more complex and far-reaching than the boundaries of my brain. What brings me to write is a story about the human need to understand experience – to reflect on reflection – and to express that, variously, in creative form. The story of our attempts to understand our experience may be the story of Everyman, and is a fitting narrative with which to link with Aidan Shingler's experience.

UNREASONABLE DISCOVERIES

It is all too often, and easily, forgotten that we would not be here today, or at least would not be enjoying our present lifestyle and culture, were it not for the influence of people who were, at least, a little *mad* (sic).[1] Such an observation depends greatly on our definition of madness, to which I shall return later. There is an emerging body of evidence, however, that some of the shapers of our culture, if not of all cultures, were – by definition – explorers of the farthest reaches of human nature (Maslow 1973). Not all these 'shapers' were artistic – in the classic sense of devoting their lives to painting, poetry, music or literature. When he was asked *how* he came to invent the electric light, Thomas Edison replied that he had ten thousand teachers. We might well ask, *who*, but a madman, would try ten thousand and one times to make something?

Although conforming, fitting in, and otherwise knowing the rules of the social game can be useful, it gives people an opportunity, only, to repeat, or rehearse, well established patterns of social living. Those people who *see* a way forward, who develop a *vision* of a better life are, by definition, deviants. It was clearly an 'outsider' who intuited the potential of the

'we would not be here today, or at least would not be enjoying our present lifestyle and culture, were it not for the influence of people who were, at least, a little *mad*'

wheel in stone-age times. Although we value logic and reason, it was never reasonable to think that a piece of stone could propel us with ease down a hill, nor that a later development of that wheel would propel a camera taking pictures of the surface of Mars. Anyone who ever thought that such things were possible, clearly was not thinking reasonably. At this very moment, some problem is being unlocked by a (non-)rational mind, which recognises that when the answer is *known*, the problem will be to translate that answer into rational terms, for uptake by a society founded on logic.

Although it is taken for granted that artists – if not all aesthetes – are unconventional or eccentric, this is true also of many scientists. Poincaré struggled for 15 days to develop what later were called the Fuschian functions. One evening, contrary to his custom, he drank black coffee, could not sleep and experienced ideas which 'rose in crowds' and which he 'felt collide until pairs interlocked, so to speak, making a stable combination'. By the next morning, he had established the hypergeometric series and 'only had to write out the results, which took but a few hours' (Poincaré 1924).

Kekulé's discovery of the benzene ring also came to him as he dozed in front of the fire, and saw in his 'mental eye' that the six atoms of carbon formed a ring (Findlay 1948). Loewi believed that the nerves of the autonomic system acted by releasing noradrenaline or acetylcholine at their nerve endings (Pickering 1974) but knew that this was unsupported by empirical evidence. One night he dreamt the idea of the crucial experiment. He woke up and immediately wrote it down but, on awakening in the morning, could not read his handwriting. Fortunately, he had the same dream the following evening, woke immediately and went to his laboratory to conduct the experiment (Ingle 1963).

Perhaps the most famous example lies in Einstein, who had a mental breakdown as a teenager and was viewed, retrospectively, by Storr (1972) as a schizoid personality. Einstein was mentally slow and unsociable as a child and was forever adrift in what his parents thought were foolish dreams (Goertzel & Goertzel 1964). In adulthood he maintained that it was as important for him to improvise on the piano as it was for him to work on physics. This was only the beginning of his eccentricity. He became indifferent to his physical appearance, at times falling silent and becoming motionless, or wandering off in the midst of conversation, being viewed by those around him as 'unreachable' (Vallentin 1954). The similarity to schizophrenic behaviour is self-evident. Yet despite this pattern of 'eccentricity', Einstein 'discovered' the theory of relativity. What is most surprising is that his discovery was made entirely through thought. His famous book contained no references and little mathematics and it was to take more than sixty years before scientists could demonstrate the accuracy of his formulae in space. In Pickering's view (1974), Einstein's teenage breakdown was a mental catharsis, during which he shed the conventional – but restrictive – faith of Judaism and ultimately developed his own notion of a cosmic religion, which was consonant with the most advanced scientific view of the universe of the day.

At the time of their *discoveries* none of these great minds was working in a classically rational mode. Or rather, all of them may have been encountering the 'ah ha' experience described as long ago as Archimedes, when he saw what he had been searching for in his bath. Indeed, all such discoveries were so eccentrically achieved as to be indistinguishable, in form at least, from some kinds of delusional thought. These scientific discoveries have in common, lapses of rational consciousness: drifting off into sleep, night-dreaming or day dreaming. Perhaps, in these lapses of rational processing, these scientific pioneers moved into a mode of 'hyper-reason'.

ORIGINALITY AND THE CREATIVE MALADY

All highly developed cultures, based on scientific and aesthetic achievement, are a function – at least in part – of the influence of eccentrics who, by definition, lay beyond the inner circles of normal thinking and feeling about the world and the human condition. Indeed, the mere exercise of logic is rarely sufficient to effect a satisfactory outcome, in human terms. The common expression 'the law is an ass' is often used to convey dissatisfaction with the outcome of logical inquiry. Some of the people who have played significant roles in shaping the development of civilised society were viewed as deranged (or ass-like) in their day. Perhaps today, even more might be classifiable as mentally disordered in some sense.[2] Rather than treat *all* of these manifestations of extraordinary thought, feeling or belief as madness (sic), we might consider celebrating *some* such people as those who might, with hindsight, be part of that group of human inquirers who might lead us towards some kind of human enlightenment.

This is no idle speculation. I have been reflecting on the relationship between eccentricity, madness and creativity for over thirty years. A distinguished body of literature on the inter-relationship of these themes is now, at last, beginning to appear (*cf.* Gooch 1980, Schildkraut & Otero 1996). Initially, my inquiries were based on the assumption that creativity and madness was limited to the classic aesthete: the writer, poet or artist. Over the past two decades, however, a burgeoning literature has emerged, which suggests that even some scientists – those final arbiters of the taste of logic – may have been predisposed to 'creative unreasonableness' (*cf.* Pickering 1974). For some of them, their logical work may have been fuelled, paradoxically, by distress or psychological 'differences'. The most recent example to emerge involved Charles Darwin, who was offered a posthumous diagnosis of panic disorder, in a recent issue of the *Journal of the American Medical Association*. Barloon & Noyes observed that:

> *'From the writings of Darwin himself, as well as biographical materials, we conclude that he may have suffered from panic disorder with agoraphobia' (1996).*

Darwin appeared to show nine of the thirteen symptoms of panic disorder listed in the DSM-IV. He was afraid to go anywhere, and this fear interfered with his work and social life. Nevertheless, he married, fathered 10 children, lived into his 70s and wrote *On the Origin of Species* over a 22 year period. Barloon & Noyes do not consider whether Darwin would have been more prolific if he'd been diagnosed and treated. Instead, they suggested that his panic disorder might have been an asset. Had it not been for this illness, his theory of evolution might not have become the all-consuming passion that produced *On the Origin of Species*. This is only a new version of an older hypothesis. In Pickering's (1974) view, the obscure illness from which Darwin suffered for most of his life was not Chagas disease, picked up in the tropics, but was undeniably mental, and served to protect him from the trivialities of social intercourse. Illness provided the solitude and leisure necessary to develop and support his revolutionary concept of evolution.

Pickering (1974) offered an original model for distinguishing the form and function of the 'creative malady'. In some cases, illness provides the condition necessary for the creative work to be undertaken: Darwin and Florence Nightingale being two classic examples. In their case, the experience of illness was not unlike that of the prison experiences of John Bunyan and Bertrand Russell. It afforded them the privacy and time to attend to their intellectual vocation. In others, the illness appears to be an essential part of the act of creation: Joan of Arc, Mary Baker Eddy, Sigmund Freud and Marcel Proust being outstanding examples.

THE LADDER OF TRANSCENDENCE AND THE ENIGMA OF MELANCHOLY

The people mentioned so far, clearly were not crippled by their illness, although this is a difficult (retrospective) judgement to make, given their eccentric lifestyles and behaviour, which were tolerated in every case – except the fated Joan of Arc. However, even more debilitating forms of mental distress are also represented in the 'creative malady'; not least in the case of melancholia: where the relationship between spirituality, creativity and mental distress is particularly well documented (*cf.* Barker 1992, Panofsky 1955).

Durer offered the most famous, and arguably the most misunderstood, image of melancholia in his mysterious engraving. The winged figure of Melancolia, in Durer's famous engraving, sits immobilised by sorrow, her head resting on a clenched fist, eyes fixed in a glassy stare. Her hair and clothing is manifestly dishevelled. She is surrounded by the symbols and tools of the creative process but appears to be suffering from what Panofsky called the 'tragic unrest of human creation' (Panofsky 1955), destined in her paradoxical union of genius and despair to lose her competition with God, the ultimate creator. This is commonly seen as the spiritual self-portrait of Durer, who was inspired by celestial influences and eternal ideas but who suffered all the more deeply when he failed to ascend the ladder – depicted in the background of the image – which would allow him to transcend the human condition. This is, arguably, the received view of Durer's most enigmatic work (*cf.* Schildkraut & Otero 1996). I offer an alternative interpretation: that Durer, rather than being debilitated by depression, recognised a superior form of melancholy, characteristic of thinkers and artists. Rather than an image of despair and

'Rather than an image of despair and bottomless sadness, Durer's engraving suggests inspired listening, and sensitivity to the mysterious language of the imagination'

bottomless sadness, Durer's engraving suggests inspired listening, and sensitivity to the mysterious language of the imagination, compared with which, the instruments and other pieces of scientific apparatus which litter the scene are of little importance (*cf*. Barker 1992, Knappe 1965). From this perspective, the image may be read as a challenge to materialism and all other 'false gods' which might serve as diversions from the chosen path (enlightenment), which is symbolised by the ladder: the means by which it will be possible to be connected to a higher plane of existence in this world, rather than a means of escape into the next.

In a slightly later engraving, Jacob de Gheyn depicted an old philosopher atop a globe beneath which the Latin inscription reads: 'Melancholy, the most calamitous affliction of soul and mind; often oppresses men of talent and genius'. The mere fact that these early images *celebrate* melancholy suggests that the artists recognised the basic human need to relate to the infinite. Since time immemorial, people have sought to understand, manipulate and manage material existence, ostensibly to create a 'better world'. Often they find, only, that the material world is ultimately unsatisfying – discovering the need to detach or dissociate themselves from the material world, in an effort to feel part of 'something bigger'. Today, the spiritual questing growing around us is dismissed as some kind of millennial fever. Yet, similar examples of spiritual renaissance are scattered down history, and correlate highly with periods of scientific or technological achievement (*cf*. Storm 1991, Barker 1996).

The search for meaning is not restricted to melancholic artists, shuffling towards the eventual release of this mortal coil. Indeed, through scientists like Newton, Darwin and Stephen Hawking may be traced a fascination with the relationship between the rulers of the universe and humanity's lowly station in the 'grand design', irrespective of how that fascination is expressed.

Durer's symbolic ladder reappears as a recurrent theme in the work of the modern Spanish artist Juan Miro. In his *Carnival of Harlequin*, Miro described how he produced this painting 'during the period of my great hunger that gave birth to the hallucinations recorded in this painting'. This painting included the image of a 'gentleman whose fasting ears are fascinated by the grace of a flight of butterflies musical rainbow eyes falling like a rain of lyres a ladder to escape the disgust of life' (Rowell 1986:164) The 'rain of lyres' to which Miro referred was a stylised ladder in the painting, an image which he had used in earlier – more representational – paintings of farmyards, and which he confessed first was plastic, 'then nostalgic at the time of painting *The Farm*; [and] finally symbolic' (Rowell 1986:208). It might be asked, 'symbolic of what?'. Perhaps the ladder represents the process of ascending to some higher realm, or perhaps an escape from the disgust of life. In either case, Miro continued to use the same visual metaphor for transcendence deployed by Durer, four centuries earlier.

DYSFUNCTION AND CREATIVITY

There is now little doubt that some of the creative minds which have shaped civilisation have operated beyond the boundaries of what would commonly be called normal experience. Studies undertaken by Redfield Jamieson (1996) and the Ariskals (1996) and others in the USA, and Post in the UK (1996), attest not only to the high representation of mental illness in creative people, but also in their family members. All that remains to be established is exactly how many is *many*. In Andreason's view such co-occurrence reflects:

> '*an underlying personality and cognitive style which predisposes to both creativity and mood disorder. [This] is characterised by traits that make an individual original, open and exploratory, but also leaves them vulnerable to suffering. These traits … include a lack of ego boundaries, intellectual openness, intense curiosity, intense concentration, obsessionality, perfectionism, high levels of energy, adventuresomeness, rebellious, individualism and sensitivity. … such traits tend to be both highly original and highly productive, but they also tend to be physiologically and emotionally vulnerable' (Andreason 1996).*

In a more poetic vein, Byron – acknowledging his own possession of such traits – described them as contributing toward his 'fearful gift: what is it but the telescope of truth, which brings life near in utter darkness, making the cold reality too real?' (Barker 1992:13).

The full extent to which writers experience what might reasonably be called *madness* is more difficult to establish. Post's (1996) recent inquiries suggest that a formidable number of western novelists have been depressed, often suicidal, and many disguised their distress through alcohol and drug abuse: William Styron being one example of an 'insightful' melancholic (Styron 1991). How many of these authors travelled to the outer reaches of the human experience remains less clear, perhaps due to the novelist's tendency for elliptical story-telling.

Ironically, full human awareness – at least as understood within meditative traditions, such as Zen Bhuddism – may bring the person closer to what in religion might be called God, and what in science might be described as the essence of the universe. Indeed in Buddhism and Taoism – if not also in the fullest understanding of Christianity – god and the infinity of the space–time continuum are one and the same thing, only represented in different language. When the activity of visual artists, specifically, is considered, it could be hypothesised that they are merely re-*presenting* – metaphorically – the universe and the human experience within it.

ALTERED STATES AND CREATIVITY

Goethe – who was a noted scientist, as well as poet and dramatist – experienced paranormal visions and auditory hallucinations. Nicolson (1947) believed that writers, especially poets, tended to display their eccentricities, rather than have actual experiences of mental illness. He recognised, however, that Goethe, despite being 'a man of the most Olympian calm and sanity' did see specters and hear voices calling and, on one occasion, 'met himself riding along a road on horseback' (Nicolson 1947:171). Despite Nicolson's reservation, few having read *Faust* could fail to appreciate that here was a man who had personally and profoundly experienced both sides of the human equation, and had personally suffered the agony of what Laing (1960) would later call the 'divided self' (Gooch 1980).

It is commonplace to assume that 'altered states' differ from psychosis, but share a dissociation from both the material world and the material body. In Goethe's case, his ability to split himself off from the consensual reality, afforded him an insight into the meaning of the world, which has been treasured ever since.

An even more curious example exists in Isaac Newton, the godfather of physical law, who appeared to experience a similar psychological crisis and subsequently spent much of his later life writing religious treatises (Gooch 1980). Newton's discovery of universal laws pre-dated this religious phase. Perhaps, he became aware of the true significance of infinity as he began to sense the edge of the universe, now being touched (theoretically) by Hawking and other contemporary physicists (Hawking 1988). Recently, I received a letter from one of Stephen Hawking's staff advising me that he had read one of my recent papers (Barker 1996) in which I had misunderstood his frequently quoted observation that:

> 'we shall all ... be able to take part in the discussion of why it is that we and the universe exist. If we find the answer to that, it would be the ultimate triumph of human reason – for then we should know the mind of God' (Hawking 1988:175).

Professor Hawking observed that I had failed to note his atheistic irony and was in danger of falling into mysticism (personal communication). I reread my paper and the section from Hawking and replied that, should Hawking – or indeed any physicist – ever reach that point of understanding infinitude – what Beckett frequently referred to as the *ineffable* (Esslin 1965) – then he may well have come to know the mind of god, since 'god' and the 'ineffable' are (arguably) the same concept framed in differing terminology.

If I had understood him correctly, Professor Hawking's efforts to distinguish the material universe from what might be called the symbolic representation of the universe, may lie at the heart of the matter. The artist travels, metaphorically, to places within the human condition ruled out-of-bounds by conventional society. *Why* the artist might wish to do this has long been an intriguing question within psychoanalysis. *How* the artist does this has become a minority interest for neuroscience (*cf.* Obiols 1996). These interests in no way reflect attempts to glamorise mental states, such as psychosis. Even artists themselves might challenge any effort to ignore the inherent distress of the creative process. As Byron observed:

> 'I can never get people to understand that poetry is the expression of excited passion, and that there is no such thing as a life of passion any more than a continuous earthquake, or an eternal fever. Besides, who would ever shave themselves in such a state?' (Marchand 1978).

The interest in 'why' and 'how' creativity is expressed, represents two dimensions of the recognition that genius, on any level, is a complex process. As Jamieson has noted, the controversy surrounding ideas of the 'mad genius' versus 'healthy artist' arises from a confusion about the nature of madness (Jamieson 1996). Despite Pickering's (1974) observation that Van Gogh's later work showed evidence of his slide into psychosis, he could never have been mad in the sense understood by Jamieson – where true psychosis involves a deterioration of personality (Jamieson 1996). Even his final works betray a lucidity of expression that is incompatible with the state of disorder associated with true madness.

This is not to say that Van Gogh was not 'mad' in another sense: existing 'beyond the pale' in human, experiential terms. The available research evidence suggests that creative people are characterised by a paradox not evident in so-called normal people. The creative type is at one and the same time psychologically 'sicker' – scoring higher on measures of psychopathology – *and* psychologically more healthy – showing elevated scores for self-confidence and ego strength (Andreason 1996). This may represent the true distinction between 'ordinary people' and those who have *exploited* the experience of the 'divided self' or have *purposefully* extended their tours of the farther reaches of human nature. Those who have extended their human boundaries are not ordinary, in any sense of the word. The greater the engagement with the creative process, the more the person passes beyond the ordinary into a world which is not already here – manifest reality – and is, therefore, *extra*ordinary.

> 'The available research evidence suggests that creative people are characterised by a paradox not evident in so-called normal people. The creative type is at one and the same time psychologically 'sicker' – scoring higher on measures of psychopathology – *and* psychologically more healthy – showing elevated scores for self-confidence and ego strength'

THE LORDS OF DISCIPLINE

Creativity cannot be a function of disordered thinking – rambling and incoherent. This is true of scientific *and* aesthetic creativity, otherwise we would not have built public and private temples of respect (e.g. museums, art galleries, theatres) down the ages. The work of art, in particular, attracts us – whether in words, images or sounds – for we recognise that the curious novelty, even idiosyncrasy, of the work is also a function of discipline, will and, paradoxically, a supreme effort of rationality. Of Goethe, Thomas Carlyle wrote:

> 'This man rules, and is not ruled. The stern and fiery energies of a most passionate soul lie silent in the centre of his being; a trembling sensitivity has been inured to stand, without flinching or murmur, the sharpest trials. The brightest and most capricious fancy, the most piercing and inquisitive intellect, the wildest and deepest imagination; the highest thrills of joy, the bitterest pangs of sorrow; all these are his, he is not theirs' (Carlyle 1971:37).

Freud encouraged us to think that the act of creation was some kind of mechanical displacement of energy, albeit deriving from a complex psychic history (Freud 1947). There seems little doubt that people draw upon formative experiences, or somehow 'work' them into their act of creation. The full horror of some such enactments – such as Plath's confrontation of her own death wish in *Lady Lazarus* – have all the characteristics of taboo, attracting and repelling us at one and the same time. But the discipline which is required to create may be acquired by an even more tortuous route than that assumed by Freud. Picasso was but one of many supreme creators who believed that he was little more than a vehicle for his art – that he was driven. This was not the wild imaginings of passionate youth. In his 80s, he observed: 'Painting is stronger than I am. It makes me do what it wants' (Berger 1965:29). Similar sentiments were expressed by poets like Keats, and musicians like Menuhin, both of whom were prodigies. Certainly, Picasso took the view that his creativity was more valuable than what he created. The effort to understand art – perhaps even to deconstruct it – is, in Picasso's voice, a hindrance, if not a threat:

> *'Everyone wants to understand art. Why not try to understand the songs of a bird? If only they could realise above all that an artist works of necessity, that he himself is only a trifling bit of the world, and that no more importance should be attached to him than to plenty other things which please us in the world, though we can't explain them' (Berger 1965:29).*

Is Picasso being unreasonable or simply pointing, like the Zen master, to the inherent paradox of understanding: that we should not confuse the finger pointing at the moon with the moon itself? Picasso appeared compelled to use visual paradox – like a Zen koan – to reveal the truth of the matter. In his notebooks, Leonardo had recorded: 'do not reveal if liberty is precious to you' (Taylor 1960:217). Four centuries later, Picasso could not understand the importance given to the word *research* in modern painting: 'In my opinion', he wrote, 'to search means nothing in painting, to *find* is the thing' (Berger 1965:30). We should not forget that Picasso was also a great showman, full of what now would be called soundbites: 'I used to paint like Raphael, but it has taken me a whole life to learn to draw like a child' (Gardner 1982). Psychoanalysis floundered in its attempts to explain *why* anyone would want to draw like a child; neuroscience is only now beginning to be interested in *how* the artist, within all of us, might do that.

Neuroscience is finally expressing an interest in *how* people exercise creativity. Chaos theory is being used to help us understand how the brain might bring a beautiful, or meaningful order out of chaos. The brain appears to have a spontaneous drive toward self-organisation, in much the same way as clouds represent the spontaneous drive towards organisation of air and water. Obiols (1996) has proposed a tentative model to explain the creative process. When the central nervous system experiences low levels of activation (such as sleep and unconsciousness), it brings mental states into the 'chaotic zone' – this is best characterised by night dreaming. High levels of activation (excitement, manic states) cause a similar kind of cognitive destructuring, precipitating a related chaotic mental state. This model may eventually help us to appreciate how – through natural dreaming, or practised day dreaming, meditation etc. – artists, writers and scientists derive their *inspiration*. In

'the transitional state between alertness and tiredness (hypnagogia) and the transitional state between normal alertness and excitement (hypomania) might be the doorway to the act of creation'

Obiols' view, the transitional state between alertness and tiredness (hypnagogia) and the transitional state between normal alertness and excitement (hypomania) might be the doorway to the act of creation. Here the chaos of the universal mind is ordered by the natural ordering processes of the brain. These hypotheses may help us clarify our understanding of the *method* by which inventors, scientists, artists, poets and writers 'discover' or 'see' their eventual work. Despite this neuroscientific theory, the riddle remains: what is the chaos out of which the muse of inspiration emerges?

WHOLES OR PARTS: IMPLICATIONS FOR PSYCHIATRIC NURSING PRACTICE

It seems axiomatic to suggest that, *of course*, the chaos from which is drawn all our understanding, whether aesthetic or scientific, *is* the universe. Some aspects of our processes of gaining knowledge imply an effort to transcend, or at least, to try to control that which we aim to know. The striving for knowledge is difficult to separate from the striving for power over a world in motion, and is – arguably – the grandest of all the human neuroses. We feel so overwhelmed by the beauty and wonder of all that we survey that our inherent inadequacy compels us to try to develop a means of setting parameters on our knowledge. Within those parameters we hope to find a rationale for separating out anything which appears not to fit our narrow construction of reality. Hence our reluctance to accommodate forms of knowledge which might be deemed intuitive, rather than logical in either form or function.

As the end of the 20th century approaches, it would be easy to assume that humanity is on the brink of knowing almost all that there is to know about life on earth. We need only decide, once and for all, whether or not there is life elsewhere in the universe. In the field of psychiatry, the knowledge base has shifted, within less than fifty years, from the assumption that the many variants of the human personality are largely a function of lived experience, to the assumption that the *mind* is largely a function of genetic influence. The best-known of the neo-Darwinians, Dawkins, argues that human life is no more than a function of: 'a concatenation of inane events whose only connecting thread is the propagation and survival of limited structure-carrying systems such as genes'. Polkinghorne describes this as a bleak view of the meaningless character of life on earth (1996:1). Increasingly, we are encouraged to take the view that the phenomena representing the *content* of the experience of psychosis – hearing voices or unusual beliefs – are also meaningless, the mere outcome of one biochemical or neurophysiological anomaly or another. To suggest that all people who 'hear voices', for example, are in any way the same, seems problematic. Some people described as 'suffering from schizophrenia' report hearing voices that tell them to lead the world to god or, as in the case of the blues musician Peter Green, to give away all their money. Others hear voices urging them to kill people or, as in the case of Peter Sutcliffe, only women. As Boyle (1990) has observed, this suggests that if these people are indeed 'ailing' from something they have very different ailments indeed.

No less an authority than Francis Crick – who was part of the team which deduced the structure of DNA – has asserted that 'you – your joys and your sorrows, your memories and your ambitions, your sense of personal identity and free will, are in fact no more than the behaviour of a vast assembly of nerve cells and their associated molecules' (Crick 1994:4). This view of the *mind* is problematic on a number of levels, as Polkinghorne, the particle physicist, has noted:

> *'At the material pole of reality, if you split me apart into my constituents, you will just find quarks and gluons and electrons. You will also have destroyed me. The self resides at the other, holistic, pole of reality. That explains its elusiveness in the reductive analyses of materialism or computer functionalism … signs that one is looking in the wrong place, scrabbling around among the pieces for what can only be found in the whole' (1996:72).*

Polkinghorne concludes his reflection on the 'disappearing mind' by arguing that:

> *'We have to be realistic enough, and humble enough, to recognise that much of what is needed for eventual understanding is beyond our present grasp' (1996:73).*

I have found myself wondering what are the implications of these ideas, assertions and hypotheses for me – as a person – and also for my discipline of psychiatric nursing. Is there room enough within psychiatric nursing, I wonder, for a similar humility about what might be involved when people 'hear voices' or 'hold strange beliefs'? The assumption that such complex phenomena are no more than the late outcome of some genetic or biological insult seems woefully flawed.

The growing literature on creativity presents an intriguing challenge to the received wisdom concerning psychic distress. The development of the human genome mapping programme has brought the promise of a 'brave new world' which will be free of the physical and mental ills which have troubled humanity, and which are passed down generations by genetic transmission. Schizophrenia and manic-depressive psychosis are two of the more 'serious and enduring mental illnesses' which are assumed to be determined by genetic transmission and may, therefore, ultimately be erased from the map of the human condition. This review of the creativity literature suggests that some of the ancestors of today's scientific pioneers were at the very least eccentric, and potentially might have been classifiable as mentally dysfunctional. The attempt to homogenise the human race has been described by the physicist and Nobel laureate, Joseph Rotblat as science out of control: genetic engineering could result in 'a means of mass destruction' (Artlidge 1996). In the context of the discussion here of creativity, such engineering may ultimately kill the goose which has laid some of humanity's golden eggs.

'The attempt to homogenise the human race has been described … as science out of control: genetic engineering could result in "a means of mass destruction" … In the context of the discussion here of creativity, such engineering may ultimately kill the goose which has laid some of humanity's golden eggs'

Increasingly, nursing and nurses define their practice as 'holistic'. Although little consensus may exist as to the full meaning of this term, it implies that people are more than patients with disorders or illnesses. Indeed, even within the limited context of interpersonal relations theory, the 'patient' might be viewed as having a relationship with her/his disorder, illness, etc. However, within the broad concept of holistic nursing have emerged specific theoretical developments such as the notion of nursing as a compassionate force (Brykczynska 1997) within a spiritual dimension (Farmer 1996). Both these approaches – although they represent much the same *attitude* towards needs for care and caring activity – recognise the inherent 'transcendent quality of human existence' (Frankl 1964:38). Mental health (sic) nursing has, for generations, expressed an interest in *who* are patients and *how* they exist within the various modes of psychic distress. There appears, now, to be a very real danger that the extant psychiatric (sic) nursing philosophies of care may be supplanted by a postmodern view of the patient (sic) as no more than a 'concatenation of inane events', which are nonetheless primarily biological with some social influences.

The creative genius is, without doubt, an exception to almost every human rule, and is a resident of a tiny community whose defining characteristic may be the alienation each member feels from the rest of humanity. There may be some value in considering the extent to which the creative genius may serve as a model of the transcendence discussed by Frankl (1964). We struggle constantly to refine, improve and 'better' the human machine, from aerobics to the human genome project. There may already exist a way – indeed that way (Tao) may well have been known for thousands of years (Barker 1996) – to accept the chaotic irregularities of the human condition and, through that acceptance, to transcend the psychic distress associated with worldly experience.

At the exposition to which I referred at the start of this chapter, we were fortunate to be able to hear a first-hand account of a young artist who brought his own reflections on his spiritual journey, teasing out hypothetical relations between himself and the cosmos. The human canvas which Aidan Shingler set up for us showed how how he is engaged in seeking and finding himself, within the various stories of his experience and all the stories which have gone before him. I hope that we might all find ourselves in there also.

NOTE

This chapter is based on a paper presented at the 'Aidan Shingler Exposition' held at the University of Newcastle, on 19 February 1997.

1. The author is discussing 'madness' here as an *idea* only. As Szasz (1987) has commented: 'The *Dictionary of the History of Ideas* has no entry for it [insanity] or for any of its synonyms, such as *madness* ... This remarkable omission points to an important phenomenon, namely, that insanity is now considered to be a fact, not an idea.
2. The 4th edition of the *Diagnostic and Statistical Manual* employs almost three times as many classifications of mental disorder as the 2nd edition, only thirty years ago.

REFERENCES

Andreason N C (1996) Creativity and mental illness: a conceptual and historical overview. In: Schildkraut J J, Otero A (eds) Depression and the spiritual in modern art: homage to Miró. Wiley, Chichester

Ariskal K K, Ariskal H S 1996 Abstract expressionism as psychobiography: the life and suicide of Arshile Gorky. In Schildkraut JJ, Otero A (eds) op. cit.

Artlidge J 1996 Scientists able to create human clone. The Guardian 26 February p 6

Barker P 1992 Severe depression: a practitioner's guide. Chapman and Hall, London

Barker P 1996 Chaos and the way of Zen: psychiatric nursing and the 'uncertainty principle'. Journal of Psychiatric and Mental Health Nursing 3(4): 235–244

Barloon TJ, Noyes R 1997 Charles Darwin and panic disorder. Journal of the American Medical Association 277(2): 138–141

Berger J 1965 The success and failure of Picasso. Penguin, Harmondsworth

Boyle M 1990 Schizophrenia: a scientific delusion? Routledge, London

Brykczynska G 1997 (ed) Caring: the compassion and wisdom of nursing. Edward Arnold, London

Carlyle T 1971 Goethe. In: Shelston A (ed) Thomas Carlyle: selected writings. Penguin, Harmondsworth

Crick F 1994 The astonishing hypothesis. Simon and Schuster, New York

Esslin M 1965 Samuel Beckett: a collection of critical essays. Prentice-Hall, Englewood Cliffs, NJ

Farmer B 1996 (ed) Exploring the spiritual dimension of care. Quay Books, Salisbury

Findlay A 1948 A hundred years of chemistry. Duckworth, London

Frankl V 1964 Man's search for meaning. Hodder and Stoughton, London

Freud S 1947 Leonardo Da Vinci: a study in psychosexuality. Random House, New York

Gardner H 1982 Art, mind and brain: a cognitive approach to creativity. Basic Books, New York

Goertzel V, Goertzel M G 1964 Cradles of eminence. Constable, London

Gooch S 1980 The double helix of the mind. Wildwood House, London

Gournay K 1995a New facts on schizophrenia. Nursing Times 91(25): 32–33

Gournay K 1995b Schizophrenia: a review of the contemporary literature and implications for mental health nursing theory, practice and education. Journal of Psychiatric and Mental Health Nursing 3(1): 7–12

Hawking S 1988 A brief history of time: from the big bang to black holes. Bantam, London

Ingle D J 1963 A dozen doctors. University of Chicago Press, Chicago

Jamieson K R 1996 Mood disorders, creativity and the artistic temperament. In: Schildkraut J J, Otero A (eds) op. cit.

Knappe K A 1965 Durer: the complete engravings, etchings and woodcuts. Thames and Hudson, London

Laing R D 1960 The divided self: a study of sanity and madness. Tavistock, London

Maizels J 1996 Raw creation: outsider art and beyond. Phaidon, London

Marchand L A 1978 Byron's letters and journals, Vol 8. John Murray, London

Maslow A 1973 The farther reaches of human nature. Penguin, Harmondsworth

Nicolson H 1947 The health of authors. The Lancet ii: 171

Obiols J E 1996 Art and creativity: neuropsychological perspectives. In: Schildkraut J J, Otero A (eds) op. cit.

Panofsky E 1955 The life and art of Albrecht Durer. Princeton University Press, Princeton, NJ

Pickering G 1974 Creative malady: illness in the lives and minds of Charles Darwin, Florence Nightingale, Mary Baker Eddy, Sigmund Freud, Marcel Proust, Elizabeth Barrett Browning. George Allen and Unwin, London

Poincaré H 1924 The foundations of science (trans G B Halstead). Science Press, London

Polkinghorne J 1996 Beyond science: the wider human context. Cambridge University Press, Cambridge

Post F 1996 Verbal creativity, depression and alcoholism – an investigation of 100 American and British writers. British Journal of Psychiatry 168: 545–555

Schildkraut J J, Otero A (eds) 1996 Depression and the spiritual in modern art: homage to Miró. Wiley, Chichester

Rowell M 1986 Joan Miró – selected writings and interviews. GK Hall, Boston

Storm R 1991 In search of heaven on earth. Bloomsbury, London

Storr A 1972 The dynamics of creation. Secker and Warburg, London

Styron W 1991 Darkness visible: a memoir of madness. Jonathan Cape, London

Szasz T S 1987 Insanity: the idea and its consequences. Wiley, Chichester

Taylor P 1960 The notebooks of Leonardo Da Vinci. Plume Books – New English Library, London

Vallentin A 1954 Einstein. Weidenfield and Nicolson, London

Commentary

Mark Radcliffe

Antonia is rich, articulate and an artist. She has also experienced depression. Her diaries published last year detail her struggle to shake off her dark moods and get on with her life. Her first novel, about a rich articulate and funny young woman struggling with depression, met with rave reviews. *Tatler* praised its pathos, its tragedy, its humanity. 'Antonia is a creative force to be reckoned with' it said.

She also sculpts and has an upcoming exhibition in a small but significant gallery in North London. Her quite remarkable little lumps of clay seek to depict the existential terror at the root of Antonia's profound depression. She herself comments 'nobody can really understand what I went through when I was depressed. I rarely went out, sometimes I hardly ate and I would cry sometimes even when no-one else was there. I did some paintings at the time. A lot of them used green which represented a place I wanted to be and it was surrounded by black which was a place I felt I was in. I can only hope people get the symbolism which is quite deep'.

For those of you who don't get the symbolism, Antonia has made a thirty minute film; she shot it herself, when at her lowest ebb. It is to be shown on BBC2 soon. The film also features her friend Rupert, another depressed person with a public school education. Rupert is a poet, 'not unlike Shelly', he says: 'Sensitive, too delicate for this world'.

Rupert has a sister, Corrine, who has, she says, 'difficulties'. 'Madness, I suppose you'd call it', she spits, at no-one in particular, not that anyone ever has called it madness, except Corinne. She is a performance artist. She uses mime to convey her experiences. She says 'to me I am my art, my experiences my mime is my art, I and my art are the same, my madness is my mime is my art is me is my madness'. Corrine says she reminds herself of Sylvia Plath. 'Sylv', she says, 'would do a lot of mime if she were around today'.

The romance, the illusion, the privilege of a sensitive near-sacred soul. The blessed may claim madness as a gift, whilst the cursed suffer for it.

I nursed for 11 years in and around inner London. My patients were rarely blessed, not in any economically viable way anyway. If they painted or wrote or moulded or mimed they did it through a veil of medication and deprivation, brutal and without charm. If they were to make art for us, it would be a gritty realistic Channel 4 drama. Except it probably wouldn't quite work. There would be no resolution, no social meaning. Maybe that in itself is romantic. Television, the great disposable medium of the late twentieth century, portraying disposable lives for disposing eyes. Mind you, what do I know. I have a chip on my shoulder the size of Birmingham, but no mental illness.

I believe in transcendence and beauty and the art and science that Phil talks of. But I loathe the romance that it has bred. In literature and poetry, and the therapy culture, where for some, madness is a fancy, a fear, a neurosis perhaps, but not a disability. Who invented the psychotherapy culture? An articulate neurotic. And who peopled the drug trials? That'll be the ones doing the finger painting in the corner.

One day I will write a book, I have the plan. It will be about a singer with a beautiful voice who writes songs with wonderful words. He may be mad or he may be strange. He will have a fragile temperament perhaps, the moods and demeanour of an artist. When he writes he will pour his heart and soul into words that lie at the very edge of him, and when he sings, he will almost bleed for the world. But to the audience it will just sound like shit. Laughable and embarrassing. There is no living to be made. We demand excellence, universality of sorts, transcendence that corresponds with our bounds, not his. Let him suffer for his art, but don't expect us to buy it. The key, may still be in the commodification of what the madman makes and perhaps increasingly in the romance of a mild and innoffensive madness itself.

A final cultural nuance. May 'we' in our clinical ordinariness become jealous of the successful, creative, effective madman? Of course we are not likely to envy the frightened psychotic with tardive dyskinesia and a bedsit in Kings Cross. He says he still hears voices, and his CPN agrees. The kids on his estate steal his money, call him names. We won't envy him, but the rich ones? The articulate, seemingly talented ones? So different but still mad. As an itinerant (diagnosed schizophrenic) patient of mine said on finally receiving his backdated Disability Living Allowance, 'I'm in the money; that means I'm not mad any more, I'm eccentric.' Those who have created for themselves a space to explore and a reason to defy logic, to be strange at the end of a century where most strangenesses have been manifested, marketed, and then murdered. We may envy those, we may be jealous of their mad ideas and their insane art. And we may crave the validation they find in their otherness.

Here are some of my fears. Those beliefs about madness, how it is itself a symptom of genius, how it informs transcendence and art and an otherness we all secretly crave, belittle the experience, the mundanity and the disablement of most of the people I ever worked with. The ones without enough of themselves left from their journeys to make art or objects or labour that we happen to value.

I am unsettled by a culture that revels in the products of some kinds of madness, and reviles others. And what makes some madness attractive? Maybe we have made madness into a narrative and we prefer our narratives grand. We want insight and resonance. We have come to expect resolution and heroism. The lunatic's struggle is different from the madman's. It is uglier, more crippling. It does not inform us, it embarrasses us. There is no romance in lunacy; it dribbles and stutters and makes no fucking sense. Those qualities that make some kinds of madness almost glorious are the same as make some kinds of art, art.

Mental health in the new millenium: dreams of a new age of enlightenment

9

INTRODUCTION

Let us pause to consider the voice of experience:

> *'There is a spirit which I see in the eyes and hearts of others who are in recovery from psychiatric disabilities. It is a force which drives the recovery of us all if we can connect with the life we are all part of. It is an inspiration. We emerge from the shadows with a message for all humanity. The time has come to unite in the greatest struggle we as a people have ever encountered. It is a struggle to set aside our prejudices and see if we can continue our interrupted evolution towards being human, whole, and connected with each other and with the world. Our journeys are uniquely our own. There are however certain themes, principles and values which continually emerge. The three I will emphasize here are* hope, humanity and voice' *(Fisher 1994:64).*

This chapter is based on a keynote address to a conference focused on the mental health service consumer's voice. It was a great honour to address the conference since, although I have had my share of distress, I shall not pretend to have experienced the distress commonly called mental illness. Members of my family have had such experiences, and a dear colleague committed suicide. But, for the moment, I stand in God's sunshine, rather than his shadow. And, wherever or whatever God is, I thank him for this blessing which, clearly, he has not conferred on all his subjects.

I have chosen Dan Fisher as the best 'voice' to open the chapter. Dan Fisher is a community psychiatrist and the Director of the National Empowerment Center in Massachusetts. He is also someone I know personally, which introduces another dimension to his words, at least for me. Dan Fisher is, as he would say, 'a person in recovery from psychiatric disability'. I take great comfort from the apparent agreement that exists between us, despite our differing professional and personal backgrounds. We appear to be speaking with the voice of unity. I hope to bring, today, something of that unanimity of voice and spirit to bear upon my thoughts about mental health beyond the millennium.

A WORLD GONE MAD

I have been a psychiatric nurse for almost thirty years. My entry to the field was entirely serendipitous: I intended that my position as an attendant at the local asylum would merely tide me over until employment more appropriate to my qualifications and aspirations, materialised. However, within a few hours I became fascinated; within a few days I became absorbed; and within a month I was captivated: I wanted to know 'what exactly is going on here'. I became interested in what the plight of the so-called mentally ill might mean for me. Very much as a second thought, I considered what I might be able to do to help them deal with their distress.

If there is a 'story' of my professional career, this is my story. I remain largely unchanged. I remain fascinated, absorbed and captivated. What has changed is that I think I now know what the plight of the mentally ill means for me; and I am also aware of what I might do to help them deal with the distress, stigma and alienation which are the very real boundaries of their experience.

'What has changed is that I think I now know what the plight of the mentally ill means for me, and I am also aware of what I might do to help them deal with the distress, stigma and alienation which are the very real boundaries of their experience'.

In this chapter, I hope to convey, through a few simple ideas, what needs to be done to advance our mental health care systems. What I have to say about mental health care beyond the second millenium is highly personal, spoken in no other voice than my own. However, what surprises me is that my continuing *mission* in mental health care has remained largely unmodified over three decades. As a young man, I learned two things which shaped my life: first, *the personal is political*; and second, that *everything is connected to everything else*. I have spent the past thirty years shaping and polishing these two ideas, and with each passing year have found that they both reflect and illuminate some of the basic needs which lie at the heart of all our human distress.

I speak also in a voice coloured by the experience of professional caring. Although nurses have feared redundancy for as long as I can remember, there is no reason to believe that, even if we dispense with nurses, we shall ever dispense with the need for nursing. The past thirty years have witnessed much debate over the definition of 'mental illness': what we should call people in mental distress as well as those who care for them. I have little interest in these academic questions. The distressed people of whom I am thinking are flesh-and-blood. All are so disabled and disadvantaged that it is *as if* they are ill, or otherwise bereft. If mental illness is a metaphor (Szasz 1987), then this illustrates the awesome power of metaphor.

Despite the growth in our human understanding, and the sophistication of our technologies of treatment, each year brings more and more people who either are, or believe themselves to be, mentally distressed. All managers know that the more services they make available, the more they will be used. If the world is not progressively going mad, it clearly is becoming less able to cope.

Many of us believe that the world is a more dangerous place; it may be more dangerous than we imagine. As Seligman observed:

'In American society, we now live in the age of the individual. What is the long term future of individuals? What is the long term future of the psychology of personal control, which has become quite fashionable in the last two decades? I suggest that both the future of individualism and, consequently, the future of the psychology of personal control are quite limited' (Seligman 1990:8).

Seligman's concern over individualism stemmed from the statistics on depression, which are not exclusive to American society. They show that the lifetime prevalence of depression in young people now exceeds, *by roughly a factor of ten*, the prevalence rates for young people fifty years ago. The explanation, though complex, involves the waxing of the individual and the waning of the commons. By contrast, communities which have maintained traditional forms of attachmnt and identity, have not suffered this tenfold increase in depression. Rural communities in Canada, the Old Order Amish in Pennsylvania, and primitive tribes, like the Kaluli in New Guinea, are examples of communities which have had little experience of change, and show no change in the rates of clinical depression. The moral, so far, appears to be that progress is bad for us! But what is it about progress?

By shifting the location of our explanation of our 'selves' from the environment to the individual, we have lost many of our anchors, and have turned up the heat in the process.

President Reagan used the term the 'Age of the Individual' in the first term of his presidency; and Prime Minister Thatcher echoed him by denying that there *was* any society, only responsible individuals. Four historical themes serve to create the Age of the Individual (Seligman 1990):

'the lifetime prevalence of depression in [American] young people now exceeds, *by roughly a factor of ten*, the prevalence rates for young people fifty years ago. The explanation, though complex, involves the waxing of the individual and the waning of the commons.'

- *Firstly, in the 1950s when I grew up, there was little choice. A radio was a wireless, and there was virtually only one kind. We didn't have a fridge, but those that existed were all economically painted white. Machine intelligence opened the way for customisation: of clothes, cars, and even fridges. To sell these products advertising shaped the notion of individual choice and, for those who can afford to buy, there is almost limitless choice. Many who cannot buy, steal; rather than risk alienation from the individualised ideal.*

- *Secondly, when I grew up in the 1950s my father rose at 4.30am, took two buses to begin work, at 6.00 and returned home at 6.30pm. The old joke that the working class man don't suffer stress; 'they have to get up for work in the morning' may have a grain of truth. I have no recollection of my father talking about stress, far less how he felt. He had a minimal self, which had remained unchanged down generations: a self which was preoccupied with living, rather than reflection on life. General prosperity and wider access to information has cultivated the 'Californian' or maximal self; strongly focused on pleasure and pain, success and failure and the whole rich business of feeling. The popularity of ideas like self-esteem and self-efficacy, derive almost wholly from this Californian self.*

- *Thirdly, my adolescence was characterised by assassinations: especially the deaths of the Kennedys and Martin Luther King, and along with them the death of the ideal of curing human ills, through social action. The Vietnam war virtually killed off youth's commitment to patriotism. The collapse of national institutions – like the ignominious fall of the House of Windsor in my country – nudge people further into looking for satisfaction in their own, individualised lives; despite the fact that the 'rules' for such individuality are framed by television and advertising*

- *Finally, who today intones the old adage that 'the family which prays together, stays together?' Those intertwined institutions – religion and the family – also have been eroded. In my youth, when the going got tough, we turned to the family, for support, or to God, for salvation. Today when the going gets tough, the tough get going – or go under!'*

As we depart from the natural path, so we seem to become more distressed. WHO data published late last year provided further confirmation of Seligman's gloomy forecast. By the year 2020, major clinical depression will be the second most important burden of disease in the world. Truly, we have entered a new age of melancholy (Barker 1992).

There are also some near-invisible problems which, possibly for ageist reasons, escape our popular attention. I am talking of the epidemics of mental distress among younger and older people. Our concerns for mental health services are focused often on adults, or more narrowly on adults with schizophrenia. Beyond this group exists many young and aging people, whose problems risk being dismissed as *merely* a function of their development or decline. Both these groups may, of course, be people who have suffered most from the waxing of the individual and the waning of the commons (Barker & Jackson 1996, 1997, Barker et al 1998). Perhaps it is time we drew back from our narrow focus on the individual in distress, in an attempt to see the bigger picture. Perhaps we need to be more sensitive to the powerful use of language – both professional and secular – to marginalise or territorialise areas of mental ill-health.

The only constant is change. As we stand on the threshold of the 21st century, almost every field of human inquiry – from physics and biology, to economics and medicine – is gripped by a paradigm shift, or feels the support of their old paradigm shaking beneath them. As Capra (1983) observed fifteen years ago, we are at a 'turning point' in history and few will escape the rising tide of change.

In *The Awakening Earth*, Peter Russell suggested the significance and profound nature of this rising tide:

'And the changes leading to this leap are taking place right before our eyes, or rather, right behind them – within our own minds' (1988:vii).

One sign of this change is our readiness to embrace the concept of mental health, another facet of the 'Californian self'. As my English colleague David Smail remarked:

'it is assumed that people should *be happy,* must *be competent to reach goals determined by their social position,* must *get on well with others,* should *be sexually adjusted and* should *enjoy sex' (Smail 1978, Barker 1990)*

Although these observations are twenty years old they are probably truer today than ever. The media would implode if it lost its franchise for exploiting our acculturated weakness for fulfilling these *shoulds* and *musts*. Indeed, this contrived social anxiety now affords plastic surgeons a new field of endeavour – providing women with silicone breasts, men with penile extensions and, more recently, fixing the epicanthic folds on the eyes of people with Down's syndrome so others would not stare at them! These may well be subtler signs of a world gone mad.

Of course, our ideas about what is a change for the 'good', has always been dependent on cultural paradigms – how we understand the world. It is only within recent history that we have redefined such influences as science.

The scientific paradigms developed down the ages make different interpretations about the human condition which, ultimately, ring out much the same tune. The *biological sciences* suggest that 'I' am the product of my genetic make up. Any problems I have, I 'got' from my grandparents. The *social sciences* suggest that I am a function of my upbringing. Any problems I have I 'got' from my parents. And finally the *environmental sciences* suggest that my problems are part of my everyday world – any problems I have I 'got' from my spouse, my family or friends. Remember that bumper sticker – 'Mental illness is hereditary: you catch it from your kids!'.

Different people use different versions of these models to explain, or perhaps excuse, themselves. We use them without even knowing that they were once theories. They *explain* why we did this or that, or why this happened rather than that. All three are, however, victim models: explaining how your grandparents, your parents or the whole wide world, got you into this mess. I know people use such excuses if only because I have heard myself using them over and over again down the years.

'Well I'm sorry but I can't help it … it (this problem) runs in the family…!'

'If you had had to put up with what I had to put with as a kid you wouldn't think it was so damned easy (to do whatever hasn't been done).'

'Oh, I'm sorry, its just that things are really difficult at home (or work, or in the neighbourhood, or in class or wherever) right now!'

These theories of causation are invariably applied only to our *mis*fortunes. These grand explanations are generally reserved for 'how shit happens'. We rarely say:

'Uh huh, I got my degree (or this job or this award) because my intelligence and commitment and hard work is programmed into my genes … I just can't HELP being successful!'

'That's right, I am very happy and contented, but then that isn't so remarkable, my folks brought me up to be happy and contented.'

'Gee another award …! This success is all due to the love and support I have received from my family, my friends and everyone at the office!'

Alternatively, if we took a more oriental view (Reynolds 1983), we might buy the paradigm that the meaning of life is to be found under our very feet, or in our very hands: in the living of it. My father, sweating in his iron foundry, and my father-in-law a mile underground, hewing coal, were virtual Zen masters in this respect. Emotional experience is largely tangenital to 'experiential reality' – what we do in our lives.

How do we begin to balance, or choose between such disparate world views. Truth – like the air we breathe – is already here and very close at hand.

We are only now beginning to let go of the old 'Cartesian – Newtonian' world view, which led us to believe that life was a random, meaningless accident – that we lived in a cold, harsh, clockwork universe. And since life (and the universe) comprises only material building blocks, all that awaits us is death. The so-called 'common sense' reality of the Cartesian–Newtonian paradigm is at least thirty years past its sell-by date. The 'new physics' (Capra 1976, Bohm 1980, Talbot 1988) demolished the myth that the world is made up of separate objects – rather, everyone and everything is interconnected in patterns of dancing energy (Zukav 1980). We are all parts of the whole, or as we Scots say – we are all Jock Tamson's bairns: all children of, and connected to God or Gaia (the good earth). Moreover, the new physics helps us to understand how consciousness not only has an impact on physical reality but also might help to create it (Davies 1982:13, Talbot 1988:180–182)

We are beginning to shift from a physical to a metaphysical vision of reality – from seeing the world and our place within it in a fragmented way, to a more wholistic vision. This is necessary, since health means whole. We cannot offer a health-related service without accommodating the whole person; without being (w)holistic.

What are the implications of this paradigm shift for mental health? The 'old paradigm' of traditional psychiatry was largely conservative: aimed at restoring people to 'normal' functioning; dislodging irrational thoughts, feelings and behaviour; encouraging conformity to some fashionable idea of sanity; plastering over the cracks, so that the person might 'cope' again. Normality and coping are seen as desirable or even optimal states: patients exchanging mental distress for ordinary misery. The old paradigm also values hard facts, often ignoring the potency of people's story-telling (Barker 1992), use of metaphors (Szasz 1987) and the poetics of their subjective experience (Mair 1989) – like a back-street mechanic, trying to find a fault under the bonnet, which he fixes as quickly as possible, using the cheapest materials, to get the car back on the road, knowing it will be break down again next week. There are more complex and more expensive versions of this paradigm, but all appear to share the same world-weary view of patients-*as*-patients.

'The 'old paradigm' of traditional psychiatry … [is] like a back-street mechanic, trying to find a fault under the bonnet, which he fixes as quickly as possible, using the cheapest materials, to get the car back on the road, knowing it will break down again next week'

Over the past one hundred years, we have moved through psychoanalytic, biological, behavioural, sociological, humanistic, cognitive and finally, neuroscientific representations of what it 'means' to be mentally ill. Today, the neuroscientific orthodoxy appears to suggest, almost, that the 'I' who experiences psychic distress is little more than a complex of physiological processes operating to the dictates of a genetically engineered programme. Little wonder that so many people want to recover what they see as their intellectual property – taking charge again of the 'I' that is 'me'. We feel the need to free ourselves, to recover – as Dan Fisher says – our*selves* and our *worlds*. We have waited a long time for Jung's prediction to come true:

'sooner or later, nuclear physics and the psychology of the unconscious will draw together as both of them, independently of one another, and from opposite directions, push forward into transcendental territory' (Jung 1951:ii).

Although we speak of mental health care, our everyday focus often remains fixated on resolving illness; and health is not simply the absence of illness. Drugs, ECT and, in the last resort, psychosurgery, can

'Although we speak of mental health care, our everyday focus often remains fixed on resolving illness, and health is not simply the absence of illness'

be life-saving, but are clearly means of dealing with *illness*. However, since we have drifted towards talking in more whole terms, we may be admitting that mental *health* is a more complex business. More importantly, the linguistic emphasis on 'health' rather than 'illness' suggests the human potential in all of us; *where* we might be going in our lives, despite the disorders, dysfunctions and other disabilities which appear to restrict or restrain us.

Our old psychiatric paradigms were almost exclusively negative: focused on what is *wrong* with people, their *illness*, *conflicts*, past *trauma* and *slights*, whether personal or social. They largely ignore, or subjugate, exploration of people's strengths, assets, talents and disguised (or perhaps obscured) potential. As Maslow suggested, thirty-five years ago:

> '*Freud supplied to us the sick half of psychology and we must fill it out now with the healthy half*' (Maslow 1962:7).

To explain people as wholes we need to move beyond concepts like 'treatment' or 'therapy'. We need to develop new ways of viewing one another. Perhaps our relationship should be akin to that of an architect or a tailor: I need to use my skills and knowledge to design something that meets the needs, and matches the personal tastes, of the customer.

This suggests a 'dynamic interaction. It implies a need for people to be cared 'with' rather than cared 'for' or otherwise 'treated'. This is no simple play on words – this is a powerful paradigm shift.

Caring 'with' might result in shedding some light on what it means for both of us to need one another, albeit for different reasons. In that sense, it might involve a new kind of enlightenment. More than twenty years ago, Alan Watts (1975) suggested that the common ground between eastern 'ways of liberation' and western psychotherapy was the transformation of consciousness and the release of the individual from cultural conditioning. Watts was thinking expressly, even then, of a new paradigm of western psychotherapy. It was – and remains – an interesting comparison. We might move from being 'therapists' or 'fixers' to 'fellow pilgrims': joint collaborators, exploring through some effective alliance, some of the stages on the life quest; helping one another to work out what – exactly – was the point of our being here; offering each other support on the journey to wholeness. The spiritual progress of all humanity involves a journey in search of the divine source, the sacred centre. The very notion of the whole suggests that, at its core, lies the sacred centre.

Sadly, little has been written about the benefits accrued by professionals, like me, as a result of spending a long time working with people in mental illness. Much has been written about how stressful it is; how ungrateful patients and their families are; how great is our vocation to care for or treat the mentally ill. People with whom I have worked down the past thirty years – as a nurse and as a psychotherapist – have changed me, for the better, far more than I have changed them. I did not always recognise this, but now know that this is the secret of all our successes. When we begin to care *with* one another, we all have a chance to change; for the better.

I need to establish what the consumer might *need me* for. In this situation the 'client' becomes the expert. This approach carries some powerful assumptions. It assumes that life is a spiritual journey, is meaningful (for everyone) and is purposeful. Although all human distress is meaningful, this should not stop us from asking for help to deal with it. However, I do say *deal with it*. I do not say get rid of it, or prevent it. Life for all of us can be difficult but, as Epictetus said over two thousand years ago: 'difficult circumstances do not so much enable a person, as reveal him'. And we are more likely to make such revelations by sharing our experience of difficult circumstances, than by any other method.

'Although all human distress is meaningful, this should not stop us from asking for help to deal with it. However, I do say *deal with it*. I do not say get rid of it, or prevent it'

I am talking here of a philosophy for living; a philosophy for a new age; a philosophy with simple yet powerful values, which will lead to powerful actions.

In the time we have left, we need to promote: love, trust, joy, creativity, cooperation, wisdom, compassion, intuition, humility, courage, vulnerability, caring, intimacy, respectability, harmlessness, integrity, humour, authenticity, uniqueness.

And, as we look back on our adolescent strivings, we need to forget how once we valued: competitiveness, domination, exploitation, fragmentation, blind reason and detached objectivity.

In these postmodern times, I remain comfortable declaring myself a humanist. My psychiatric philosophy is a humanistic philosophy. When Gary Zukav wrote his best-seller about the new physics he could not resist drawing an analogy between the rhythmic nature of pure matter and our life in the wider world of human affairs. The model for effective human agency can be found in the dancing molecules which are the essence of the universe:

> '*We see that when the activities of life are infused with reverence, they come alive with meaning and purpose. We see that when reverence is lacking from life's activities the result is cruelty, violence and loneliness*' (Zukav 1980:22).

- Dare we embrace this kind of harmonious collectivism?
- Dare we think that, if we believe it, we shall see it?
- Dare we risk developing a more optimistic model of true mental health?
- Dare we adopt an abundance mentality, believing that, like Hannibal, if we cannot find a way, we shall make one?
- Dare we risk believing that if we put our emotional and intellectual potential to the test there is virtually nothing which we might not achieve?
- Dare we develop a life *mission* based on our dreams and our desires, rather than on some arid scientist *model* based only on our basic needs?

When John F Kennedy told his people in 1961 that they would put a man on the moon by the end of the decade, the USA had neither the technology nor the knowledge to drive the Apollo rocket. Mission Control became a buzzword. JFK set a goal with no evidence that they could reach it, but in July 1969 Apollo 11 touched down and the moonwalk became history. How could a nation muster behind such a mission, for such an obscure end, but individual people and families and communities rarely have such life-enhancing missions to shape and develop their own lives on this Earth?

If a small proportion of the readers of this book developed such 'personal missions', the whole structure of mental health care would experience a seismic paradigm shift. If only 10% of you put down the book, dreaming of a new age of enlightenment, and kept dreaming of it by day or night, it would surely materialise, the product of our collective consciousness raising. The strangest secret is, that people become what they spend most of their time thinking about! Our scarcity mentality, with its assumptions about lack of resources and socially conditioned fear of failure, holds most of us back from that simple, yet profound act of becoming personal and corporate missionaries.

You already know this in your hearts. You are put off from acting on this knowledge by people waving statistics. Another strange secret is that nobody here *is* a statistic. Even stranger, is how many people accept statistical predictions as fact and act on them and prove the predictions right.

We should not focus entirely on ridding ourselves of illness – history shows that it will always return, often in a more virulent form. What we should be concerned with is healing: helping people become whole again, despite their illness or disability. To do that we need to help people to become explorers and makers of new maps. This is of course much more demanding than being simply a psychological tourist, simply following the map already prepared for you (Mair 1989:37). Of course, some will say that we need structure, we need protocols, we need frameworks for practice; and so we do. But these props are like tickets or transport. But, as Casey Stengal the former coach of the New York Yankees used to say: 'If you don't know where you're going you'll likely end up some place else'.

Although I have disparaged the notion of predicting the future, I feel – intuitively – that the experience of psychic distress beyond the millennium will become a story of all our journeys, rather than simply the journeys of those whom we artificially define as the mentally ill. I expect us to rediscover the wisdom of the ancients. I expect all of us to remember, daily, that for all of us, life is a short journey; and that we must give ourselves up to the realisation that the only thing we *really* know is that we must take this journey. We all must take that journey with no idea of where we shall reach or when. In that uncertainty, might exist a paradox of certainty. As Hughes observed:

> *'I prayed to God to break down the barriers of my certainty, security, respectability, my systems, rules and categories ... I wanted to be a pilgrim all my life long, a wanderer, uncertain of my destination, certain only that God is faithful and if I search for Him, He will find me'* (Hughes 1989:123).[1]

If I search for Him ... He will find me. That, dare I say, is the voice of recovery! I have offered you a highly personal account of what I hope will materialise over the coming decade. It is not a reasoned account in the sense that it employs the traditional 'masculine' voice; indeed, to some ears it may sound as if my heart has led my head. If this is so, I offer no apology. I wait patiently for any form of wisdom and have no intention of turning away the wisdom of the heart should I be so lucky as to be offered that prize.

I have no doubt that in the next ten years neuroscience and artificial intelligence will continue to amuse and astound us. As I noted earlier, however, despite our amazing stories of progress, we are in a bigger psychic pickle than ever before. Who is telling us what, exactly? For those of us who are not neuroscientists, what shall we do with our feeble *human* knowledge?

I have decided that I shall devote myself to joining with the people in my care; learning more from them about the business of being human; learning more about my own weaknesses; and through discovering their great resources and boundless assets, may come to realise some of my own.

As I completed the address on which this chapter is based, at home in England, quite unexpectedly, I received an essay from Sylvia Caras in the USA, the owner of the 'Madness' list on the Internet, and also an invitation to review a book by the British research psychiatrist, Phil Thomas. It was as if Sylvia's essay and Phil's book had been sent, through the power of some universalised intelligence, expressly to provide a validation of the simple message at the heart of my address.

In a message to all parents, Sylvia, the psychiatric survivor, wrote:

'I want you to see my potential, and to stop sensationalising the family despair [of mental illness]. It stigmatises your loved one, me, all of us. Instead – Listen. Instead of discussing medication and non-compliance as an inability to understand one's condition, listen to your loved one's objections. Instead of thinking how you gain, think of what, with medication, your loved one loses. Instead of forcing your loved one into unwanted treatment, attend to what is wrong with services, attend to why services are refused. For just a moment, become selfless. Listen. Pay attention to the flair, the ingenuity, the craft. See the worth, not the disease'.

And, in the conclusion to *The Dialectics of Schizophrenia*, Phil Thomas wrote:

'We must allow ourselves to be moved by others. Psychiatry has lost touch with this ability, indeed it is questionable whether it ever possessed it in the first place. Each step into the spurious certainty of neuroscience is a step away from matters of human concern. If we are to deal with the loss of certainty implicit in post-modern thought, we must be truthful with ourselves and others. We must allow ourselves to be ourselves with others'.

My dreams of a new age of enlightenment are stimulated by just these kind of appeals for conjoint human action. People like me who offer mental health services can learn from and be enriched by the experience of the people deemed to be in my care; and – I hope – they will learn from me and be enriched in the process. Together, we may represent a radical model for the kind of alliance that finally will deconstruct and dismantle the power structures that have bedevilled psychiatry, and all social services associated with it.

I began with Dan Fisher and will close with his voice:

'There is inside of me a self, a spirit, which is becoming more aware of me and others. That self is becoming my guide. It encompasses all that I am. My self includes, but is greater than, my chemicals, my background and my traumas. It is the "me" I am seeking to become in my relationships, in that creative uncertainty when I make contact with another'.

By developing true alliances between people in mental distress and all those who might care to help them, we might all come to value that creative uncertainty. It might form the basis for developing new ways to 'be human' in often 'inhuman conditions'.

NOTE

This chapter is based on a keynote address to the Australian National Association for Mental Health (ANAMH) Conference: 'Life chances and mental health – forging ahead to the new millennium',
Old Parliament House, Canberra, Australia, 14 August 1997.

1. I am grateful to my colleague Eileen Inglesby from the Department of Religious Studies at the University of Newcastle, for drawing this reference to my attention.

REFERENCES

Barker P 1990 Blind in one eye: the ethics of psychotherapy. Changes

Barker P 1992 Severe depression: a practitioners guide. Chapman & Hall, London

Barker P, Jackson S 1996 Seriously misguided. Nursing Times 92(34): 56–57

Barker P, Keady J, Crooms S, Stevenson C, Adams T, Reynolds B 1998 The concept of serious mental illness: modern myths and grim realities. Journal of Psychiatric and Mental Health Nursing 5(3): 213–220

Bohm D 1987 Unfolding meaning. Routledge and Kegan Paul, London

Capra F 1976 The Tao of physics. Fontana, London

Capra F 1983 The turning point: science, society and the rising culture. Fontana, London

Davies P 1982 Other worlds. Sphere, London

Davies P 1984 God and the new physics. Penguin, Harmondsworth

Fisher D 1994 Hope, humanity and voice in recovering from psychiatric disability. Journal of the California Alliance for the Mentally Ill 5(3): 13–15

Hughes G 1989 In search of a way. Darton, Longman and Todd, London

Ikehara H 1995 Creative resolution: an alternative philosophy for nursing practice. Asylum 9(2):24–26

Jung C G 1951 Collected works, Vol 9. Van Nostrand Reinhold, New York

Mair J M 1989 Between psychology and psychotherapy: a poetics of experience. Routledge, London

Maslow A 1962 Towards a new psychology of being. Van Nostrand Reinhold, New York

Reynolds D 1983 Playing ball on running water. Sheldon Press, London

Russell P 1988 The awakening earth. Arkana, London

Seligman MEP 1990 Why is there so much depression today? The waxing of the individual and the waning of the commons. In: Ingrams RE (ed) Contemporary psychological approaches to depression: theory, research and treatment. Plenum Press, New York

Smail D 1978 Psychotherapy: a personal approach. Dent, London

Szasz TS 1987 Insanity: the idea and its consequences. John Wiley, New York

Talbot M 1981 Mysticism and the new physics. Bantam, New York

Thomas P 1997 The dialectics of schizophrenia. Free Association Books, London

Watts A 1975 Psychotherapy east and west. Vintage, New York

Zukav G 1980 The dancing Wu Li masters. Fontana, London

Commentary

Catherine Conroy

The Australian writer Elizabeth Jolley (1993) observes in *Central Mischief*, 'There is a connection between nursing and writing. Both require a gaze which is searching and undisturbedly compassionate ...'. Nursing and writing, unreserved loves of Phil Barker, reflect a gaze that is 'searching and compassionate'; indeed Phil's abiding belief in the importance of empathic and deeply compassionate relationships is central to mental health and remains the kernel of the creative exploration in this chapter.

The chapter is solid, provocative, built up with layers of interesting and stimulating facts and ideas. At times, its creative and meandering nature demands close attention; however, the notion that psychiatry is losing its human relevance is strongly apparent in the ideas expressed. Phil speaks of the effects that breakdown of traditional forms of 'attachment or identity' have on society and just what the loss of 'our anchors' has meant in relation to mental health. He quotes Seligman, who says, 'In American society we now live in the age of the individual'. In becoming a consumer society, western society has its eyes on goods and services, rather than the people around them.

Strong warnings of the result of such disconnection are heralded by many. In the video *The Global Brain*, Peter Russell says 'We are more than just biological organisms bounded by skin. We are also unbounded, part of a greater wholeness, united with the rest of the universe. If we are to fulfil our role, no longer will we perceive ourselves as isolated individuals. We will need to change, in the most radical way, our attitudes toward ourselves, others and the planet as a whole'.

Phil recognises that 'we are all parts of the whole, all children of and connected to God'. How much is this a shared psychiatric practice of understanding? Reports from consumers about their mental health treatment and their therapeutic relationships, constantly suggest there is the use of medication, and medication alone. *Relationship* and its deepening development for a true 'I and Thou' relationship seems rare. Our 'psychiatry cannot afford to ignore or dismiss millennia of religious and philosophical thought about the very essence of human nature, reality and existence'. And so Phil Barker underlines the metaphysical vision of reality, accommodating the whole person.

There is a strong sense of acknowledgment, a deep humanity in Phil's perception of the person. He says: 'I have decided that I shall devote myself to joining with the people in my care; learning more from them about the business of being human; learning more about my own weaknesses; and through discovering their great resources and boundless assets, may come to realise some of my own'.

His grateful recognition is that 'in giving we receive' and that we too, most importantly, have the capacity to awaken the potential within the other as 'the other' awakens the potential within us.

In many respects, it seems like simple stuff! We should not be misled. It is the stepping stone to the building of community – *a community* that over time has been so dangerously eroded; and at the same time it is the development of a constancy of belief in the unwell and the anguished so that there may be some passage along the journey of recovery, the journey to finding self-value.

In speaking of the 'new physics' Phil gives a sense of what the evolving consciousness of man means, its impact on physical reality and our part in the creation of it. Phil has grappled with many important issues and ideas. I would like to quote Theodore Roszak whose attributed words echo the beliefs of Phil, the beliefs that would mean such profound change if comprehensively adopted for people with mental health problems:

> *'Responsible work is an embodiment of love, and love is the only discipline that will serve in shaping the personality, the only discipline that makes the mind whole and constant for a lifetime of effort. There hovers about a true vocation that paradox of all significant self-knowledge – our capacity to find ourselves by losing ourselves. We lose ourselves in our love of the task before us and, in that moment, we learn an identity that lives both within and beyond us'.*

As a mental health consumer advocate I think of the consumers I represent and I find myself reflecting deeply on who I am. I must face my responsibility in being a person with a mental illness. Am I to blame? Oh that I could detach myself from the ferocious claws of such a state. Where did things go wrong, why me, how this?

The empathy, compassion and care that is part of Phil Barker means much to a consumer advocate. To awaken the heart of deep care in the mental health worker is problematic. The system in Southern NSW, Australia, does not sufficiently encourage nurture, it does not recognise value in the 'heart to heart', nor work as an embodiment of love.

From my fellow consumers I hear over and over a deep longing for communication. The service should grow to value such communication and recognise how it uplifts the spirit of the person, confirming individuality and engendering self-acceptance and love.

REFERENCES

Jolley E 1993 Central mischief. Penguin, Harmondsworth
Russell P [video] The global brain.

Commentary

David Brandon

Like Phil Barker I came into psychiatric nursing (but never trained professionally) in the late 1960s and became fascinated, even hooked, on its many mysteries and paradoxes amid the horrific treatment of people – both patients and junior staff. It was like being in some crazy asylum army. My Dad had been a longstay mental patient, and later I followed him in becoming what is now fashionably called – not a lunatic – but a mental health survivor.

Phil is right to identify individualism and the 'creation' of stress, linked with the invention of self, as a major and recent problem. It is an immense spiritual problem which takes us away from any experience of unity towards an eternal fragmenting. I once experienced a famous Zen Master interviewing eighty people twice a day for a week and, as his attendant, saw no visible signs of any stress. Living on the edge of a coal-mining community I saw no stress, in the way we now understand it almost as a commodity, but a lot of heavy drinking and violence.

But Phil's reminiscences, like mine as I get speedily older, err on the romantic, and, as is usual with social scientists, tend to very considerably underestimate the influence of genetics (Pinker 1998). He is also dangerously attracted to the slushier, mystical and semi-numerate end of physics and biology. He needs purging with more hard-edged materials which are an astronomically long way from Capra, Zukav and Woodstock joint smoking (Hawking 1988, Dennett 1995, Dawkins 1997). A few pages of reading on copulating millipedes would do him the world of good and provide him with enough dancing energy to last a whole lifetime.

I can dance along with him when he proclaims how negative the interventions and understanding of our professional generation have been. Maslow was quite right. But professional people make considerable monies out of human despair, hardly ever out of their happiness. There is a mountain of money to be made in raising the achievement high jump bar for Homo Sapiens. Chinese doctors who you pay when you are well are the stuff of ancient folklore. It would be wonderful if true, but, like all those supposed Inuit (Eskimo to the non-politically-correct) words for snow, it is just a fantasy. There is payment when we believe we are ill – hence the cosmological proliferation of syndromes. I fully expect the imminent invention of 'Normal Syndrome' in the near future. I must tell you privately that I don't suffer from it at all and neither does Phil.

In the latter part of the piece Phil turns to tiresome moral exhortation – railing against the world. I am very familiar with this sermonising. As a Zen Buddhist monk, it is my stock in trade, but I am not so deluded to think that it works. I recognise a fellow John the Baptist syndrome sufferer. We have our own popular website. Religions, just like economists (the dismal science) have a vested interest in being gloomy. For the most part, I am on the side of Philip Larkin, whom once I knew at Hull University. His classic poem on death expresses the scepticism well.

This is a special way of being afraid
No trick dispels. Religion used to try,
That vast moth-eaten musical brocade
Created to pretend we never die…

(Larkin 1988).

I don't know whether I hate all that positivism – Cartesian dogmatism – more than New Age mushy peas. Do I really have to choose between Jeremiad philosophical rantings and crystal swinging and aromatherapy? They both stink. Our spiritual leanings have their own profound problems, wandering through forests of candy floss. They can become yet another form of object – taking on the shape of spiritual materialism. Wilkinson (1996) provides a strong antidote. He concentrates on commonalities rather than individualising. He comes up with some possible, even likely structural, ways of changing our society which don't involve sitting on a rock in a lotus posture for forty years.

So what does all this guff really amount to? Phil is right in seeing the so-called breakdowns as often forms of breakthrough. Lunatics not only have to take over the asylums but become our professional teachers. Grof & Grof (1991) are helpful in explaining (usually rather exotically) about spiritual crises. His techniques of breathing, rebirthing and beginning to understand different states of consciousness are constructive in taking us away from the autocracy of DSM-IV and the psychiatric megalomaniacs, in climbing the asylum wall.

This will pressure some of us to become Shamans – wounded healers. Our wounds can become a potent source of healing. Presently, the professions erect high barriers, especially in nursing, to those who know or have known depression and treatment, so-called psychosis (Walsh 1990). We desperately need a lot more of these sorts of students with their valuable knowledge of psychological impermanence.

We need more ordinary systems of understanding what is happening. It is more than forty years since Russell Barton, a really great psychiatrist, said we needed landladies much more than psychiatrists. The current resistance to the application of the principle of normalisation to mental health services does not bode well. Fear and dogmatism are firm bedfellows (Brandon 1991).

REFERENCES

Brandon D 1991 Innovation without Change? Macmillan, London

Dawkins R 1997 Climbing mount improbable. Penguin, Harmondsworth

Dennett D C 1995 Darwin's dangerous idea – evolution and the meanings of life. Penguin, Harmondsworth

Grof C, Grof S 1991 The stormy search for self – understanding and living with spiritual emergency. Mandala, London

Hawking S 1988 A brief history of time. Bantam, London

Larkin P 1988 Auhade. In: his Collected poems. Faber & Faber, London, pp 2–9

Pinker S 1998 How the mind works. Allen Lane, Harmondsworth

Walsh R 1990 The spirit of shamanism. Putnam & Sons, London

Wilkinson R 1996 Unhealthy societies – the afflictions of inequality. Routledge, London

Part 3
Reflecting on practice

Much academic literature appears to distance itself from practice, obfuscating through its arcane language and theorising, rather than clarifying the complex phenomena which we encounter in the 'real world' of practice. Although we are faced now with a burgeoning research and theoretical literature, in psychiatric and mental health nursing, the issues we study appear almost timeless. The changes, which sweep through practice, often appear bewildering in both their effects and momentum. Yet, once the dust of the change process has settled, much appears as before. Everything changes but most things remain the same.

One of the changes in contemporary practice has been the move towards considering the 'patient' as a 'consumer'. We often act as if this is a radical concept, or even a novel one. Our professional and academic literature is replete with references to advocacy and consumer-advocacy: the whole rag-bag of patient-empowerment. Almost twenty years ago, Annie Altschul presented a 'Winfred Raphael Lecture' entitled 'The consumer's voice: nursing implications'. In the lecture, Professor Altschul talked of 'patient advocacy [being] certainly the major growth area'. Altschul noted that although it appeared 'respectable to listen to researchers who go around asking patients for their views' it appeared less respectable 'to listen to patients directly … [especially] when they regale us with their experiences in person when we meet them'.

Altschul's struggle to grasp the nettle of consumerism, and to clarify the nature of some of the problems which might result from 'listening to patients', could be seen – with hindsight – as breaking new ground. What is clear is that, twenty years on, we continue to grapple with many of the same problems. How we listen to people who appear to be having experiences which are 'beyond our ken' – as in psychosis, is one such problem. How we support nurses – through supervision – when working with such people, or indeed in working closely with any group of patients, is another of the issues Altschul addressed all those years ago. These issues are problematic perhaps because they are so fundamental to the nursing task – working closely with people, trying to identify and respond to *their* needs. Such issues belong to the territory of ethics and philosophy, which, in the simplest possible sense, underpin this whole text. I have chosen these thorny areas of practice as the most appropriate way of concluding the book. These chapters represent areas of practice which have long exercised my conscience as well as my intellect: how exactly do I hear what people might *really* be saying, and how might I continue to doubt that I have all the answers to the problems which people bring to care?

REFERENCE

Altschul A 1982 The consumer's voice: nursing implications. In Denton P F (ed) *They speak for themselves: the Winfred Raphael Memorial Lectures – 1981–1990.* Royal College of Nursing, London

The nurse's psychotherapeutic role in caring for people in psychosis

10

INTRODUCTION

The manifestation of psychosis takes many forms, both organic and functional. Traditionally, however, the term has been used to exclude physical illness and neurosis and to refer to specific illnesses (sic) or symptoms where the patient's basic competence *as a person* is called into question (Davis 1987). The person who is defined as 'psychotic', in general, betrays a misapprehension or misinterpretation of the consensual reality. Although the term is often used to denote the severity of the illness, in some instances, psychosis may be less serious than other forms of psychiatric disorder. For the purpose of this paper, I shall emphasise its experiential nature, assuming that by psychosis we mean:

> *'the experience of transformation which results in a specific and dysfunctional way of relating to self and others and of interpreting the world'.*

The term psychosis is used, invariably, to designate a severe or 'major' psychiatric disorder. For more than twenty years, various writers have described the difficulties, both practical and theoretical, in using severity as the governing criterion of psychosis, or vice versa (e.g. Arieti 1974). Clearly, however, some forms of psychosis may be much less serious, from the point of view of the sufferer or society, than other (arguably more minor) forms of mental disorder. *Psychosis* invariably is equated with insanity, and incompetence – in a legal sense – suggesting the need for special control and supervision. When 'in' psychosis, the person undergoes, predominantly, a symbolic transformation and not only deals with the world in a defective way, but believes that there is nothing wrong in living in accordance with that symbolic transformation (Arieti 1980). This kind of definition lends itself, however, to justified criticism because it 'implies that we know what is reality and what is unreality. Many philosophers would promptly indicate to us how naïve we are in assuming that we have such knowledge' (Arieti 1980:59). However, a person who is depressed to a psychotic degree, undergoes such a severe emotional transformation that he believes that his feelings are appropriate to his life circumstances. Whereas the person with a 'neurotic' depression complains about his emotional distress, the person in a psychotic depression does not attempt to fight the distress, but lives with it: accepting this as no less than appropriate. This *acceptance* of a version of 'reality' which most people would attempt to deny or oppose, appears to be the key to distinguishing the experience of psychosis.

> *'acceptance* of a version of "reality" which most people would attempt to deny or oppose, appears to be the key to distinguishing the experience of psychosis'

Given my interest in the *experience* of psychosis, I shall not refer at any length to the various ways open to us for classification and categorisation of such experiences. However, given the importance of the classification of the psychoses for modern psychiatry – not least the method for distinguishing the psychoses from the neuroses – I offer a brief synopsis of the history of classification and its relevance for the nursing approach to the person in psychosis.

THE ORDER OF MADNESS

Although all forms of classification have their drawbacks, any system that allows us to consider how apparently disparate symptoms or patterns of behaviour might be related, clearly is of some value. Over the past one hundred years, various ways of grouping, thematically, the phenomena of psychosis have been proffered. Despite the disagreements and irreconcilable differences which these various schema have stimulated, at least a common ground has been established, from which more meaningful disagreements have emerged.

Kraepelin (1896) first grouped a number of differing mental conditions under the heading of *dementia praecox* in the 1890s, this provisional classification being developed further by Bleuler, who emphasised primary symptoms and the splitting process (Bleuler 1959; see also McGhie 1969, Stone 1980). Given his emphasis of the splitting which occurred (psychically) within the individual, Bleuler renamed this group of conditions, *schizophrenia* (literally, *split or cut mind*).

NATURE AND NURTURE

Increasingly, it is asserted that the most common forms of psychosis – schizophrenia and manic depression – are rooted in some biological pathology. However, the hypothetical causes of schizophrenia, for example, range from genetic influence (McGuffin et al 1994), through trauma at the intra-uterine stage of development (Eagles 1992), to various brain abnormalities (Gournay 1995). Developments in neuroscientific technology – such as positron emission tomography (PET) – have suggested the possibility of monitoring, biologically, psychotic phenomena – such as auditory hallucinations (Toufexis 1995). These claims are, however, beset by controversy. Contemporary research is more focused in view of the great strides made in developing the technology of exploration. However, the claims made today are remarkably similar to the claims that have been made by way of explaining psychosis for the past one hundred years. Various 'environmentalist' researchers and theorists have argued that many of the biological–genetic claims are confounded by other variables. Alterations in the environment (such as stress or the quality of relationships) can have major affects on body chemistry. Indeed, in his original polemical work, Szasz argued that learning a foreign language was sufficient to alter the chemistry of the brain (Szasz 1961). More recently, Deutsch's (1983) study of separation from parents suggested how disturbance of a key relationship might hold possibilities for triggering psychosis in some children.

Although various propositions about the putative causation of psychosis have been made from a stress–diathesis perspective – 'high expressed emotion' (Leff and Vaughn 1985) being the most significant contemporary theory – these appear to involve some kind of revisiting of Freud (1940) and, more recently, Laing & Esterson (1964). Freud did not deny the possibility of a physical basis for mental illness and even envisioned basis psychological structures that would 'develop according to an innate timetable but would require specific environmental conditions to unfold (Eigen 1993)'. Winnicott (1974) later referred to these conditions as 'maturational processes and the facilitating environment'. Indeed, Freud was torn between an 'innatist' and an 'environmentalist' position throughout his life. Initially, he believed that actual sexual trauma in childhood was involved in causing neurosis. Later, he emphasised the role of an innately programmed fantasy life, but never ceased to write about actual trauma. Although it has been argued repeatedly that Freud 'suppressed' his knowledge of the importance of actual trauma (e.g. Masson 1985), the complex nature of his theory allows for the influence of both actual trauma and fantasy – environmental *and* innate factors. Laing's view of the role of power in relationships, especially within families, represented what might be seen as an extreme environmentalist position when he spoke of the politics of the family, describing deeply rooted imbalances in power relationships that could result in madness (Laing 1970). However, Laing may have been anticipating the views of numerous environmentalist writers who also argued that the prevalence of madness among the poor and powerless is a function of political disadvantage, on a general political level as well as within interpersonal relationships.

More recently, Peplau has argued that much of the contemporary research confuses the study of the brain with the study of the mind. Although it may be possible to monitor the *process* involved in 'hearing voices', the *content* of voices which say, for example, 'don't act stupid', in Peplau's view, must surely 'have their origin not in brain cells but in words used by persons in the patient's interpersonal milieu' (Peplau 1995). This echoes Freud's final conclusion that no amount of physical or biological knowledge could replace the study of experience for its own sake: 'experiential knowledge would always be necessary' (Eigen 1993, Freud 1940: 157–159).

Peplau's assertion is central to the thesis of this paper, and acknowledges both the importance of the interpersonal relationship and powerlessness in, at least, maintaining the state of psychosis. Although nurses' interventions include drug administration and the support of other forms of physical investigation and treatment, their core role involves addressing the everyday, often changing story of the patient's life. In the case of the person in psychosis this involves addressing the manner in which the patient enacts his[1] life story in accordance with the symbolic transformation which he has undergone. It seems axiomatic that the nurse's interest is not in the possible causes of the psychotic state (which is the province of psychiatric medicine), but is focused on the patient's understanding and interpretation of everyday experience – including psychotic phenomena – and the *meanings* developed as a consequence of those shared reflections. The sharing of such reflections, in the form of some kind of 'everyday psychotherapy', lies at the very heart of the nurse's psychotherapeutic role.

INTERPERSONAL RELATIONS THEORY

The contemporary psychotherapeutic role of the nurse has a long pedigree, originating in Peplau's development of a theory of interpersonal relations for nursing practice in the early 1950s (Peplau 1952). Peplau's work stimulated interest in the development of formal one-to-one working, theory-based appraisals of the ward milieu (Peplau 1989) and the dynamics of group work (Lego 1996) and more general functions within nurse–patient interactions (Altschul 1972). The discrete processes involved in individual working with psychotic patients were first described by Peplau (1952) and Schwartz & Shockley (1956) over forty years ago. These were developed further by Travelbee in the late 1960s, when she described the interpersonal style required of the nurse when relating to patients in, for example, a delusional state. Travelbee appears to have been one of the first to suggest the method by which nurses might use Socratic inquiry to 'create doubt in the patient's mind' concerning, for example, delusional beliefs (Travelbee 1969:201). This interpersonal method was developed most famously by Peplau, who has outlined the kind of questions which might be used to maintain the distinction between the nurse's and the patient's experience, and to promote the patient's examination of his 'here-and-now' experience. Various other authors have described how the nurse's psychotherapeutic *function* in psychosis can range from providing support through clear, unambiguous communication (Fleming 1988), to enabling 'the curative process of self-disclosure' (Lego 1996:37). Nurses have now begun to extend this psychotherapeutic work to community settings, especially to work with families, emphasising, in particular, the provision of information about psychotic illness and helping the patient and family develop coping mechanisms for dealing with discrete positive symptoms – such as auditory hallucinations or delusions (Baguely 1995).

ORDINARY PSYCHOTHERAPY – THE ARRAN RELATIONSHIPS MODEL

Much of nursing practice takes place within ordinary settings – whether in hospital wards, in day care centres or in people's own homes. Such settings are characterised by a flow of events, which are part of the patient's 'lived experience' (Parse 1995) and from which the patient derives his sense of personal meaning. Such settings may easily be distinguished from more formal 'therapy' settings. In more formal therapeutic interaction, the patient is removed from the everyday living context to allow exposure to a time-limited, highly structured and, often, carefully controlled interaction with the psychotherapist, who may be a nurse, psychiatrist, psychologist or any other member of the mental health team.

At the University of Newcastle, my colleagues and I have developed a model for the exploration of the interpersonal relations context of the patient's everyday 'lived experience'. This model was designed to promote the everyday psychotherapeutic function of nurses, as an adjunct to more formal psychotherapy, conducted by clinical nurse specialists.

The *Arran Relationships Model* was first developed within an intensive rehabilitation unit for people described as suffering from treatment-resistant psychosis. The model was developed within a cooperative inquiry research paradigm (Heron 1996) over a one-year period, during which the participating nurses synthesised common themes drawn from an analysis of their individual casework (Barker et al 1997).

The model (Figure 10.1) assumes that the 'person' is characterised by several core concepts, including: autonomy, self concept, self esteem and values. These develop as a function of personal and interpersonal experience, and involve a continuous – and reflexive – relationship with discrete aspects of his 'lived experience'. Within the context of this model, five dimensions of the lived experience have been identified as relevant to the person in psychosis. These are:

- the relationship with *self*, including the person's view of himself, personal strengths or assets, and presentation of self in everyday life
- the relationship with *others*, including the perception of others, patterns of interaction, formal relationships and membership of groups
- the relationship with the *world*, including role in society, dreams and ideals
- the relationship with *health*, including exercise, diet drug use
- the relationship with *illness*, including risk of self harm, medication and discrete manifestations of mental illness.

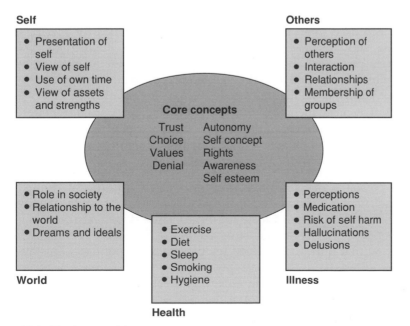

Figure 10.1 The Arran model.

The emergent model acknowledged that the 'proper focus of nursing' (Barker et al 1995) was:

'the diagnosis and treatment of human responses *to actual or potential health problems' (American Nurses Association 1980:9 emphasis added).*

The nurse is concerned, in effect, more with *how* the patient relates to any phenomenon embraced by the five dimensions of experience, than with the phenomenon itself.

The model assumes that the patient's exercise of autonomy, choice, trust, etc. is influenced, at least in part, by his relationship with each of these five dimensions of lived experience which influence one another and, in turn, are influenced by the exercise of the core concepts. Meanings, which the person develops about himself and his life, are an holistic function of this complex of inter-relationships.

PREPARING THE NURSE FOR PRACTICE

To help the patient grow and develop – on a human level – the nurse needs to help the person extend his awareness of the personal meanings he has attributed to specific experiences and how these relate to his 'whole lived experience' within consensual reality. The long-term nature of such an exploration of the patient's experience is well documented within the nursing literature (*cf.* Peplau 1996), as are the necessary qualifications to offer such psychotherapeutic support (*cf.* Lego 1996). In the UK, nurses receive only limited preparation for psychotherapeutic work, as part of the basic education. Typically, the practice of psychotherapy in nursing is dependent on specialist post-registration training. To help nurses with limited experience of psychotherapeutic nursing use the Socratic method of the ARM, a focused interviewing technique was developed for specific use in working with the psychotic patient (Barker 1997). To help promote the necessary emotional and cognitive 'distance' from the psychotic phenomenon, nurses are trained, initially, to interview the patient (within a role play) without knowing the nature of the problem. A 'fear of being poisoned', or reports of 'hearing the voice of a dead person or God', are simply described as 'X'. Within the context of the therapeutic interview, the nurse is taught to explore any or all of the following eight dimensions of personal experience:

1. 'So when did you first notice X?' (Origins in time): This question invites the person to set his present experience in a historical context. The person who is 'hearing pejorative voices' today, which are causing distress, is offered an opportunity to retrace his steps, recalling the first experience of this phenomenon; recalling what was happening in his life around that time, that seemed relevant to the experience. This question is predicated on the assumption that the experience is inherently meaningful – that 'hearing voices' or 'feeling paranoid' possess some human meaning for the individual.
2. 'How did 'X' affect you at first?' (History of problem function): The nurse is interested primarily in 'how' the problem works: what does it

do, and not do, in terms of disturbing the person or disrupting the person's life? This question offers the person an opportunity to describe the function of the problem, recalling how it affected the person at first, which may be different from how things are now.

3. 'And how did you feel about that?' (Past emotional context): Our experience is invariably described in emotional language – how we process our experience at the most abstract level. By inviting the person to recall how he felt when he first experienced the problem, the nurse allows the person to begin to map the emotional canvas of his experience. What kind of feelings did he have *then* about the problem, which might be different from the feelings he has now?

4. 'In what way has that changed over time?' (Developmental history of problem): The nurse now summarises the story so far. 'When you first experienced X (this) and (that) were happening and you felt (this way and that) about things. That was all (so long) ago.' The nurse now invites the person to describe what has changed and what has remained the same since then.

5. 'How does "X" affect your relations with others?' (Relationship history): The experience of serious distress invariably shows itself by disrupting relationships. People in psychosis may find it difficult to make or sustain relationships, or experience the immediate fracturing of established relationships when problems of a psychotic nature become manifest. How does the person experience such relationship disturbance? What does the person think has happened to his relationships that might be traced to the original problem?

6. 'And how do you feel about that?' (Current emotional context): It is always important to gain an appreciation of how the person's feelings have changed over time. It is vital, however, to establish how the person feels now, comparing and contrasting those feelings with earlier feelings. The feelings the person might have *now*, might not simply focus on the problem, but might include feelings about other people's attitudes towards the problem, or lack of support they get in dealing with the problems.

7. 'And what does that mean for you?' (Holistic content): The nurse now summarises again, the practical, relationship and emotional developments which have occurred in relation to the 'problem', and invites the person to interpret the core meaning. The person might suggest that this 'means' that they are being 'punished by God' or 'being let down by their family,' or are 'a bad person', or have 'been chosen'.

8. 'And what does that say about you as a person?' (Holistic context): The nurse is primarily interested in 'who is the person who is the patient?' (Barker 1997). This final question aims to establish what kind of *personal* meaning is attached to these experiences, all of which are associated with the original experience of 'problem X'.

A CLINICAL EXAMPLE

A thirty-year-old man, who had been hospitalised frequently over a ten-year period is detained under the Mental Health Act in a 'special care' ward for patients requiring close supervision and intensive rehabilitation. He is hostile towards staff, disruptive of other patients' activities, and has poor personal hygiene. Frequently, he presents with paranoid or grandiose delusions, describing either how the staff are conspiring against him or how he is supremely intelligent and the descendant of an ancient English king and the rightful leader of his people.

The ARM assessment found that he was defensive when discussing his relationship to *Self*, and appeared to hold grandiose ideas when discussing his relationship with *Others* and his *World*. In an interview focused on his interest in playing the guitar he described how he intended to 'get a band together', hire a local football stadium and 'play some gigs for my fans'. Increasingly, nurses employ cognitive therapy methods, to 'challenge' the evidence supporting 'delusional' ideas in psychosis. This approach is a development of Travelbee's original Socratic method (Travelbee 1969). Rather than explore the 'evidence' of the quality of his guitar-playing, far less his 'fans', in this case the nurse addressed the meanings he attached to this (delusional) story. A different picture emerged of a young man, disabled early in life by schizophrenia, who was 'forgotten' – as a result – by his friends and family and who felt a great need for respect. He believed that by playing 'to a stadium full of fans' they would 'look up to me!'. What this meant for him, as a person, was that: 'I will be important, everyone needs to feel important!'.

This exploration suggested that the patient's needs were focused on self esteem and self concept. Viewed from this perspective, his intrusive and hostile behaviour could be read as inherently meaningful – in part, acting out his disappointment – but also in creating negative relationships which would confirm his low sense of self.

THE FUTURE OF THE PSYCHOTHERAPEUTIC ROLE OF THE NURSE

A growing body of literature suggests the possible diversity of psychotherapeutic roles and functions which might be fulfilled by nurses providing that they receive appropriate training and clinical supervision (Beeber 1994, Winship 1997). The model of everyday psychotherapy suggested here is only one of the many forms of psychotherapeutic nursing which might be appropriate for people in psychosis. Indeed, it may prove especially appropriate for the patients who are enduringly psychotic, and who tend to be viewed, from a wholly pathological perspective, often depicted as little more than the pathology attributed to them. In this regard, Peplau has recently issued a call to 'personalise' the nursing of patients with a diagnosis of schizophrenia. She noted the popularity and primacy of 'advocacy for patients, consideration of their needs and interests as persons having dignity and worth'. In keeping with such claims, she argued that such an attitude might help nurses:

'recognise such (psychotic) behaviours as problem-solving actions emblematic of difficulties arising within interpersonal relationships. Their highly personal meaning can be retrieved and understood by that patient as an outcome of

psychotherapeutically-oriented sessions within the nurse-patient relationship. Such a nursing model is different from yet complementary to the prevailing biomedical-psychiatric model of treatment' (Peplau 1995:3 emphasis added).

The method suggested in this chapter involves extending the traditional supportive psychotherapy approach to allow greater attention to be paid to the *personal* and inter*personal* experience of psychosis. By teaching nurses how to explore problems in the abstract (as 'problem X' rather than as 'hallucinations' or 'delusions') the nurse may acquire a helpful curiosity about the person's experience. By their very nature, psychotic experiences can be distracting – leading the nurse off into a fantastic universe, where she loses the original point of the inquiry. The person needs to explore his experience constructively. The format we are presently developing in Newcastle helps nurses to provide a structure for the exploration of psychotic experience which both validates the person's experience, but also offers the person an opportunity to learn more about the experience. Through that validatory learning, the person may come to 'know' something fresh by way of experience. That 'knowledge' may help the person understand the human significance of his voices or delusional beliefs. By validating the inherent meaningfulness of the person's experience of dysfunction, nurses may begin to address their patients primarily as *persons*.

NOTE

This chapter is based on a paper presented to the Psichosis Conference, Palencia, Spain, 18 April 1997.

1. For convenience patients are referred to in the male gender throughout.

REFERENCES

Altschul A T 1972 Patient–nurse interaction: a study of interactive patterns on acute psychiatric wards. Churchill Livingtone, Edinburgh

American Nurses Association 1980 Nursing: a social policy statement. ANA, Washington, DC

Arieti S 1974 Interpretation of schizophrenia. Basic Books, New York

Arieti S 1980 The manifest symptomatology of depression in adults. Ch 3 in: Arieti S, Bemporad J Severe and mild depression: the psychotherapeutic approach. Tavistock, London

Baguely I 1995 Evaluation of the Tameside Nursing Development Unit for psychosocial interventions. In: Brooker C, White E (eds) Community psychiatric nursing: a research perspective, Vol 3. Chapman and Hall, London

Barker P 1997 The assessment of the experience of psychosis: tales from the underworld. Ch 8 in: Barker P J Assessment in psychiatric and mental health nursing. Stanley Thornes, Cheltenham

Barker P, Reynolds W 1996 Rediscovering the proper focus of nursing – a critique of Gournay's position on nursing theory and models. Journal of Psychiatric and Mental Health Nursing 3(1): 76–80

Barker P, Davison M, Turner J 1997 The development of a heuristic model for the nursing assessment of people in psychosis: a co-operative inquiry approach. Unpublished manuscript

Barker P, Reynolds W, Ward T 1995 The proper focus of nursing: a critique of the caring ideology. International Journal of Nursing Studies 32(4): 386–397

Beeber L 1994 The one-to-one relationship in psychiatric nursing: the next generation. In: Anderson C A (ed) Psychiatric nursing 1946–94: a report on the state of the art. Mosby-Year Book, St Louis

Bleuler E 1959 Dementia praecox or the group of schizophrenias (trans J. Zinkin). International Universities Press, New York. First published 1911

Davis D R 1987 Psychosis. In: Gregory R L (ed) Oxford companion to the mind. Oxford University Press, Oxford

Deutsch S 1983 Early parental separation in children at risk for schizophrenia. Unpublished doctoral thesis, Yeshiva University

Eagles J 1992 Are polio viruses a cause of schizophrenia? British Journal of Psychiatry 158: 834–835

Eigen M 1993 The psychotic core. Aronson, Northvale, NJ

Fleming L 1988 Thought disorders: disruptions in the communication process. Ch 10 in: Krebs M J S, Larson K H (eds) Applied psychiatric-mental health nursing standards in clinical practice. Wiley, New York

Freud S 1940 An outline of psycho-analysis. Standard Edition 23:141–207

Gournay K 1995 New facts on schizophrenia. Nursing Times 91(25): 32–33

Heron J 1996 Co-operative inquiry: research into the human condition. Sage, London

Kraepelin E 1896 Psychiatrie: Ein Lehrbuch für Studierende und Ärzte. Barth, Leipzig

Laing R D 1970 Knots. Tavistock, London

Laing R D, Esterson A A 1964 Sanity, madness and the family. Penguin, Harmondsworth

Leff J, Vaughn C 1985 Expressed emotion in families: its significance for mental illness. Guilford Press, New York

Lego S 1996 Psychodynamic individual psychotherapy. Ch 3 in: Lego S (ed) Psychiatric nursing: a comprehensive reference, 2nd edn. Lippincott, Philadelphia

Masson J M 1985 The assault on truth: Freud's suppression of the seduction theory. Penguin, Harmondsworth

McGhie A 1969 Pathology of attention. Penguin, Harmondsworth

McGuffin P, Owen M, O'Donovan M 1994 Psychiatric genetics. Gaskell, London

Parse R R 1995 Illuminations: the human becoming theory in practice and research. National League for Nursing, New York

Peplau H E 1952 Interpersonal relationships in nursing. Putnam, New York

Peplau H E 1989 Thought disorder in schizophrenia: corrective influence of nursing behavior on language of patients. In: O'Toole A, Welt S (eds) Interpersonal theory in nursing practice: selected works of Hildegard E Peplau. Springer, New York

Peplau H E 1995 Another look at schizophrenia from a nursing standpoint. In Anderson CA (ed) Psychiatric nursing 1974–1994: a report on the state of the art. Mosby Year Book, St Louis

Peplau H E 1996 The client diagnosed as schizophrenic. Ch 34 in: Lego S op. cit.

Schwartz M S, Shockley E L 1956 The nurse and the mental patient: a study in interpersonal relations. Russell Sage Foundation, New York

Stone M 1980 The borderline syndromes. McGraw-Hill, New York

Szasz T S 1961 The myth of mental illness. Harper and Row, New York

Toufexis A 1995 Brainwork; pictures shed light on the mystery of schizophrenia. Time 186(21): 101

Travelbee J 1969 Intervention in psychiatric nursing: process in the one-to-one relationship. F A Davis, Philadelphia

Winnicott D W 1974 The maturational processes and the facilitating environment. International Universities Press, New York

Winship G 1997 Establishing the role of the nurse psychotherapist in the United Kingdom. Perspectives in Psychiatric Care 33(1):25–30

Commentary

Professor Gloria Novel

This excellent chapter causes me to think about a number of things, but first I should like to thank Phil Barker for giving me the chance to put down on paper what is so often in my mind, but which I dare not say: the question, 'Is what I think normal?'.

Phil Barker says in his introduction that psychosis can be defined as 'The experience of transformation which results in a specific and dysfunctional way of relating to self and others and of interpreting the world'. In fact, when we talk about 'experience', we are really placing the illness in its correct setting, because it is precisely this component of experience that makes the individual 'act' in a way incomprehensible to society. And when this happens, the subject is marginalised for being 'incomprehensible', for not following the social norms of living together and/or in connivance.

Of course there are many types of patients diagnosed as psychotic. However, I am not going to mention here those (few) who live peacefully with their illness, or those (also few) who remain stable because they live in an accepting family environment and accept the need for medication to neutralise the voices and the frequently aggressive instincts. I am thinking, rather, of those who live alone and confused. Those whose families find it hard to accept and look after them. Those who wander the streets begging because their chronic state prevents them from living in our world in any other way. Those who are serving sentences in a psychiatric prison. What kind of care can we provide to those people? Are we able to 'understand' their experience at a deep level? Or rather do we treat them as demented, low down on the social scale, marginalised, unrecoverable? Are we able to care for the person or do we treat her/his incurable illness in an irremediably passive way? A colleague who works in a prison told me the other day that a warder was complaining because his sick inmate had insulted him. He took this as something personal and unjustifiable. The psychiatrist answered him with that phrase so typical of counselling: 'OK … so what?' Thank goodness! Sometimes we all rush in like a bull to a red rag.

Furthermore, I sometimes wonder: Is there really such a thing as absolute reality? What does sane really mean? I recall the book *The Stormy Search for Self* (Grof & Grof 1990), which introduces the idea of 'spiritual emergence' to describe a phenomenon that any psychiatrist would brand as psychosis. This book mentions mystical-type experiences, voices, physical and emotional pain caused by the awakening of the Kundalini, and in no case catalogues it as problems of mental or physical health. Likewise, in everyday situations, I see aggressiveness, sometimes contained, sometimes not (car drivers, especially men, coming to blows in the middle of the street for the most trivial incident), the behaviour of supposedly sane persons who show a clearly paranoid streak (remember that the characteristics of a good executive as measured by certain tests indicate a high sensorial level, albeit with a low score when it comes to taking action), absolutely excessive competitiveness, which means that for some, *things* are more important than *people* (for example this often translates into grave and complicated problems of relating to family members or workmates) and thus the capacity continually to hurt the other – to assault – which cannot be compared to the behaviour of a psychotic patient. I ask myself: is this normal? If we define psychosis as the incapacity to be in reality, then do these kind of people (who could sometimes be ourselves ...) live in reality? Or, put another way, in what kind of reality do they/we live? Because reality as an isolated entity does not exist, but is made up of all those signifiers and signifieds that we attribute to it in any given society. Perhaps then, *the question is not so much how we live, how we experience our reality, but how we express it.* The psychotic manifests him/herself the way s/he feels, with no control, not caring less about whether the result is pleasing or not. The non-psychotic expresses this with care, in line with social rules, in a controlled way. This does not necessarily mean, however, that the feeling of one is more adequate than that of the other. Nor is the thought necessarily different. Anyone experiencing a spiritual emergence who realises the consequences of showing it, will not mention it to anyone apart from those who understand. Anyone who competes excessively believes deep down that s/he is a god in his/her own field; but they make very sure not to show it without control, in a clear way. The aggressive person only hits in certain circumstances and, if possible, hits the weakest one, never the stronger, and in certain circumstances can put off the blow until they find the person who will do best (the wife, the children, the elderly: someone suitably weak) ... In any case, it is only a question of control, of manifesting things at the appropriate time and with the appropriate people, in order to be part of so-called 'normality'. But people's internal experience does not always have healthy qualities.

Fortunately, not everyone keeps themselves in this 'normality'. Some do not interpret the world as a hostile place. Some act in such a way as to spread harmony around them. Some people think that, all in all, people are more important than things. Some have a philosophy of life that includes the universe and those who live in it. Some master the demons inside them and let the best of themselves shine through. The interesting thing about this matter is that there are two sides of the same coin. And those of us involved in care can help the best part of ourselves and of the other come to the surface.

Commenting on the Arran model of relationships, Phil Barker says 'I recognised that the main role of nursing ... consisted of diagnosing and treating human *responses* to real or potential health problems'. And in the section: 'The nurse's preparation to carry out her practice', Barker suggests a means of action that gives an answer to precisely that, helping the person to understand, to find meaning in their experience. This is a type of therapeutic intervention that I at the time called 'of instrumental or material support' (Novel 1997, 1998). One can observe its therapeutic effects when the patient is capable of saying 'Listen, I'm going to come along because I think I'm not well. I thought I was Jesus Christ again'. This means that we are able to help her/him to live with it, with her/his demons, like other mortals. It means that we have been able to care for the person in a holistic way, meaning when *the important thing in nursing care is the person (the patient) more than the thing (the illness)*: a great change and a great challenge.

REFERENCES

Novel G 1997 Psychosocial nursing and mental health, 2nd edn. Masson-Salvat, Barcelona

Novel G 1998 Psychosocial intervention in nursing: a structural model for holistic care. In: Baldwin S (ed) Needs assessment and community care: clinical practice and policy making. Butterworth-Heinemann, Oxford, Ch 11, p 140

Grof C, Grof S 1995 La tormentosa búsqueda del ser: una guía para el crecimiento personal a través de la emergencia espiritual. Los Libros de la Liebre de Marzo, Barcelona [Spanish translation of The Stormy Search for Self]

An overview of clinical supervision

INTRODUCTION

The concept of clinical supervision is now well accepted within nursing. There remains some doubt, however – which in some quarters may be considerable – as to what is or is not 'supervision'. More importantly, there exists much doubt as to how supervision might or should operate within different nursing settings. These concerns, in my view, are wholly appropriate at this stage of our professional development.

Here, I shall attempt to sketch the background to the development of the concept of supervision in clinical nursing practice, outlining something of its origins and saying something about the models of implementation distilled to date. I shall also say something about 'how' supervision might operate at the *human* level: what might it mean for supervisor as well as supervisee. I shall end by expressing some reservations – 'what are the limitations of the concept, and how might the problem-solving nature of supervision become a problem in its own right?'.

TOWARD A DEFINITION

Several definitions of supervision exist but all share, of necessity, an emphasis on the *meeting together of at least two people with a declared interest in examining aspects of the work of at least one of them* (see Wright 1989). This definition, which is the most *liberal* of all the definitions, is the starting point for my guided tour. This definition of supervision is not specific to nursing, but has proven meaningful across the whole range of professional and technical disciplines. It is the definition which marks the working relationship between the master craftsman (sic) and the apprentice, the business guru and his acolyte, the consultant physician and the registrar. The uses to which this relationship may be put are many and various. It may be an *educational* endeavour, aimed at promoting learning; or it may be a means of *maintaining clinical standards*; or it may be aimed at *identifying the processes that might assure good practice*. The applications of this supervisory relationship are potentially limitless. At present we can enumerate a number of ways in which it is used. This should not be confused with the *potential* of supervision, which is as wide as we might wish to make it.

I shall assume that this simple definition will prove acceptable to this audience. Before moving forward I aim to offer one example of the value of supervision which is often overlooked and which is in-built to the examples of the master–pupil relationship, which can be developed to suit our needs in a changing health care environment.

Many nurse practitioners have traditionally assumed that, on qualifying, their education is complete and that they have reached the end-point of their professional development. The downside to this assumption is that having self-actualised – professionally speaking – it is no longer appropriate for them to seek advice or counsel. They reach a point of professional 'aloneness' which – speaking as a professor who remains a practising nurse – I find frightening. The value of supervision – which I still appreciate as a practitioner – is that one is never alone, or at least not for long. We shall return to that point shortly, when we address the practicalities of supervision in practice.

ORIGINS OF SUPERVISION

Clinical supervision is a purposeful activity – people meet together for a specific purpose. It focuses on thinking or reflecting – or even recalling reflections from outwith the supervision sessions – and then talking about these thoughts and reflections. Supervision begins and ends, therefore, with a relationship (Barker 1992). Much of what I have to say here is about relationships: how they develop, what are their functions and what might be their outcomes. And of course, within the supervisory *relationship* we find the origins of clinical supervision as we understand it today.

'Supervision begins and ends... with a relationship'

Clinical supervision – both in terms of its principles and process – draws from the relationship between the analyst and the anlysand in traditional psychoanalysis. Those psychotherapists who intend to become psycho-analysts are required to undergo a similar analysis process to that of the patients whom they hope to analyse. Although this 'training analysis' is fundamentally an experience of therapy for the prospective psychoanalyst, within this experience lies a key ingredient of all forms of clinical super-vision. By *submitting* themselves to exploration and examination of their work – which will in many instances involve their *human* relationship with the patient and/or family – the nurse gains some appreciation of what it may be like to be the patient or family. The supervisee's direct experience of having decisions, reasonings and actions 'opened up' by the supervisor, may help her[1] appreciate (directly) what such experiences might mean for the person who is the patient. Such experiences may help the supervisee toward a different appreciation of both the inherent threats and potential rewards of the nurse–patient relationship. As Hawkins & Shoet (1992) observed, such an experience will help caring agents to 'take care of them-selves', staying open to the possibilities of continuous learning, if not ongo-ing self-development. And, at a more fundamental and practical level, as Burnard (1989) has observed, by exposing themselves to 'active listening and the experience of empathy' within the supervisory relationship, nurses may find it easier to enact similar therapeutic exchanges with their patients.

These short notes on history make clear that I recognise the origins of clinical supervision to be in psychotherapy and counselling. Readers might be forgiven for thinking that 'I would say that', as a psychotherapist and counsellor myself. I hope that my acknowledgement of these historical roots betrays honesty, rather than territoriality. However, the origins of the psychotherapeutic relationship extend much further back than psycho-analysis. Counselling and therapy are part of that broad church of activity which we once called pastoral care, and which was embedded within the supervision of the religious flock by its pastor, or shepherd. And shepherding may be a useful metaphor, since the last thing the shepherd wants to do is to scare his sheep. I recognise that one of the issues which concerns many nurses when the psychotherapeutic and counselling roots of supervision are teased out, is a quite reasonable concern that they do not want to be 'therapised'. As I proceed, I hope to clarify my acknowledgement of those concerns and, more importantly, my recognition that therapy of the nurses is, by no stretch of the imagination, necessary.

THE ASSUMED FUNCTION OF SUPERVISION

If we assume that we know what supervision is, and where it came from, what is its *function*? What is it intended to achieve? Other disciplines have used supervision for many years as a means of clarifying the nature of their work and of maintaining some standards of practice. Social work, in particular, has emphasised in its core training, the need for a 'life long tutorial' (Westheimer 1977), although that ambition has often proved both unpopular and impractical. An example closer to hand is midwifery, which has enshrined a longstanding tradition of supervision as a statutory mechanism in its code of practice, which provides a useful definition of the *function* of the supervisor, who acts:

> 'as a supportive colleague, counsellor and adviser ... to promote a positive working relationship which is conducive to maintaining and improving standards of practice and care' (UKCC 1991).

This relationship acts as 'an effective communication mechanism' within which problems may be shared and resolution sought at the earliest oppor-tunity.

Three main functions have been identified within supervision, which I shall discuss individually and shall relate, later, to different models of supervision in practice.

1. Supervision may fulfil a *formative* function within which the supervisee's skills and understanding are developed. This is essentially an educational function and is perhaps most often described as part of the teacher–pupil relationship. The supervisee reflects on and explores – both analytically and creatively – her work with a particular patient, and is supported throughout by another more experienced practitioner. A wide range of benefits might be gained from such a formative relationship: increased awareness of the patient's needs; enhanced awareness of the nurse's own skills, attitudes, prejudices or weaknesses, whether technical or psychological; and awareness of alternative means of addressing the patient's needs. The nurse may also acquire an awareness of her role relationship with other members of the interdisciplinary team, and how that might be further developed.

2. Supervision may also fulfil a *restorative* function, when the supervisor focuses on the emotional needs of the supervisee. Nursing across all fields carries a range of emotional demands. The most common demand involves the way in which nurses are drawn into an appreciation of the nature of the patient's distress, whether this be physical or psychic pain, or the experience of loss – including the prospect of death. The intimate nature of nursing brings nurses closer to these human experiences than do many other health care disciplines. That closeness can be rewarding but it can also present challenges, which require careful exploration, if only to save nurses from themselves.

Nurses working in the emotional hothouse of 'caring' face two common problems. Firstly they may get so close to their patients that they cannot distinguish their feelings from those of the patient. Such over-identification can lead to reduced proficiency and efficiency: the nurse may become so 'distressed' by the patient's distress that she is no longer able to provide the support needed by the patient. The second problem may be an extension of the first. When nurses can no longer face the distress of their patients or the distress evoked within them of working with people in great distress, they may feel the need to turn away, or develop blocking mechanisms to shield themselves, psychologically, from the patient and their distress. At its most pronounced, this phenomenon is called 'burn out', when care staff become blunted to their patients' distress, and no longer appear to have the capability to *care* (Maslach & Jackson 1982).

'When nurses can no longer face the distress of their patients or the distress evoked within them of working with people in great distress, they may feel the need to turn away, or develop blocking mechanisms to shield themselves'

The *restorative* function of supervision focuses on the emotional needs of the individual nurse. How does caring for people affect the nurse? How does the nurse feel about the patient who is abusive, or who appears to be harming himself? How does she feel about the family who visits the child who is seriously ill or may be dying? The emotional impact of nurses' closeness to either difficult people, or demanding situations, results in truly unique experiences for individual nurses. The supervisor's function is to help the nurse restore some emotional balance, thereby allowing her to continue to face such challenges efficiently and effectively.

3. The third function of supervision is *normative*: helping to maintain the highest possible standards considered desirable within the discipline or service. I have alluded already to some of the possible weaknesses or prejudice, which we all possess to varying degrees. When the supervisor exercises the normative function, he helps even the most experienced nurse to become more aware of her weaknesses, blind spots and vulnerabilities. For most of us, this is the most challenging dimension of supervision. Only the vain and misguided use the mirror as a means of self-worship. My mirror tells me each day that I am getting older and greyer. I am not unduly concerned about these facts. They are, if you like, messages from reality. We all need another kind of mirror to bring us other kinds of messages from

reality. These will help us to see through the blind spots, or perhaps even recognise how our practice is sagging or growing weak, where once it was robust and dynamic. Although it is commonly asserted that the normative function of supervision is painful, and to be avoided, this need not be the case. As we shall see, it all depends on how this mirroring is conducted, and on the person who helps us to see ourselves stripped of our pretensions and make-up.

This summary suggests that supervision might provide an opportunity for us to *learn* something through the formative process; to be *supported* through the restorative process; and be *managed* through the normative process. Although I have teased these out as three discrete functions, clearly they are linked and, within the supervisory context, may need to blend in with one another.

PRECEPTORSHIP AND MENTORING

Having determined what are the functions of supervision, we need to consider *how* these functions might be exercised. Before I proceed to consider some models of supervisory practice, I should like to review some of the characteristics of the supervisor. What kind of animal is this? What makes a supervisor? Might there be more than one kind of supervisor?

The clinical supervisor is often distinguished from the *preceptor* and the *mentor* on the assumption that these titles refer only to the practice of student nurses in clinical settings. This is an unfortunate distinction, since on one level it involves a corruption of the traditional concept of the mentor (for instance) and more importantly suggests that clinical supervision is a wholly different kind of activity, which may not be the case (see Barker 1990).

The key distinction between *preceptorship* and clinical supervision is the level of supervision involved. Where there is a need for a preceptor, one nurse is deemed to be the novice, student or incomer. The other is more expert, more established in the setting and generally more *au fait* with the organisational process of the care setting. When I joined my last clinical setting, despite being the Professor, I needed a preceptor, who turned out to be a staff nurse with almost fifteen years less experience than I, but who could orient and guide me in developing my role within the ward. In keeping with the received wisdom of preceptorship, we had a formal contractual relationship, which defined what I needed and (more importantly) what was not part of the preceptorship package. As we consider what are the boundaries of clinical supervision, we might need to consider where supervision ends, blurring into preceptoring; and where both might enjoy a relationship with *mentoring*.

The role of the *mentor* has been narrowly defined in Britain as a concept, which only applies in student circles. This is unfortunate in my view. One of my mentors is Annie Altschul, the Professor Emeritus in Edinburgh. Another is Hildegard Peplau in California. That both are geographically distant, and could also be counted as friends, is an irrelevance, as I hope to illustrate. Their status as mentors is conferred by me, and the mentoring relationship – how it is negotiated, its boundaries and limits and its practical workings – is determined by both of us informally, but no less effectively.

I am moving the discussion here to a consideration of *who* is this animal who might function in a formative, restorative or normative fashion. Those of you who are preparing to become supervisors and those of you responsible for organising and managing the institution of clinical supervision within your practice areas, need to know the answers to this question, *above all others*.

The traditional definition of the *mentor* – as distinct from the more recent educational definition of this role – will help us determine the qualities of the person who might fulfil these demanding supervisory functions. In Homer's *Odyssey*, Odysseus entrusted Telemachus to the care of Mentor, when he went to fight in the Trojan War. The relationship between Mentor and Odysseus and Telemachus has come to characterise the example of commitment to development, which is not commonly present in preceptoring or indeed in any other role model. I shall consider here briefly what characterises this commitment and why I believe these features are central to our understanding of clinical supervision.

The mentor has been described as a combination of a good parent, trusted friend, godparent, rabbi or coach (May et al 1982). Mentorship is a voluntary activity, often conducted outside of the natural role boundaries of the person, and confers no financial incentive for the mentor. The mentor–protégée relationship is dependent on:

- the mentor possessing the knowledge and perhaps reputation needed to meet the protégée's needs
- the presence of mutual respect for goals and past accomplishments
- the mentor's willingness and capability to open up the protégée to significant growth
- a matching of ideals and aspirations.

A nurse might well have more than one mentor – as I have. The protégée who knows what are her needs will seek out a mentor who is:

- confident, possessing the qualities necessary to form good relationships
- has a clear self-concept
- commands respect
- is willing and able to give of herself
- has a personal interest in the protégée's self-development.

The protégée is, therefore, *attracted* to the mentor, whom she admires and desires to emulate in some way. The mentor must have the potential for the kind of *action* which will be necessary for the protégée to realise her development. The mentor must also have the same kind of *positive feelings* toward the protégée as the protégée shows toward the mentor. Without this mutuality, the respect, encouragement and support, which is essential to the supervisory relationship, will not develop.

Each of you can think of at least one person whom you would not want to recruit as your mentor, if you had the choice. You might not be *sufficiently attracted* toward that person. Or, you may not believe that they possess the energy and motivation necessary to fulfil the demands of the supervisory relationship. Or, you may believe that they do not feel sufficiently positive toward you, and might even be antipathetic toward you. If you would not be happy with this person as your mentor, would you be happy with her/him as your clinical supervisor?

Of course, here we are considering the issue of choice and self-determination, which seems to me to be fundamental to professional development. I am aware that many will say that choice and self-determination are logistically impossible and that supervision will need to be a more organised and 'top down' affair. Hannibal is reputed to have said that if he could not find a way, he would make one, which is a robust way of saying that 'faint heart never won fair lady'. When we come to consider the logistical challenge of organising clinical supervision within our services, we might care to remember that the biggest limitation which we face is our own preconceptions as to what is or is not possible.

SUPERVISION AND PRACTICE

What are the possible roles that might be undertaken by the supervisor in a practice setting? The supervisor might:

- *monitor* the practice, helping to maintain professional standards
- *manage* the practice to ensure that the goals of the organisation are realised
- help *educate* the practitioner through bridging the theory–practice gap
- serve as a *mentor*, providing personally meaningful support
- act as *counsellor*, helping the nurse resolve her personal and interpersonal difficulties
- help *analyse* the intricacies of the caring relationship
- provide *training* in some specific practice method
- *audit* the overall care process
- *facilitate* the nurse's identification and resolution of professional stress
- serve as a *role model* for the pursuit of the 'life long tutorial'.

The common denominator of all these supervisory functions is the *development* of the individual nurse or of the nursing service as a whole. The most informed supervisory system aims to develop both concurrently. As noted earlier, there is little agreement as to how, exactly, these goals might be achieved, at least in terms of a specific method of supervision. This doubt may ultimately prove to be our greatest asset, allowing the development of a range of methods which will be geared to the specific needs of individuals or settings. A catholic diversity is likely to be more personally satisfying – and organisationally effective – than a singularly rigid ideology.

The developmental nature of supervision emphasises, of necessity, the exploration of the individual case, and perhaps also the context of care within which that case is located. As I have noted, the most widely accepted paradigm of clinical supervision is drawn from the fields of psychoanalysis, psychotherapy and counselling – all of which are focused upon the processes of identifying and meeting the needs of an individual, through the medium of another individual: the analyst, therapist or counsellor. It seems axiomatic that in all areas of 'need-meeting' – whether defined as health-care, social-care or psychotherapy – the raw material is the relationship between the person-in-need and the helping agent. Viewed from this angle there are two ways of considering the operation of supervision. We may:

- examine the *process of caring* – exploring what is being done in the name of caring, through observed practice, care plans, case notes or other recordings of nurse–patient interaction; or
- examine the nurse's *experience of caring* – expressed through her reflection on and recollections of her relationship with the patient.

The first is clearly a more *technical* process, whereas the latter is manifestly more focused upon the *emotional* or 'human' dimensions of the caring relationship. I shall now consider each of these briefly in turn.

The process of caring

There exist at least three possible options when we consider how we might explore the *process* of caring.

1. We might focus on the patient's needs: the core content of the nursing process; what the person needs from the nurse and from nursing. This first approach emphasises 'the *what*' of nursing.

2. We might focus on the content of caring: what the nurse has done, to date, to attempt to meet the needs of the patient. This second approach emphasises 'the *how*' of nursing: how the nurse is currently aiming to meet needs, what alternatives might exist and how she might come to decide between one approach and another.

3. The supervisor might focus on what is *going on* 'within' and 'around and about' the nurse–patient relationship. This approach can be facilitated by asking the simple – yet profound – question, 'So, what do you make of it?'. The emphasis within the question is clearly on the 'make', since the nurse who perceives the caring process to be 'working' is 'creating' – at least in her own mind – a successful care plan. The nurse who perceives difficulties may be constructing a failure. Either way, the supervisor is inviting the nurse to *defend* or deconstruct her view of the care process. This may involve the softest – although often most accurate – form of represen-tation, the metaphor. One of my PhD students is presently studying the process of clinical supervision.[2] She invites the nurses to define their experience, specifically, in metaphorical terms. Despite its abstract nature, this appears to be the most evocative of media: human experience is often best described in metaphorical terms – 'She sees right through me', or 'I feel so desolate', or 'It's like I am hiding behind something, why?'.

This kind of exploration has been described as an examination of 'what happens around the edges' of the interpersonal process (Hawkins & Shoet 1991). I prefer to take the view that this is the very *heart* of the care process. Even in the most hi-tech of environments – such as intensive care – what the nurse *makes* of the care process will ultimately determine its effectiveness.

'Even in the most hi-tech of environments – such as intensive care — what the nurse *makes* of the care process will ultimately determine its effectiveness'

The experience of caring

The emphasis on 'what is going on' within the care process can be taken an important stage further by focusing on the nurse's *experience* of the care process. Again, three options are possible.

- The supervisor may focus on how the nurse is *mirroring* the experience of caring for the patient within the supervisory session. Where the patient appears to reject the efforts of the nurse, the nurse may mirror this by appearing to reject the facilitation of the supervisor.
- Secondly, the supervisor may focus on material that the nurse appears to be 'carrying over' from the clinical contact with the patient. The emphasis here is very much upon the nurse's 'unconscious' life: her deepest feelings about the patient, expressed through her attempts to deal with specific difficulties in meeting the patient's needs.
- Finally, the supervisor might be brave enough to address her own experience of the supervisory process. This third dimension involves examining the supervisor's feelings, which have emerged as a result of dealing with the supervisee's thoughts, feelings, metaphors and images. This dimension is clearly the most subtle and sophisticated, involving the supervisor's feelings about caring for the nurse, who is involved in caring for the patient.

MODELS OF SUPERVISION

I am advocating the widest range of possibilities, within the broad concept of clinical supervision. I am emphasising – at least implicitly – also the need to tailor the focus of the supervisory process to the needs of the individual nurse, and the capabilities of the individual supervisor. It would be folly to suggest that a supervisor who was not comfortable with examining *her*… own feelings about the supervisee and the nurse–patient relationship, should be required to examine these feelings, openly, within the supervision session. On the other hand, where the nurse is uncomfortable about addressing her feelings towards the patient – especially where he might be defined as a 'difficult patient' – it might be necessary to help the nurse, carefully, towards addressing the dimensions of that relationship. Wherever we are required to consider what might be the *best* option, or what *should* we do in a given situation, we are required to confront ethical dilemmas, which rarely allow easy answers. Knowing that making such decisions is intrinsically difficult, may provide some reassurance to those nursing supervisors who are required to determine what are the most appropriate supervisory processes for this or that nurse, or this or that clinical situation.

I shall now consider some of the possible *models* of supervision, which might conceivably express the processes that have been outlined so far.

The least intrusive model may be *peer group supervision*. Here, practitioners review, analyse and deconstruct their care plans and processes within a 'sharing and caring' environment. The individual nurse may feel 'enabled' to undertake the necessary emotional soul-searching and technical investigation because she feels supported, at least implicitly, by fellow practitioners who face similar dilemmas and challenges. The classic criticism of this approach is that it may maintain the *status quo* through the operation of conservative values, and group-ego defensive strategies, which may be wholly unconscious in origin. The group may well merely serve to reinforce its own prejudices about the difficulties of developing quality care in *this* setting, or of the demands imposed by this particular patient or family.

Individual supervision with another clinician may provide the nurse with an opportunity to explore – in depth – the process of care and its associated emotional content, with someone who appreciates the demands being made of the nurse. Many options are possible for the fulfilment of this role.

- The senior nurse or team leader might provide this service to all primary nurses or keyworkers, as part of her role as 'lead clinician' or 'nurse leader'.
- A network of individual supervision might be established within a unit or service area.
- Supervision might be provided by an independent lecturer/practitioner from an academic department.
- A senior nurse, with a specific remit to develop practice within a defined clinical area, might lead the supervisory process.

These options are diverse and potentially 'developmental' in the sense that they involve more independent examination of the care process. It is clear, however, that the selection of the supervisor is critical, as nurses might feel that *their* developmental needs might be sacrificed in favour of meeting organisational needs. This is especially the case where some hierarchical process is involved – as in the power-based relationship between a senior nurse and primary nurse. If we take seriously the issues raised earlier, regarding the values of mentoring, it might seem obvious that nurse clinicians should *choose* their own supervisor. There exists in many quarters a resistance to this on the grounds that nurses might choose the least-challenging or most supportive person. This anxiety, which may derive from the hierarchical and militaristic traditions within nursing, need not present insurmountable problems.

Group supervision with an independent facilitator was first popularised by Hildegard Peplau, and is a cost-effective system allowing individual nurses to learn from one another, whilst learning about themselves (see Peplau 1994). Despite its obvious utility, this particular group process appears under-used. Here again, a number of practical options are possible. The group might focus only on the emotional context of caring, functioning as a *staff support group*. Alternatively, it might function as a *care plan surgery*, exploring week by week the development of individual care plans, and the responsible nurse's expertise, decision-making and emotional attachments. Here also, various permutations of facilitation are possible. The facilitator may be a nurse from another area of practice; or a practitioner from another discipline; or a lecturer/practitioner. In my clinical role I provide group supervision to nurse colleagues both within areas in which I practise *and* in areas which I merely visit, as an external supervisor.

Individual supervision with a practitioner from a different discipline: this process is best suited to the exploration of personal and interpersonal conflicts, which are common within all the helping disciplines. Where the supervisor is not a nurse, difficulty may be encountered in presenting any critical analysis of the content of care, the discrete elements of which may be foreign to the independent supervisor. This independent status may, however, allow the supervisor to act as a true 'devil's advocate' when exploring the general organisation of care and, especially, the human undercurrents of the caring process.

LIMITATIONS OF CLINICAL SUPERVISION

These are the most commonly accepted models of supervisory practice. How they are implemented in practice allows for great diversity.

- How often should supervision take place: weekly or monthly?
- Where should supervision be held: in the nurse's area of practice, in the supervisor's office or on 'neutral territory'?
- What should be the composition of a group: all nurses, a mix of disciplines, different levels of experience and proficiency?
- Need supervision always be face-to-face: is telephone supervision possible, or supervision by correspondence, or by exchanging audio-tapes?

These few questions about the organisation of the supervisory process suggest the range of approaches possible. These might allow the needs of individuals or organisations to be better accommodated.

What are the limitations of supervision? It seems clear that any approach can only achieve what it sets out to achieve, but that goal is by no means guaranteed. If the supervisor and the nurse do not agree to negotiate the aims of supervision, one or other or both may end up dissatisfied. If the nurse is looking for support with personal development, and the supervisor is trying to maintain general standards, then conflict may result.

Perhaps the greatest danger presented by the *concept* of clinical supervision is that of unrealistic expectations. Nursing has a tradition of developing concepts *outside of practice*, which are then introduced *into practice*, with a view to resolving some problem that may not necessarily be amenable to this novel intervention. There appears to be an assumption that clinical supervision will serve as an effective means of *developing* the individual clinician, *assuring* the quality of a service and *reducing* the stress indigenous to the care setting. Clinical supervision may realise all these ambitions, but we should not be surprised if its success is limited.

'Perhaps the greatest danger presented by the *concept* of clinical supervision is that of unrealistic expectations'

Other initiatives – such as quality assurance or total quality management – were introduced with a view to raising the standards of service provision and have, more recently, been supplemented by others such as clinical audit. PREP[3] has been introduced as an overarching system for nursing practice to foster the 'lifelong tutorial' noted earlier, within which individual nurses will be responsible for their ongoing professional development. All these initiatives were struck with a view to improving services. Their success will be determined only partly by the motivation of individuals or even of organisations. Logistical problems require to be overcome if the resources – both financial and human – necessary to support the operation of these intiatives are to materialise.

These reservations must apply to clinical supervision also. Even the best organised supervisory structure may fail to deliver if the distress felt by the team is a function of inadequate staffing, or their lack of specialist skills is at least partly a function of inadequate funding of necessary training. Everyone concerned with the development of clinical supervision in practice must beware of adding a further layer of stress – whether intellectual or emotional – to the everyday business of care provision. If supervision 'works' it will bring nurses together, allowing natural networks of support and professional growth to develop. If it does not work, it will be divisive and may contribute further to the demoralisation process seen by many to be endemic within some areas of practice.

The key supplementary concept to the success of supervision, which risks becoming merely another buzzword, is the concept of *empowerment*. If nurses feel that their needs are being met, even when those needs might be to address challenging technical or emotional problems, nurses will feel that they are truly being *enabled*. The supervisory process is helping to take the individual nurse, and the care system she represents and expresses, to where they both need to go: in pursuit of excellence. However, if nurses feel that their needs are not being met, they may feel a degree of uncomfortable empathy with some of their patients, who have been patronised, cocooned or controlled by the care process. It may not be a bad thing for nurses to experience both 'good' and 'bad' clinical supervision, since such an experience may help sensitise them to the enabling or disempowering potential of nursing care from the patient's perspective.

NOTES

This chapter is based on a paper presented to the conference 'Clinical supervision' at The University of Wales College of Medicine and Cardiff Community Health Care Trust, on 22 May 1996.

1. For convenience, the female gender is used throughout for nurses.
2. I am grateful to my doctoral student, Eileen Graham, for helping me to appreciate the importance of specific metaphors in clinical supervision.
3. Post-Registration Education and Practice (PREP)

REFERENCES

Barker P 1990 Professional networking. In: Cormack D F S (ed) Developing your career in nursing. Chapman and Hall, London
Barker P 1992 Clinical supervision in psychiatric nursing. In: Butterworth C A,

Faugier J (eds) Clinical supervision and mentorship in nursing. Chapman and Hall, London

Burnard P 1989 The role of the mentor. Journal of District Nursing 8(3):8–17

Hawkins P, Shoet R 1992 Supervision in the helping professions. Open University Press, Milton Keynes

Maslach C, Jackson S E 1982 The measurement of the experience of burnout. Journal of Occupational Behaviour 2:99–113

May K, Meleis A, Winstead-Fry P 1982 Mentorship for scholarliness: opportunities and dilemmas. Nursing Outlook 30(1):22

Peplau H E 1994 Clinical supervision. In: O'Toole, Welt (EEls) Hildegard E Peplau: selected writings. Macmillan, London

United Kingdom Central Council 1991 The scope of professional practice. UKCC, London

Westheimer I J 1977 The practice of supervision in social work. Ward Lock, London

Wright H 1989 Groupwork: perspectives and practice. Scutari, Oxford

Commentary

Dr Mami Kayama

I was impressed by the concept embodied in the word 'mirror' in this paper. Dr Barker pointed out that clinical supervision brings the supervisee face-to-face with reality. Sometimes reality is too painful to confront. In clinical practice, nurses often feel themselves to be powerless. It causes them to bring fear and anger to their own practice. It will reduce their commitment to patient's needs and rights.

Dr Barker has explained that the function of supervision is not to provide magical problem solving, but to become sensitive to our own weakness and strength. Because it is painful to see reality, we demand magical problem solving from our supervisor. But the way to solve the problem is not in the other person. It is in reality. When nurses become brave enough to see the mirror, which is shown to them by their supervisor, they will discover the way to solve the problem not from the supervisor but within themselves. Dr Barker mentioned the similarity between clinical supervision and psychoanalysis. When the person is empowered in the therapeutic relationship, they will become braver and more willing to accept reality.

I was fortunate to have Dr Barker as my supervisor for a three-month period in 1997. From him I received my 'lived experience', which I want to report on here. When I first met Dr Barker, I felt as if I were looking at a still mirror. At that time I had only been in England for three months. It was my first trip to England. My self-esteem was low. He had some questions about my own specialty, psychiatric nursing. These I could answer with confidence. Soon, I regained my self-esteem. It was as if we were having a discussion in my own office. During his supervision, he didn't support me emotionally. All of his insights stemmed from knowledge and wisdom. I have learned that insight drawn from wisdom and experience is free from norms. Sometimes too much knowledge will be threatening to the peace of mind of the inexperienced person. But I never felt myself to be threatened by his supervision. On the contrary, I felt relaxed and thought: 'I will be able to practise here as my real self though this is not my own country'. Wasn't this a great outcome for supervision overcoming culture shock?

In Japan, for a long time, we have had a very paternalistic way of administrating nursing. We had rigid norms, and it was assumed that nurses should be self-sacrificing, as if they didn't have their own emotions. Nursing supervision only meant labour management. Nursing preceptors trained young nurses to make them adhere to an ideal of self-sacrificing. Nurses had been educated within a strong medical model curriculum. In such a paternalistic hierarchy, the bosses were the MDs. They provided 'supervision' in a medical context, rather than through a nurse supervisor.

In the 1980s, burnout syndrome among caring professionals was first perceived. At that time, many nursing scholars returned from America after having received nursing degrees. They established postgraduate nursing programmes as leaders. They initiated research programmes from nursing perspectives.

Today, all nursing education programmes in Japan are constructed from a nursing perspective. Now, we have a number of nursing supervisors with nursing degrees. Nurses are in touch with their own feelings during their daily work, without unnecessary guilt feelings. To develop a knowledge of nursing, it seems that we have fostered a freedom from strong norms. To feel powerlessness, anger, over-identification, emptiness, and other types of negative feelings, is considered reasonable. Liaison nurses are working to deal with emotional problems between nurse and client. Some directors of nursing also serve as hospital vice presidents. They consider that employing liaison nurses provides satisfactory results. However, further study is needed.

The other stream of clinical supervision in Japanese psychiatric nursing is the continuous case conference. Miyamoto et al (1995) reported on the continuing professional education which originated in group psychotherapy. To assure the quality of care, we have been using the group method. When I asked about empowerment, Dr Barker suggested that the concept might not fit Japanese culture. He thought that when the person became empowered, the person would be more individualistic in outlook.

Traditionally, Japanese people value harmony above individualism. However, to advocate an individual's right, we can't always give priority to harmony. Today, in my generation, we are already aware of our identity as individuals rather than only as group members. This trend has caused conflicts with the old system. Miyamoto (1985) described how continuous group supervision could be helpful to the person within the group. Because nurses provide care by team, I believe that it is important to know weakness and strength in the group dynamics.

Now we must seek a new paradigm of nursing for the next century. I feel that I am in the tempest. In the windstorm, people need a beacon from a lighthouse for guidance. The lighthouse is nursing wisdom drawn from daily experience. I wish we could see Dr Barker's warmhearted beacon, even from Japan.

REFERENCES

Barker P 1992 Clinical supervision in psychiatric nursing. In: Butterworth C A, Fauguier J (eds) Clinical supervision and mentorship in Nursing. Chapman and Hall, London

Miyamoto M, Komiya K, Hirose H, et al 1995 A methodological study of continuing professional education for psychiatric nursing – an analysis of case conferences. Journal of Japanese Academy of Psychiatric and Mental Health Nursing 1:1–11

Where care meets treatment: common ethical conflicts in psychiatric nursing

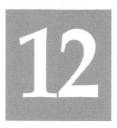

Nursing may be a relatively insignificant part of the psychiatric empire, but nursing – through nurses – has always been the closest, most consistent and enduring branch of mental health care, as far as the patient and the patient's family are concerned.

'nursing – through nurses – has always been the closest, most consistent and enduring branch of mental health care, as far as the patient and the patient's family are concerned'

The public may most readily think of psychiatrists, psychotherapists and psychologists, when 'the mind' comes to mind. It is not a judgement to say that these disciplines, although important, are fleeting images of psychiatric provision. There is a constancy about nursing which may render it almost invisible in the public consciousness.

Such proximity only *might* be a good thing. The ease with which nurses gain access to the patient's self and private world, can be exploited for ill as well as good. The essential nature of the nurse's relationship to the patient confers special privileges. Those privileges, in turn, bring responsibilities. Judging how to respond to those responsibilities brings an ethical and moral dimension to nursing, which may distinguish it from other branches of the psychiatric service.

This paper concerns some of the commoner ethical dilemmas that face psychiatric nurses in the course of their everyday work. Such issues in nursing are increasingly thrust into centre stage as the roles and responsibilities of the nurse change, and the consensus view on mental illness and health shifts dramatically (Barker & Baldwin 1991). At the beginning of this century a nursing authority observed that ethics:

> 'teaches men [sic] the practice of duties of human life and the reasons for what they do and for what they should leave undone' (Robb 1915).

The assumption that ethics could ever *teach* us our duty would, likely, today be seriously challenged. Nursing at the beginning of this century was primarily about implicit, unquestioning obedience. Today, nurses are expected to exercise careful thought, if not abundant reasoning, before deciding what actions they ought to take in the name of care. Although making ethical choices *can* be difficult, ethics need not be viewed as an albatross weighing heavily on our hearts and minds. Rather, we might view ethics as the basis for *choosing* the kind of professional life we believe we should lead, so that we need not look back with regret in the future.

'we might view ethics as the basis for *choosing* the kind of professional life we believe we should lead, so that we need not look back with regret in the future'

Psychiatric nursing has been transformed, almost overnight, into *mental health* nursing, suggesting that the focus of nursing has shifted. Whether this shift is real or imaginary – part of a serious philosophical initiative, or deriving from political 'spin-doctoring' – is unimportant, since it does at least prompt us to consider what *is* the proper focus of nursing?

Many commentaries on the development of psychiatric and mental health nursing tend to emphasise *what* nurses are doing, or could be doing in the name of care. Here, I am concerned with a much less certain topic:

- To what extent are we offering the *right kinds* of care?
- What is the *most fitting* form or context for such care?
- How do we *establish* what is 'right' or 'fitting' anyway?

These questions do not possess any absolute answers. There are no prescriptions for care, only (perhaps) general principles that might help us determine what needs to be done and how we might do it.

The field of psychiatric care is fraught with complex ethical problems that nurses, and other disciplines, need to deal with on an everyday basis. The history of psychiatric care is replete with records of the serious and recurrent abuse of people's rights to appropriate care and treatment. Britain in the late 1960s and early 1970s provided a bulging catalogue of such abuse (DHSS 1969, 1971, 1972, 1974). I do not intend to address such blatant examples of breaches of human rights, which were as much criminal as unethical in form and function. Instead, I shall focus attention on some of the subtler ethical dilemmas which emerge from the core of psychiatric nursing practice. By examining the principles which might be infringed, I hope to begin to clarify the nature of such ethical conflicts, and how we might resolve them. I shall desist from offering instruction in the *specifics* of ethical practice. Ethics may be studied but there is no award for ethical conduct. To paraphrase a Taoist saying: there is no way to ethical practice, ethical practice *is* the way.

We cannot begin to consider the nature of such ethical conflicts without considering briefly the nature of nursing: what is nursing and what is it for?

It should be apparent that nursing is concerned with human distress which others, most notably doctors, might define as mental illness, disorder, dysfunction, etc. Nursing does not deal with such illness directly – since they are no more than a special class of ideas. Instead, nursing deals with people's human responses to illness, disability or dysfunction.

Nursing addresses such human responses through the relationship between nurse and the person-in-care. The goal-directed nature of nursing demands that certain steps, actions, operations, negotiations or performances that occur between the nurse and the person, confirm the interpersonal nature of nursing. This suggests the *substance* of nursing; its core characteristic.

What goes on within those relationships suggests that we are organising the conditions which facilitate the forward movement of personality and other human processes in the direction of creative, constructive and productive personal and community living. This human growth and development is what nursing, in general, aims to achieve. This provides us with some idea of the nature of nursing: how it works. Nursing is a maturing force by means of which individuals and communities can be aided to use their capacities to influence living in desirable ways.

These observations – all from Hildegard Peplau – are the closest thing we have to universally accepted definitions of psychiatric nursing practice. Given that ethics represents the closest thing we have to universal principles of *moral* behaviour, such a definition of nursing guides us in our enquiry into the nature and function of ethical practice.

THE NATURE OF ETHICAL DILEMMAS

Psychiatric nursing is, fundamentally, a moral or ethical pursuit. It is *moral* in the sense that it is based upon standards of behaviour governing what is considered appropriate, by the profession if not by society at large. It is *ethical* in the sense that there are ways of monitoring these standards, all of which contribute to our notions of appropriate professional conduct. Ethics is a branch of moral philosophy and, by definition, is not a science, far less an exact one. Whenever nurses spend any amount of time, in any situation, considering whether they *should* do this or that, they are, of necessity, involved in ethical enquiry. In essence, ethics involves thinking or reasoning about morality: deciding what we *ought* to do (Rowson 1990).

Although many of our traditional concepts about nursing and caring have been reframed as quasi-medical, psychological or sociological concepts, at the most fundamental level, nurses are involved incessantly in making judgements about what they *should do* in very specific contexts. We attempt to use general principles, or overarching theories of human conduct, as guides for our actions. However, ultimately, our decision-making about what we should do, in relation to another person, is often bounded by our power structure. Given that nurses have, for so long, been construed as a subordinate – or at best *semi*-profession (Etzioni 1969) – such decision-making is often highly complex. Nurses have often assumed that decisions about rightful conduct may be made *for* them by, for example, the responsible medical officer or, more recently, by the consensus of the multidisciplinary team. Here, I shall suggest that these ideas represent convenient ethical myths, which have outlived any usefulness they ever possessed. All our decision-making is highly specific and, therefore, each decision is fraught with its own special considerations. To paraphrase the family therapist Virginia Satir: nothing ever happens in general; everything happens specifically. When there is a conflict between different moral principles – 'what we believe we ought to do' – or between different moral values – 'what we think or feel is fundamentally good or important' – we are confronted by the ethical and moral context of everyday decision-making.

Let us consider an ordinary example. A person in a hospital ward becomes emotionally distraught. In terms of deciding *how* we should respond to this person, what are the available choices? Should we offer the person medication *to* calm him down, *or* should we sit with the person *until* he calms down? There may be countless other options, but, in every case, deciding between *doing* 'this' or 'that' involves a moral dilemma. By giving medication we may help reduce the person's emotional distress quickly. This may ease the pressure on others as well as on us. We may believe that such a course of action may also reduce the likelihood that other people-in-care will become distressed. We might consider, however, whether – by taking such action – we are only postponing the examination of the problem *or* making life easy for ourselves. We might even consider that we are denying the experience of the person in some way. We may ask ourselves to what extent are we only papering over the cracks, constructing a semblance of normal function which might ultimately have no effect (unmet need), might compound the person's problems (antitherapeutic) or might be construed ultimately as harmful (abuse).

From this perspective, the alternative – spending time with the distressed person – seems more appropriate. By listening to the person we may establish the true nature of the distress, and may begin the process of achieving true resolution. However, our colleagues may favour the anxiolytic medication option, or this might be the conventional clinical policy. If we challenge this, are we simply trying to demonstrate our own virtue? Are we quietly challenging the authority of other team members, especially our medical colleagues who, ultimately, will prescribe the medication? We might also ask if spending time discussing the problem is likely to alleviate the person's problem, or will this merely bring the person into closer contact with his distress?

The dilemmas inherent in this everyday story demonstrate the basic nature of ethical or moral decision-making. Deciding what we *should do* involves teasing out and weighing up the *values* upon which such decisions are based. All our ethical decisions are based upon recognition of the values that underlie the beliefs that, in turn, underlie the attitudes that we hold that, in turn, determine our moral behaviour. The ethical dilemma always involves the close-run race between one idea of what is right and fitting and another – and of course between the values, beliefs and attitudes which underpin such definitions. Such ethical dilemmas need to be distinguished from situations where we *know* that this or that action is in some way prejudicial to the welfare of the patient, or others. Taking such action is *immoral* in the true sense of the word. When a nurse ignores someone's call for help, *knowing* – in the proper sense of the word – that a compassionate ear would be the appropriate ('right') response, no ethical dilemma is involved. Rather, an immoral action has taken place. Many such actions are not illegal in any formal sense and may indeed be common practice. This serves only to reinforce the proposition that moral judgements and their underlying moral principles are not always the same as the codes or rules of conduct which control the activities of disciplines, such as nursing. Ethics involves the exercise of a necessarily more complex form of reasoning.

The range of ethical challenges in psychiatric care is wide indeed. I have chosen, here, three interlinked themes that reflect the core characteristics of nursing defined forty years ago by Peplau.

Firstly, I shall consider some ethical issues concerned with the *nature* of nursing:

- To what extent is the fulfilment of the nurse's role consonant with the definition of nursing as a *development* activity?

'The ethical dilemma always involves the close-run race between one idea of what is right and fitting and another – and of course between the values, beliefs and attitudes which underpin such definitions'

- To what extent is nursing concerned with helping people to grow and develop within the limitations of their personal and societal circumstances?
- What might be some of the ethical dilemmas involved in fulfilling different nursing roles? These ethical issues concern the 'what' of nursing.

Secondly, I shall consider some issues related to the *process* of nursing:

- How should we go about developing and implementing different systems of care?
- What ethical issues are inherent in the care-planning process?

Finally, I shall consider what we hope to achieve by offering *nursing*, as opposed to any other kind of care or treatment. Mental distress in its various forms weakens the person, delimiting or restricting them in their engagement with the world and the pursuit of the general activity of living.

- To what extent does nursing restore the autonomous status of the person?

Empowerment is one of the 'buzzwords' of contemporary care and treatment. In a related sense we might well ask:

- In what way does nursing realise the goal of empowerment?

THE NURSE'S ROLE

The notion of nursing as a developmental activity suggests that this is the *only* role of the nurse: to promote the person's independent functioning. Is the developmental activity Peplau discussed realised by the fulfilment of one role or many? To answer this question, we need to clarify what we mean by *role*.

The role that the nurse fulfils is how she *acts* in specific situations. Just as an actor acts in a particular way to convey a certain meaning, so the nurse acts in different ways that are meaningful in different situations. Given that people in care present themselves differently, at different times, so the nurse's role might be expected to change correspondingly. There is, however, some agreement that a range of valued roles exists, from which the nurse draws as appropriate. In organising the delivery of care, a range of sub-roles needs to be fulfilled. Among these are the parental or authority role, the technician, the teacher, the social contact, and the counsellor or therapist. Most nurses recognise the value of these different sub-roles. Ethical dilemmas emerge when nurses are faced with choosing between two or more of these roles, any of which might appear appropriate for the situation.

Consider a man living in the community who has been attributed the diagnosis of schizophrenia. He is reluctant to accept this diagnosis, which he considers to be invalid. He also rejects the offer of medication that has been prescribed to control the symptoms of his 'schizophrenia' Currently, he is managing reasonably well, and is not showing any overt signs of serious psychiatric disturbance. The consensus view of the multidisciplinary team is, however, that without medication – indeed without his acceptance of his diagnosis – he may relapse quickly and will require more intensive care and treatment at some point in the future. Which role should the nurse fulfil in this context? The psychiatrist, who has made the diagnosis of schizophrenia, has prescribed a treatment and needs the nurse to ensure the efficient and consistent delivery of the medication, perhaps by depot injection. In rejecting the diagnosis and treatment, the patient expressed the belief that no one appreciates the true nature of his difficulties. What he needs at this time is a confidante: someone with whom to share his problems; in whom to confide; someone who will believe in him as a person, rather than as a patient. Is this 'confidante' role the most appropriate role for the nurse to adopt at this stage of the relationship?

Although he has never displayed any aggression, the person's family believe they have reason to fear him. In addition to being troubled by some of the strange ideas expressed by their son and brother they have seen some alarming reports about schizophrenia on television. They need the nurse to take whatever action is necessary to make them feel secure. They would prefer if this involved coaxing him to take medication which might 'control' his illness.

The psychiatrist, the person, and the person's family all need 'something' to be done. What they each need, and their motivations for seeking the nurse's help in fulfilling the need, are, however, quite different. The values and attitudes that underlie these needs stimulate an ethical dilemma for the nurse. Which role, or combination of roles, should the nurse fulfil? Should the nurse act as a parental or authority figure, encouraging the person to 'face facts', 'see reason' and otherwise accept the inherent wisdom and usefulness of the medical diagnosis and its related treatment? This might meet the needs of the psychiatrist and family, but to what extent will it meet the needs of the person himself? Choosing and applying any of the other roles already mentioned would likely satisfy some but not all of the parties involved. The role conflict is set in motion by some of the conflicting moral imperatives that are accepted as general roles in nursing.

Nurses are expected, for example, to show 'respect' for the person, his values, his beliefs, what makes him a unique individual. Stated simply, nurses should accept the person's view of himself and the world, however much in conflict with our own that might appear.

- To what extent is the nurse expected to care for the patient as a *person*?

At the same time, nurses are expected to base their actions on values such as honesty, fairness and justice. If the nurse has reason to believe that the diagnosis is accurate (right) and appropriate (fitting), is she not bound morally to tell him – honestly – rather than deny this belief or feign ignorance? If he does indeed 'suffer' from schizophrenia, is he not entitled – by virtue of the moral law of justice – to care and treatment which is right and fitting?

- To what extent is the nurse expected to treat the person as a *patient*?

At the same time, nurses are expected to fulfil their roles for the right reasons, for the proper motives. They should, therefore, aim to bring as much benefit as possible to the person, incurring as little harm in the process, without acting immorally.

If we emphasise respect for the individual we may feel obliged to be economical with the truth, as we understand it, from a diagnostic viewpoint. If we emphasise honesty and our more objective version of what he needs – and deserves by right – as a 'patient', we may prejudice our respect for his autonomy. Careful consideration needs to be given to choosing between these options, or otherwise balancing them to ensure the greatest benefit for the least harm.

This utilitarian scenario would be complex if only the person defined as patient were involved. The situation is complicated further by the needs of the family. We need to ask whose needs will be met by fulfilment of the different nursing roles? These role conflicts are now cast on a much larger stage, as nurses are required to operate the power of recall to hospital over patients living in the community, or may be offered the opportunity, in future, to prescribe – by joint protocols – psychotropic medication. To what extent will these new roles present new ethical dilemmas? Much has been said – on both sides – about developments or extensions of the nurse's role. Little attention has been paid to the ethical dilemmas which might be inherent in such role extensions, far less that many nurses might recognise true conscientious objections to detaining, coercing or (perhaps) treating people against their natural will. The reference to conscience is by design rather than accident. In every ethical arena, we are required to commune with our consciences when engaged in decision-making. Having checked with our conscience and decided, we must live with the consequences.

> 'In every ethical arena, we are required to commune with our consciences when engaged in decision-making. Having checked with our conscience and decided, we must live with the consequences'

THE PROCESS OF CARE PLANNING

Issues concerning role, flow naturally into consideration of issues involved in care planning. We appear to remain locked in a sterile debate about nursing assessment systems and the sorts of nursing models and psychiatric theories that might inform care planning. Given the various dimensions of the debate, I shall focus only on the issues that may suggest the inherent ethical complexity of care planning.

We have moved closer to acknowledging that the person in care is the proper focus of care planning. Individual care plans, the identification of primary nurses, the named nurse and nurse keyworkers confirm this. We need to ask, however, to what extent is the person in care involved *equally* in the care planning process? Especially in the UK, psychiatric nurses talk glibly about 'working in partnership' with the people in their care. This seems – at least on the face of it – to be a disingenuous proposition. The power imbalance between the nurse and the 'patient' is often so acutely defined that to speak of partnership seems almost folly. Partnership implies mutual influence, creative collaboration and – perhaps also – opportunity for constructive disagreement. Who among us would enter into a 'partnership' with someone who might choose, or be required, to use the power of the law against us should we decide to disagree with his or her worldview? The notion of partnerships is flawed at this fundamental legal/political level. It might be more appropriate to think about the nurse–patient–family relationship in terms of a possible *alliance*, where *parties with differing motives and power bases* conjoin in an attempt to pursue shared goals. However, even such an alliance will be possible only if both the person and the nurse clarify the roles they are adopting. Although we talk about the 'patient role', there is no such thing. Some people in care are passive, others wish to be dominant, and there are many shades of grey between. If the planning of care is to be an allied affair, these roles need to be clarified. Without this clarification, either nurse or patient may stage-manage the planning, to the disadvantage of the other.

Secondly, we need to consider how free are people in care to express their needs, wants or wishes. Where nurses adopt a 'high-tech' care system with formalised assessment procedures, perhaps using 'diagnoses' – whether nursing, medical or psychological – the expression of 'personal' needs may be thwarted. We often argue that some people, especially those with more severe psychiatric problems – such as dementias or other organic disorders – cannot express themselves. This suggests a prejudiced view. Sophisticated nursing will be sensitive to the range of messages sent by the patient, Some of these will be primarily non-verbal in form, others largely symbolic or metaphorical in nature. All require sensitive handling to establish what the person might be 'saying'. This requires a most interactive form of assessment, which may be more time-consuming than following a behavioural checklist or standardised model of assessment. We need to consider whether or not such standardised forms of assessment hold any promise of a 'right and fitting' description of the person's true needs, as held at the present time.

Thirdly, it seems uncontroversial to suggest that the care-planning process should emancipate the person, freeing him to make decisions about what could or should happen to him. Such emancipation should enable the person to find his own level for happiness, freedom from pain and spiritual peace among other dimensions of his 'quality of life'. Nurses may assume that they are restrained from such emancipation by legal issues. However, as Martin Ward has argued, there are no legal restraints to emancipation in care planning, only a lack of imagination on the part of unenlightened or thoughtless nurses. *How* nurses conjoin with the person to determine the shape and function this emancipation might take, is part of the creativity of nursing, which is all too often overshadowed by respect for the rigorous replication of proven technique.

The emerging influence of political or economic external factors on the role of nurses has already been noted. Nurses have a responsibility – when they purport to adopt the role of advocate – for resolving the conflict that might exist between the needs of the organisation and those of the clientele. Where there is a conflict between the availability of resources and clinical demand, nurses have traditionally felt demoralised, have taken industrial action or resigned on principle. These actions clearly have failed to serve the people in care. We need to ask if there is a moral imperative to find new, or alternative mechanisms for resolving such conflicts: so that we can realise the greatest good for the least pain and disruption.

It has been noted already that some nursing philosophies may be in conflict with those of other disciplines within the care and treatment team. This is not a major problem. Indeed it might well enhance the service. There is a view, however, that all members of any team should not only subscribe to the same value set, but should operate within the same skills set. Short of cloning people, I fail to see how this can be realised. Instead of trying to homogenise the operations of the different members of the team, we should be considering how nursing care plans might balance – rather than echo – those offered by other team members. If nurses are implementing a care plan that is identical in shape and form to that of other members of the team, based on the same philosophy, it is probably not a *nursing* care plan. Successful teams, in any sphere of activity, have a united goal, but embrace diversity of skills and knowledge. It is within this diversity that the true strength of the team lies.

'Instead of trying to homogenise the operations of the different members of the team, we should be considering how nursing care plans might balance – rather than echo – those offered by other team members. ... Successful teams ... have a united goal, but embrace diversity of skills and knowledge'

Such a consideration leads to the next two issues:

• Have nurses the necessary capacity to advocate for themselves *and* their patients as necessary?

• To what extent does nursing (and nurses) need to change, rather than the person in nursing care?

It is commonly assumed that the person should (moral imperative!) be the focus of the change process – this is illustrated by the development of the concept of individual care plans. We need to ask, however, to what extent do the person's problems lie *within* them – at a personal level?

• Might the person's problems not be a function of family or societal relationships?

• Might the person's problems be the consequences of wider factors such as poverty, alienation or isolation?

• Might the person's problems be a function of the nursing care scenario itself?

This prompts us to ask – 'What is the true nature of the "problem" which is the focus of the care plan?'.

Nurses might consider the need to review, constantly, their attitudes and beliefs, and the values which underpin them, since these are the major factors in determining what is detailed in – and what is omitted from – the care plan. As noted already, we now talk of *mental health* rather than *psychiatric* nursing. To what extent is this a mere cosmetic change? The distinction between a mental *health* care plan and a mental *illness* (or psychiatric) care plan must be considerable. The promotion of health and the reduction of the manifestation of illness may be related, but are likely to involve quite discrete roles, functions and related care processes. Our values concerning respect for the individual, the construction of themselves and the world, may conflict with the views of family members, professionals and the world at large. This is certainly true when we consider the difficulty in gaining agreement over what *is* or *is not* a problem. When we come to consider definitions of health and how these relate to notions of care and treatment, new conflicts may emerge.

EMPOWERMENT IN THE CARING RELATIONSHIP

Before concluding, I should like to consider empowerment within the caring relationship, since this implies a certain kind of action and a highly specific ethical stance. Empowerment is in danger of becoming no more than a buzzword – an attractive expression disguising its inherent emptiness. Just as we talk casually about providing holistic care, we now talk about the need to empower the person in care. But what exactly does this mean, and how do we do it? The answers to these questions lie embedded somewhere in most of the questions that we have posed so far.

There is little doubt that psychiatry and psychiatric care have become increasingly complex. We face a renaissance of interest in, and appreciate the growing power of, neuroscience. Since the 1960s we have witnessed a proliferation of the psychotherapies. And, there exists a discrete tension between categorical systems, like the DSM-IV and constructivist paradigms in describing and attempting to explain mental distress. To what extent do these changes within the broad church of psychiatry have implications for psychiatric *nursing* practice? The face of psychiatry has changed dramatically in the past twenty years. What, if anything, has changed within psychiatric nursing? To what extent is Peplau's philosophy of nursing practice – stated forty years ago – still relevant? If, as some have suggested, Peplau's theorising is now outmoded – an anachronism – with what shall we replace it?

Those who espouse empowerment suggest that mental distress – and the loss of power involved in that process – is a core issue and determines the ethical parameters of nursing practice. We need to consider, therefore, how we go about returning the power to the person who has been disempowered. How do we 'power-up' those who still have some sense of their own power?. How do we help the person make informed, personalised choices which work for her without working against the needs of others? In considering how we *execute* this empowering action we need to consider to what extent the person is disempowered by the nature of her relationship with us – her carers – as well as by her relationship with the whole of the psychiatric process. Many of the ethical issues that have been considered so far involve reflections on the potential for disempowerment held within the institutionalised processes of nursing and psychiatric practice. How might we go about reducing their disempowering effects, without abandoning psychiatry altogether, and risking abandoning the person who is the patient to her fate? I shall refer briefly to gender and ethnic issues here, since I believe they are not only critical dimensions of the ethical debate in psychiatry, but are both linked to empowerment.

I recall one year when four women with whom I had been working – first as inpatients, who later attended as outpatients – all discontinued. Two of the women advised me at the end of the session that it was time for them to stop 'seeing me'; the other two dropped into the clinic and left notes for me, with much the same message: all within a one-month period. One night, the receptionist with whom I had worked for many years, and who knew all the women well, commented: 'I have been wracking my brains to figure out what was bothering me about those patients. And then I realised that I hardly recognised Mrs Brown, and Mrs Green had to tell me who she was before the penny dropped!'.

I too had noticed obvious physical changes in the two women I had seen. Now I knew that all four of them had physically changed. Gone were the downtrodden, miserable, angst-ridden 'selves' who had trudged in and out of the hospital for what seemed like years. The only common denominator, I realised later, was that each had either divorced, left or rejected the men in their lives. Having shed their male partners, apparently, they were now free to 'be' whoever they wanted to be.

Having spent more than a decade working closely with seriously depressed, some psychotic and most suicidal, women – like these four – I had long harboured the idea that a major part of their psychic distress lay on the other side of the marital bed, and in their disempowered status. That year I felt like starting a women's group, which I did, and ran – quite successfully – for a couple of years, until the nonsense of a man leading a women's group finally grew too much for me. That year I was confronted, however, with a new ethical challenge. Should I be 'powering up' women who were manifestly disadvantaged, abused, put upon, and generally undervalued, by restoring their 'personhood', and perhaps invalidating their marriages or relationships in the process? Or, should I be 'caring for' women who were manifestly disabled by their illness, involving their partners in supporting them during this period of 'patienthood'?

A few years ago, a colleague told me of a young Muslim man with whom he had been working. The man had a 'severe psychosis', this diagnosis being proferred by the psychiatrist who visited the man and his family at home, accompanied by the nurse. At the team meeting, the treatment plan was contrived and the nurse went out to begin the process of helping the family deal with their son and to administer the therapy. Having explained himself, and the necessary treatment, the nurse felt that he had got off to a good start with the (by now) silent patient and gently smiling family. 'Oh thank you very much', said the father, 'but we have everything in hand'. He pointed to his son's neck, where there hung a kind of necklace: 'We have made a garland of prayer beads for our son. Now we wait. Allah will provide'.

What are we to make of this situation? The family needed to 'know' what was wrong with their son, but, having gained the diagnosis, returned to their cultural tradition in search of an answer.

• If the 'patient' had wanted to treat himself with prayer, but the family wanted phenothiazines, would the situation have been any different?

- If the young man was assessed as a 'risk to self or others' but the whole family still decided prayer was the answer, would the situation have been any different?

- Finally, would it have been any different if the family had been Christian (or followers of any other faith, sect or cult)?

In all of these instances, the ethical challenge is: 'How do we *respect* the cultural tradition that serves as a critical boundary for the individual or the family?'. We are firmly established in a neuroscientific age, where we risk breeding a new nihilism concerning the human condition. However, as Dossey (1993) has illustrated, although religion may be in decline in the west, evidence for the power of prayer is growing. In the USA, David and Susan Larson (1991) surveyed 12 years of papers in the American Journal of Psychiatry and the Archives of General Psychiatry. They found that when measuring participation in religious ceremony, social support, prayer and relationships with God, 92% of the studies showed benefits for mental health, 4% were neutral and 4% showed harm. As Dossey wryly commented at the end of his book: 'Those who believe in prayer might pray for this process to continue'. These findings are scientific, but have a long way to go before they even reach the fringes of most Community Mental Health Teams, far less help frame the agenda of care plan decision-making. However, nurses cannot shirk from asking themselves 'How should I deal with this situation when it arises?'.

MANAGING AND DAMAGING HEALTH CARE

In moving toward a conclusion, I am obliged to set at least some of my observations in an appropriate context: the society to which we all belong and from which, allegedly, we get our ethical supports. This society appears less interested in moral conduct and ethical principles than was the case even twenty years ago. Many of my generation wanted to drop out, hang loose and generally have a good time. Many also wanted to ban the atomic bomb, stop the Vietnam war, abolish cruelty to animals and save the whale, before we realised that we had better save the planet for the whale. Recently, a survey of American college students found that the most popular and important hero was Clint Eastwood, with Sylvester Stallone coming a close second. As Paul Fink, Past President of the American Psychiatric Association, observed, the chosen hero figure was:

> 'not the President, not the Chief Justice, not the winner of the Nobel Prize for medicine or physics, but two actors whose claim to fame is the enactment of wanton murder and the exaltation of indiscriminate violence' (Fink, 1989).

I wonder who are our 'heroes' in health care? Are they those who can demonstrate the struggle for the greatest good, or at least the struggle to attain the emotional rescue of the most seriously mentally distressed? Or, are they those who can manage the tightest budgets, run the most cost-efficient service, or generally offer less in the hope that it might spread more?

Some years ago, the American Medical News carried a tongue-in-cheek 'code of ethics' for the medical profession, framed by medical economists. It read:

1. Practice the most cost-effective medicine possible in accordance with government guidelines.

2. Reduce hospital admissions by maximising outpatient treatment (realising that this may jeopardise their health and compromise medical judgement).

3. Shorten hospital admissions by as many days as possible. Quality of care cannot be allowed to compromise cost-effectiveness.

4. Employ outpatient and same-day treatment ... ignoring patient apprehensions and care complications.

5. Cast asunder conscientious medical judgement and employ the most cost-effective procedures mandated by the government.

6. Conserve on medical diagnostics and treatment ... allowing health insurance companies to reap greater profits ... and conserve funds so that government agencies are not embarassed by their inept management.

7. Admit only patients with current medical insurance, avoiding financial stress on the institution.

8. Accept without question the medical judgements and decisions of our esteemed senators, congressmen and other knowledgeable government executives, realising that their decisions will adversely affect patient care.

9. Consider above all the 'quality of life' and financial viability of all health insurance carriers and cause no carrier undue financial strain.

10. Accept without question the ever-increasing financial and medico-legal burdens with malice towards none.'

(Coblenz 1988).

This American ethical nightmare will increasingly haunt our dreams as the spectre of rampant capitalism erodes all the gains made by ethicists in the west since the time of Hippocrates, who, I suspect, is spinning faster in his grave. The general principles – if not the actual detail – of these awful commandments are already with us. Already nurses, who once cared for everyone who presented before them, are beginning to echo the mantra of the economists: prioritisation. The consequence is already with us, in the shape of ideas about who deserves psychiatric nurses attention and who doesn't. Next, will come a diktat detailing the specific roles and functions of the nurse in relation to the deserving patient body.

The coming years seem likely to be increasingly challenging, but mostly on an ethical front. How will nurses find the resolve to both identify and confront the ethical issues which the current upheaval in health care practice will generate. How will they safeguard the ethical principles that have served health care and nursing well throughout its recorded history. These will, ultimately, be personal questions, requiring to be answered by each individual nurse as she stands between her conscience and the new barons of health care. Margaret Thatcher was right, to an extent, when she declared that there was no society, only individuals.

- Society will not safeguard our ethical heritage – individuals will struggle alone to do so, or will band with others to do so.

- Society will not frame new ethical codes – individuals who seek election to positions of power will do so.

- Society will not be displeased with their ethical handiwork – only individuals will be so, and will challenge at conferences, meetings, in the press and through professional and lay publications, the authority of any who would risk prejudicing the ethical legacy handed down the generations from the ancient Greeks. As my generation was wont to say, 'the personal is political'. I live with the hope that that phrase may also come back to haunt us.

NOTE

This chapter is based on a paper presented to the Professional Nurse Study Day – 'Mental health nursing' – at Edgbaston Cricket Ground, Birmingham on Thursday, 18 May 1995.

REFERENCES

Barker P, Baldwin S 1991 Ethical issues in mental health. Chapman and Hall, London

Coblentz M G 1988 An oath to practice medicine the American way. American Medical News. 8th August

DHSS 1969 Report of the Commitee of Inquiry into allegations of ill treatment of patients and other irregularities at the Ely Hospital, Cardiff. HMSO, London

DHSS 1971 Report of the Farleigh Hospital Committee of Inquiry. HMSO, London

DHSS 1972 Report of the Committee of Inquiry into Whittingham Hospital. HMSO, London

DHSS 1974 Report of the Committee of Inquiry into South Ockenden Hospital, HMSO, London

Dossey L 1993 Healing words: the power of prayer and the practice of medicine. Harper, San Francisco

Etzioni A 1969 The semi-professions and their organisation. Free Press, New York

Fink P 1989 Presidential address: On being ethical in an unethical world. American Journal of Psychiatry 146(9):1097–1104

Frankl V 1962 Basic concepts of logotherapy. Journal of Existential Psychiatry 3:11–18

Larson DB, Larson SS 1991 Religions, commitment and health: valuing the relationship. Second Opinion: Health, faith and ethics 17(1): 26–40

Robb IH 1915 Nursing ethics. Cleveland University Press, Cleveland, OH

Rowson R H 1990 An introduction to ethics for nurses. Scutari Press, London

Commentary

Richard Lakeman

Barker proposes that there is an ethical dimension to the decisions which psychiatric nurses make in everyday practice. Few would argue with this position, and this commentary doesn't. Instead it proposes a complementary case for values clarification by nurses as the first step to 'being alive' to such dimensions. It suggests that the first step in this process is acknowledging, and productively channelling the tension arising from value conflict in everyday practice. It is from such work that nursing can begin to establish substantive practice-based moral positions.

The secondary definition of 'ethical' in the *Concise Oxford Dictionary* (1982) relates to that font of wisdom on pharmaceuticals, 'not advertised to the general public, and usually available only on doctor's prescription'. This definition might also describe the traditional arbiters and process of decision making about what is right and ought to be in psychiatric medicine and care. Barker suggests it is the constancy of nursing that renders psychiatric nursing 'almost invisible' to public consciousness. More likely it is that psychiatric nursing is perceived as having little power in the psychiatric decision-making process and by this virtue is perceived as the most trustworthy and helpful of the psychiatric professions. Johnstone (1989: 1) states that nurses are 'not expected to have a substantive moral position on anything significant, and are most certainly not expected to express a view publicly'. However, it is only through establishing substantive moral positions that the public trust in nursing will be justified.

As we enter a new millennium, psychiatric nursing is in a state of flux and may well be an historical artefact in the coming years. The last physical vestiges of the asylums in which the occupational identities of several generations of psychiatric nurses were formed are being dismantled. The 'decade of the brain' has delivered some modest, but significant gains in the treatment of 'mental disorder' and promises substantially more in the near future. New 'market' ideologies and 'rationalisation' have come to dominate policy in the health sector, as has the 'new nursing' (Salvage 1990) ideologies, and generic roles for nurses such as case management. With the myriad of roles that a nurse may now assume and for which others make claims, it is sometimes difficult to identify the values which bind psychiatric/mental health nurses together or set them apart from other groups.

Values are not invented, rather they are discovered (Frankl 1962), and as Tschudin (1992:31) suggests, 'values only take on significance when they are tested against someone or something'. Barker argues that nursing is fundamentally a moral undertaking and that what is good and helpful (viz. ethical) about nursing arises from interpersonal relationships and the nature of these relationships. The 'common ethical dilemmas' which he describes, arise when the values inherent in the view of nursing as a primarily interpersonal endeavour conflict with those inherent in roles which nurses choose or are required to assume. The discomfort from this conflict may be channelled into discovering what it is that we value and share. This statement in itself reflects values and beliefs about the nature of discomfort or anxiety, which also arise from the theory of interpersonal relations which views anxiety as a motivating force for learning, growth and change (Peplau 1992). No discussion about ethics may be value neutral, and any practical discourse about nursing ethics is inevitably coloured by beliefs about the 'proper focus of nursing', which Barker firmly locates in the realms of interpersonal relations.

Few people would dispute that interpersonal skills are part of the repertoire of essential skills which are necessary to function in almost any nursing role. However, is the nurse–client relationship valued as the vehicle for promoting positive change in the client? If it is, then it is hard to account for Porter's (1993) reflection that decades of studies on psychiatric nursing practice have identified that nurses tend to interact with clients in anything but a therapeutic manner. A value which is firmly held is one which is acted upon. In terms of the value clarification process (Steele & Harmon 1983), the psychiatric profession tends to wallow in the beginning stages of choosing, prizing and even publicly declaring values and beliefs, but tends to be slower in the final step of action. Salvage (1983:11) suggests that 'we tend to latch onto buzz-words which seem valuable because they hint at something we want to incorporate in our practice'. Barker identifies some of the factors which constrain the enactment of the values which underpin the 'proper focus of nursing', not least of which are the often contradicting values underpinning the many roles required of nurses. It may be rather uncomfortable to examine the everyday practice of nursing in light of the rhetoric of nursing theory, but this may be a productive sort of discomfort.

Nurses share a common adaptive trait with the rest of humanity: that of feeling uncomfortable about being uncomfortable. Discomfort provides a message that something is wrong and a cue for behaviour to minimise the discomfort. It is discomfort that leads us to identify our choice of behaviour, as posing an ethical dilemma. It is a cue that something we prize, value and believe in may be lost or compromised. This discomfort may be synonymous with the idea of 'conscience' that Barker suggests is a human part of ethical decision making. Nurses draw on a repertoire of responses to cope with the discomfort arising from the ethical dilemmas they face each day. Barker outlines how such commonplace choices in responding to a person experiencing distress might pose an ethical dilemma. For many nurses there will be no felt discomfort, no conflict of genuine values and hence no perception of a dilemma. This is not to suggest that an ethical dilemma might not exist from some hypothetical veil of ignorance, or that the choices made are not of an ethical nature. Real human responses weigh lightly on the scales of ethical rationality but are the key motivators which guide behaviour in daily life.

Barker suggests that there is a view that all members of a multidisciplinary team should subscribe to the same value set. Discarding the values and beliefs which conflict with the more dominant values and beliefs of the team may well be an adaptive response to deal with ethical conflict, although it doesn't resolve it. For example, it is an enticing position to regard human distress as arising primarily from biological mechanisms and to view the key nursing roles as assessing, monitoring and evaluating symptoms of illness. The person experiencing mental distress may be viewed as 'not in control', requiring some corrective biological intervention and the person's response requiring 'management' until it is able to be achieved. The interpersonal relationship may become little more than a vehicle to ensure compliance with medical treatment or to instil insight (which amounts to the person's adopting the same beliefs about the nature of his or her distress as the nurse). Success in these endeavours is likely to bring rewards for the nurse, whilst enactment of roles which don't further these aims might be met with negative sanctions or conceptualised as some negative type of transference. The offshoot of this for the nurse may be a constriction in the repertoire of roles she or he can draw on in a given situation, an easing of discomfort arising from conflicting values, and a selective vision which is blind to the ethical dimensions of everyday practice. In the extreme, the nurse no longer selects roles, rather the roles become nursing.

There is of course a myriad of responses that people may employ to deal with the discomfort arising from ethical choices. These are as diverse and potentially constructive or destructive as the range of ordinary human responses to anxiety. The continual migration of staff from acute inpatient services into other areas of nursing and the endemic burnout in those that remain is perhaps testimony to the ethical discomfort that can arise in these areas. Some will decry nurse education and the 'theory–practice gap', and others will theorise why such a gap exists. Barker states that nurses need to constantly review their attitudes and beliefs and the values which underpin them. This is inevitably an uncomfortable process which requires us to own, experience and reflect on the source of our anxiety. What is more, the process of ethical choice may not alleviate our anxiety.

Ethical dilemmas invariably involve choices in which one or more cherished values or beliefs are compromised. But through the process of reflection we might at least become aware of what it is we cherish and be more assured that we have made the right choices. Barker challenges us to do this and would no doubt agree with Street (1990) who suggests that rather than view practice from the high ground we should descend to the swampy lowland through the process of reflection, where messy confusing problems defy technical solution but where the realities of practice in its context may be found. It is in the swamp where the reflective practitioner can view things as they really are, complete with philosophical contradictions. It is here that the dimensions of uncertainty, uniqueness and value conflict will be visible in problematic areas of practice, and, I might add, where the solutions can be found.

REFERENCES

Frankl V 1962 Basic concepts of logotherapy. Journal of Existential Psychiatry 3: 11–18
Johnstone M-J 1989 Bioethics: a nursing perspective. W B Saunders, Sydney
Peplau H E 1992 Interpersonal relations: a theoretical framework for application in nursing practice. Nursing Science Quarterly 5(1):13–18
Porter S 1993 The determinants of psychiatric nursing practice: a comparison of

sociological perspectives. Journal of Advanced Nursing 18: 1559–1566

Salvage J 1983 What's in a name? Nursing Times 18th May:11–12

Salvage J 1990 The theory and practice of the 'new nursing'. Nursing Times 86(1):42–45

Steele S M, Harmon V M 1983 Values clarification in nursing. Prentice-Hall, London

Street A 1990 Nursing practice: high, hard ground, messy swamps and the pathways in between. Deakin University Press, Victoria, Australia

Sykes J B (ed) 1982 The concise Oxford dictionary of current English, 7th edn. University Press, Oxford

Tschudin V 1992 Ethics in nursing: the caring ethic, 2nd edn. Butterworth-Heinemann, Oxford

Prejudice and sexuality

THE NATURE OF PREJUDICE

The origins of *prejudice* are to be found in the Latin *praejudicium*, which, like most words, no longer has the meaning first intended. In its ancient sense it meant a precedent, or judgement, based on previous decisions or experience. Later, as an English word, it developed an emphasis on judgement made without due consideration of the facts – a premature or hasty judgement. For some time now, *prejudice* has emphasised the emotional context of the show of favour, or disfavour, which accompanies such unsupported judgements.

W C Fields remarked, wisely, that he was free of all prejudice: he hated everyone equally.

William Hazlitt believed that prejudice – the child of ignorance – was never easy, 'unless passed off as reason'. I wonder how many of us have become competent at such passing off. Prejudice in Voltaire's view was 'the reason of fools'. For, as John Stuart Mill said, 'he who knows only his own side of the case knows little of that'. And William Addison acknowledged the painful truth that prejudice *and* self-sufficiency naturally proceed from inexperience of the world, and ignorance of mankind. This appears to be the rub. So many prejudices put one human against another in the blissful ignorance that such divisions can ever work – that we can do without one another.

A key feature of prejudice, whether showing favour or disfavour, is that it involves a paradox. When we hold a prejudice, for or against something, this involves an act of will. Prejudice is learned – it is not instinctive. We are born with no prejudices, only animalistic fears which may feed prejudice. The sum of all our prejudices represents a major aspect of our human identity: who we are.

At the same time, however, the exercise of prejudice requires us *not* to think, *not* to be open to the evidence or experiences that might determine a different outcome. This decision *not* to think represents the paradox of prejudice. We might say that prejudice is unwarranted: without sufficient moral justification. This echoes Hazlitt's conclusion that it was born out of ignorance. As the wit noted: 'prejudice is being down on something you're not up on' (Allport 1958). This highlights a critical dimension of many prejudices – that it is so easy to be prejudiced: there is no need to think about it, it is 'common sense'. And, as Albert Einstein remarked, what else is common sense but the collection of prejudices acquired by the age of eighteen.

Anti-Semitism is perhaps the most widely recognised form of prejudice. Because of the emotional context of prejudice, we rarely consider whether being opposed to people who are prejudiced is, in itself, a prejudice. If I am deeply uncomfortable about anti-Semitism and join the Anti-Nazi League, is my hatred of people who are anti-Semitic, of itself, a prejudice? More specifically, at what point does morality enter the equation? Is it acceptable to have prejudiced thoughts, providing we don't act on them? Are prejudiced thoughts morally neutral? Who determines what are the boundaries of this moral conundrum? Where can I go to look up the answer to this riddle? How can we be sure that any conclusions we reach, or those of someone in authority who serves as our oracle, are not also prejudiced? (McLeish 1994).

The nature of prejudice may even be more complex. Essentially, prejudice involves the expression of preference. Expressing preferences is one of the most frequent human behaviours: choosing this over that. In that sense, prejudice – as preference – is normal. Or at least, as I shall discuss in a moment, it is uncommonly common.

However, the expression of preference is not without its problems. When you go for a picnic and it rains, you are disappointed, feel cheated, and become angry. You would have preferred the sun to shine. The downpour, however, saved a crop in an adjoining field. The rain, which made you so miserable, increased the crop yield and, eventually, provided food that someone else used to go on a picnic. Prejudice may be the price we have to pay for our preferences, as I shall discuss in a moment,

We often speak, casually, of our prejudices, biases and points of view *as if* these were related, if not the same. Just because we do not agree with someone's position (assumed bias) or point of view, does not render them prejudices. We should reserve *prejudice* for convictions that are formed prior to *any* examination of the evidence. In bowls, the ball has an in-built bias, which causes it to roll away from the straight line. This is a permanent feature of the bowl, but it can be recognised and offset by a skillful player (Flew 1991:208). A bias in thinking is similar, reflecting a disposition to underestimate or overestimate in a particular direction. Men who believe they are better than women at this or that, are biased, not prejudiced. Such biases can be compensated for, as prejudices may be identified and examined in an open-minded manner, but only by those who are ready, or can be encouraged to develop beliefs which – however uncomfortable – are built on evidence and are, one hopes, true. Points of view, on the other hand, merely reflect a position or direction of an observation. Depending on where we are standing, we shall – of necessity – have a restricted view. By changing our position, or being required to – as in a reverse role play, when we take the position of 'the other' – we become aware of that which was screened from us by the limits of our 'point of view'.

THE ADOPTION OF PREJUDICE

Prejudice is a social phenomenon, focused largely on our loyalties and membership of social groupings. H G Wells described this aptly:

'He has a strong feeling for systematic botanists as against plant
physiologists, whom he regards as lewd and evil scoundrels in this relation;

but he has a strong feeling for all botanists and indeed all biologists, as against physicists, and those who profess the exact sciences, all of whom he regards as dull, mechanical, ugly-minded scoundrels in this relation; but he has a strong feeling for all who profess what he calls Science, as against psychologists, sociologists, philosophers, and literary men, whom he regards as wild, foolish, immoral scoundrels in this relation; but he has a strong feeling for all educated men as against the working man, whom he regards as a cheating, loafing, drunken, thievish, dirty scoundrel in this relation; but as soon as the working man is comprehended together with these others, as Englishmen ... *he holds them superior to all sorts of Europeans, whom he regards ... (and so it goes on, potentially,* ad infinitum*)' (cited by Allport 1958).*

I could easily rewrite that as a Celtic monologue, narrowing it to cover only the lowland Scots and their famous jibe – performed as a toast: 'Here's tae us; wha's like us? Damned few—and they're a' deid'.

For prejudice is linked strongly to pride. We feel a great sense of pride in the groups to which we are affiliated. Membership of groups often leads to a feeling of superiority over those who are not members, especially those who have been excluded, for whatever reason. Superiority also breeds prejudice. There is no point in being superior without the existence of an inferior grouping; indeed it is not logically possible. Superiority requires inferiors, whether real or imaginary.

'Superiority requires inferiors, whether real or imaginary'

The various means and motivations which lead to the formation of social groupings, is a vast topic, quite beyond the scope of this chapter. One form of social grouping that has been around for at least a half-century, and is relevant to this discussion, is the *in-group*. In the 1960s, this was translated into the concept of the 'in-crowd' – reified in a song with the catchy, but banal title: 'I'm in with the in-crowd'. More recently, in England, the Sloane Rangers became a widely-publicised in-crowd, because of the purported membership by young members of the Royal family. I shall return to some of the implications of such in-crowd membership later. For the moment it need only be said that tension *between* groups of people depends, paradoxically, on similarity, rather than difference. Only when groups of people are similar – or related in some sense – do they become acutely aware of their differences. Consider the enmity between brothers and sisters; or the bitterness within families or religious sects, or for that matter, countries – like former Yugoslavia.

THE IMPACT OF PREJUDICE

One of the key effects of prejudice is its power to create the world of our fears. The assumption that – at least on a social level – there is any 'world out there' is misconceived. Instead, it seems that there is consensus that we participate in the creation of our world of reality. At least this seems true for those who have thought long and hard about it. Take this as one such example of long, hard thinking.

'the essence of existence (reality) is meaning, and the essence of meaning is communication defined as the joint product of all the evidence available to those who communicate. In this view meaning rests on action, which means decisions, which in turn force the choice between complementary questions and the distinguishing of answers' (Casti 1989:449).

Since time immemorial we have assumed that there is a world 'out there', an objective reality which exists independent of us, the observers of the world who inhabit that reality. For some time now, physicists have begun to dispute the existence of such a world 'out there', which is independent of us, the observers. My quote, above, was from J A Wheeler, the physicist, who has popularised the notion of the *contextual* as opposed to *objective* reality. I refer to these contemporary developments in physics by way of emphasising what is, in my view, the *obvious* reality: that we construct our social world, and all its associated values, beliefs, preferences and prejudices, through our participation in that contextual reality. People are neither, indeed cannot be either, 'this' or 'that', 'good' or 'bad', 'right' or 'wrong' – *as if* they had been born that way, or even occupied some fixed spot which is (territorially) far removed from the fixed spot on which we stand. Such ideas of 'fixed spots' are illusions. All our ideas about ourselves and others, which we use in our lives, are no more than that – ideas: clouds of shifting reason, the composition of which we are largely uncertain, but the shape and effect of which are evident to most of us. At least, they are when we witness such ideas enacted – as in the form of prejudice.

Fifty years ago, Robert Merton offered us the term 'the self-fulfilling prophecy' to define the countless subtle ways in which our expectation that certain behaviours *will* occur in others, serves to evoke such behaviour. This well-used expression explains why so many of us come to believe that our prejudices are no less than a recognition of a social reality – a reality which we have helped construct, through our expressions of prejudice. Shaw said that the American created the boot-black for the negro so that he could look down on him every day.

'many of us come to believe that our prejudices, are no less than a recognition of a social reality – a reality which we have helped construct, through our expressions of prejudice'

Prejudice has many effects on its victims:

- psychological consequences: when people become aware that they are being judged, universally, as inferior, they risk suffering loss of self-respect, which can in turn bring about a loss of their sense of social responsibility – why should I contribute to a society from which I have been excluded?
- loss of opportunity, reducing their capacity for joyful living
- destruction of initiative, impairment of creative and inventive aptitudes
- the risk of provocation and retaliatory action
- fracturing of society.

It was once said that civilisation is just the slow process of getting rid of our prejudices. If that is true, then civilisation has been a long time coming.

NORMATIVE TERRORISM

We attempted to address some of our difficulties with prejudice by the manipulation of language. More than forty years ago, in the USA, where political correctness was born, the traditional teaching of the *Merchant of Venice* in schools was challenged, on the grounds that if students did not study the character of Shylock sufficiently deeply, young people might develop stereotyped views of the Jewish person in American society. Around the same time, traditional stories aimed at younger people became suspect. *Little Black Sambo* was seen as portraying the black child as silly and greedy, among other things, and *Pinocchio* as potentially harmful because of the close association of Pinocchio with 'assassins'. Some of my childhood characters have also been 'cleansed' from childhood literature because of their stereotypic potential – not least Little Plum my Redskin Chum. Ironically, such cleansing may merely make matters worse. Lack of exposure to the images and narratives is seen as protecting young minds from corruption. Better, perhaps, to strengthen all our abilities to distinguish the stereotype and to acquire the critical power to handle the potential impact of such images and stories in our social and interpersonal worlds.

One of the common ways that we have of counteracting prejudice is to cite examples of famous members of the 'out-group'. In the area of sexuality there is no shortage of famous people who challenged the prejudices of their day by 'coming out' as women or men of a different sexual persuasion. A growth industry has emerged in identifying famous figures from the past who, on the basis of available evidence might have been homosexual, lesbian or bisexual. These seem to be unfortunate attempts to challenge prejudice, by demolishing its assumption of inferiority for the prejudiced group. What any minority group needs – perhaps fundamentally wants – is not the recognition that geniuses from all fields of human endeavour have been ranked among their number, but the right to have fools, rascals and complete wastrels among their number, without being condemned as a group. Geniuses and fools, altruists and philosophers appear equally distributed among most social groups. Only when perceived wrongdoers are identified among minority groups do we highlight their weaknesses. Trying to counterbalance such prejudice by highlighting the successful members of the minority group serves only to diminish the basic humanity of all the members.

VALUES, ATTITUDES AND BELIEF SYSTEMS

To what extent is it easy to challenge and modify prejudice concerning sexuality, or indeed any dimension of human behaviour. The research literature would suggest that it is not all easy, since we are trying to manipulate stereotypes which either are well-established, or ingrained; or serve some adaptive function, especially at an unconscious level (Hamilton 1981). Simply providing people with information, which does not fit their stereotypes, is rarely effective in changing attitudes towards the 'out-group'. The challenge to prejudice involves a shift in a person's fundamental assumptions, and requires to be validated through experience, as well as with the support of valid information. Information alone simply will not do. The effects of, even simple experience of in-group and out-group membership can be profound and lasting.

A teacher in a small Iowa town in the 1980s divided her class on the basis of eye colour, arbitrarily giving more privileges to one over the other. The privileged eye colour was changed the second day, so both groups had a chance to experience discrimination. Fifteen years later, the grown children testified to the powerful impact of the demonstration, claiming profound effects on their understanding and treatment of others (Janoff-Bulman & Schwartzberg 1991). Such demonstrations appear to signal the importance of validity derived from direct experience: 'emotional' knowledge that allows us to accept anomalous experience and to integrate new information with old assumptions.

Prejudice, in the context of sexuality and sexual mores, appears to possess some special characteristics: in particular, the hypothesis that homophobia – for which we might read any extreme rejection of alternative sexual orientation – derives from a death anxiety.

Thirty years ago, when homosexual relations 'between consenting adults in private' were decriminalised, the spirit of the decade allowed the establishment of a consensus of tolerance (Levidow 1989). This consensus was based on the reassuring belief that homosexuals posed no threat, since they 'formed an almost distinct subspecies, to be pitied and left in peace' (Levidow 1989:196). Thirty years on we are much less tolerant, and our patronising attitude, which was a psychic defence, has collapsed in the face of the provocation and public display of homosexuality and lesbianism, which generates an intolerable anxiety. The demands that have been mounting from gay rights groups for acceptance as equals, rather than as objects of pity, have provoked this death anxiety. In an era when the fear has been expressed that the 'normal family' may be dead, or at least dying, the challenge presented by alternative sexuality and sexual mores heightens such fears. A decade ago, we saw and heard the first arguments for 'Positive Images' of gay and lesbian people. These campaigns were, arguably, the key stimulus for the death anxiety felt by many parents, who feared that their children would be shaped into becoming gay. Right-wing politicians and the tabloid press, of course, expressed those anxieties best. Although complicated by the threat of biological death through AIDS, the threat was mainly symbolic, not actual: death of innocence, death of heterosexual identity, death of parental/adult authority, death of the natural order, even a feeling that a child turned gay might just as well be dead. As Levidow noted, 'within that psychic continuum, homosexuality doesn't simply cause disease: it *is* a disease, a deadly social disease, (Levidow 1989:186).

To the rational mind this is the height of unreason. As I noted earlier, however, prejudice is not about reason. Indeed, reason may merely make matters worse. It was reason which led gay couples to seek to adopt children. It was reason which led gay activists to assert their basic humanity, to take to the streets in numerous public displays of 'gay pride', culminating, in 1997, in the public recognition of the gay men and women who have died for their country. All these were and are quite reasonable displays in the true sense of the word. However, paradoxically, the more powerful the evidence, the greater the resistance.

The concept of resistance leads us to consider prejudice as a form of terror management. It is accepted that threats to meaning generate anxiety which, in turn, generates defences which, when enacted, reduce anxiety. Religious groups which predict the end of the world, do not disband when it does not materialise; they engage in post-hoc rationalisations, increased faith and renewal of efforts to recruit more followers to validate their group (Festinger et al 1956). This illustrates the great myth of reason – most people are simply not reasonable. When it comes to in-groups and out-groups the absence of reason also is evident. Numerous studies show how people who do not conform to our values, do not agree with our attitudes or who try to promote an alternative lifestyle, threaten our faith in the validity of our worldview. Faced with this possible crisis of

'people who do not conform to our values, do not agree with our attitudes or who try to promote an alternative lifestyle, threaten our faith in the validity of our worldview'

faith, we do not review (reasonably) the evidence for our worldview – as a scientist might – but are more likely to respond like those who failed to predict the final coming: we defend our faith, and recruit new members to offset the threat. We also tend to return the threat with interest.

It could be argued that one effect of gay liberation was an increase in anxiety levels in people who already felt vulnerable about their sexuality. The provocative, and often aggressive, tactics proposed but not always implemented regarding, for example, 'outing' of public figures, may be one example of self-defeating strategies. Such attempts to provoke an honest appraisal of the state of sexuality in contemporary society are justifiable, if one considers the double-standards, denial and deception which is being challenged. The question under consideration here is more expedient: not 'is such action right?' but 'will such action help reduce or increase the state of sexual prejudice?'. They succeeded only in reinforcing the fear concerning the threat they posed.

The current state of homophobia could be read as a moral panic in decline. Cohen, appeared to be the first to use this term in his description of public – especially media – reactions to the Mods and Rockers clashes of the 1960s. He described the media as setting the normative boundaries 'beyond which one should not venture and the shapes the devil can assume' (Cohen 1973). Such moral panics have appeared frequently: some condition, an episode, a person or group is identified as a threat to societal values or interests. In Cohen's view, the nature of the panic is presented in a stylised and stereotypical fashion by the mass media.

'The moral barricades are manned by editors, bishops, politicians and other right-thinking people; socially-accredited experts pronounce their diagnoses and solutions; ways of coping are evolved or (more often) resorted to; the condition then disappears, submerges, or deteriorates and becomes invisible. Sometimes the panic is passed over and forgotten. At other times it has more serious long-term repercussions and might produce changes in legal and social policy or even in the way society conceives itself' (Cohen 1973:9).

The witch trials in Cromwell's England and in Salem; the McCarthy communist 'witch-hunt'; the persecution of the Jews in Nazi Germany; and more recently, the exclusion of homosexuals, are classic examples of moral panics. Where are we now on Cohen's continuum? The media is no longer manning the barricades and the public anxiety may have peaked and be transforming to deal with new threats to the public self-system. The most recent moral panic has focused on the creation of the so-called 'seriously mentally ill', in the wake of the failure of community care for people with more complex mental health problems, social deprivation or both (Barker & Jackson 1996, Barker et al 1998). This panic also appears to be subsiding, its place being taken by paedophiles: 'appearing soon in a neighbourhood near you'. This, however, might merely serve to return homophobia to the top of the prejudice agenda – the assumption that homosexuality and paedophilia are the same being one of the cornerstones of prejudice.

If one accepts this perspective – and there might be several good reasons to reject it, paranoia being part of most of them – then one might conclude that the heat is off as far as the whole prejudice and sexuality issue is concerned. I suspect, however, that this is a premature conclusion. More realistically, we have merely moved to another stage of our socio-sexual development. There is still work to be done, in fostering the development of truly human (if not also humanitarian) attitudes toward sexual preference and sexual mores.

SEXUALITY, PREFERENCE AND ORIENTATION

It seems a long time since the sexual revolution of the 1960s, and yet, to a large extent, we seem still shackled to a neurotic notion of sexuality. Recently, we have seen a rather public debate over the appropriateness of billboard advertisements portraying women stamping on naked men with their high-heels. Some would argue that this is a signifier of liberation. Maybe its just about selling jeans. For some time there has been a good living to be made implanting silicone into the female breast. More recently, a new area has opened up for cosmetic entrepreneurs, in implanting fat into the male penis. Vanity, folly or neurosis: take your pick.

I mention these contemporary issues which appear, superficially, to involve sex and sexuality, but may have a deeper meaning, a subtext, concerning power, territoriality and anxiety. In a similar vein, Susan Sontag suggested that 'what pornography is really about, ultimately, isn't sex, but death'.

When I was young we used to try not to talk about sex, recognising that those who talked about it, had little experience of it. James Baldwin turned that concept around: 'money, it turned out', he said, 'was exactly like sex, you thought of nothing else if you didn't have it, and thought of other things if you did'. Of course sex isn't always a serious business. Sex can be the most fun you can have without laughing, as Woody Allen noted. And if you are fortunate enough to be attracted sexually to both sexes then it immediately doubles your chances for some fun on Saturday night.' And our ideas of what sex is all about constantly changes. As my old friend Tom

Szasz said of masturbation, 'it's the primary sexual activity of mankind. In the 19th century it was a disease and in the 20th century it's a cure'. And, although Freud saw creativity as the sublimation of deep-rooted sexual conflicts, David Lodge, the English novelist wrote recently, 'I gave up screwing around a long time ago. I came to the conclusion that sex is the sublimation of the work instinct'. Anyone who read the recent account of John F Kennedy's sexual reign in the White House might come to similar conclusions. Certainly, Kennedy and his brothers seemed to spend more time in the pool frolicking with carefully-selected sex-kittens, than overtly managing the most powerful nation on Earth. Although Nixon was commonly blamed for shafting America, it appears that Kennedy was also screwing the taxpayer, who assumed that he was engaged in sweating over Castro, rather than concubines. And here, we might find some real reason to be judgemental about sex, when it takes the form of abuse – either of people or of power.

For at least the past two thousand years we have been involved in trying to unravel sex and sexuality. It remains uncertain to what extent we are any the wiser. For a long time we have known that sex is conducted differently from place to place, as well as from time to time. As Gauguin noted, 'In Europe men and women have intercourse because they love each other. In the South Seas they love each other because they have had intercourse. Who is right?'. Malcolm Muggeridge wryly observed that the English have sex on the brain which, as he noted, was a very unsatisfactory place to have it. But what is there to think about – or rather to reflect on, apart from old glories. Sex *is*, as Gore Vidal said. There is nothing more to be done about it. Sex builds no roads, sex writes no novels and sex certainly gives no meaning to anything in life but sex itself. At the station and airport I stand bemused in the newsagent, scanning the rows of women's and men's magazines, all vying to have the catchiest headline and raunchiest picture. These publicists clearly haven't read Vidal's conclusion. Or perhaps they have. That may be why sex is such an industry. Everyone is working very hard to make something of it which was not there before and maybe will never be there. Sex as a living dream industry. This is sex as a commodity: part of the consumerist nightmare. Advertisers have long wanted us to doubt the value of our appliances, cars and cookers, so that they can sell us a new one which we really don't need. Now they have hit on the realisation that they can make us doubt the value of our sexuality and sex lives. Now they can sell us a new sex-dream.

Our prejudices about sexuality are not deep rooted: they are superficial like most prejudices, flimsy, premature judgements based on a rag-bag of assumptions. Most of the problems concerning sexuality involve little more than a chronic form of nosiness. As Evelyn Laye, the actress noted, 'sex, unlike justice, should be seen not to be done'. Paradoxically, the more we drag this best bit of fun between consenting adults into the public eye the more anxious we seem to get about it. I am waiting for the inevitable retreat of sexual behaviour and

'I am waiting for the inevitable retreat of sexual behaviour and sexuality: its return to the private world from whence it came and within which it might recover some of the potency it lost by trying to turn a private affair into a public entertainment'

sexuality: its return to the private world from whence it came, and within which it might recover some of the potency it lost by trying to turn a private affair into a public entertainment.

Although some excitement was stirred up by the prospect that we might have discovered the gene that determines sexuality, I remain doubtful. Indeed, I remain cynical about most of these genetic markers. For a long time it has been accepted that sexuality and relationships are closely connected. We use sex to express affection and anger. How we come to express more of one or the other is a developmental issue, and concerns how we become 'who' we are: our spiritual selves. How we become heterosexual, homosexual, bisexual or transsexual, clearly involves a complex interaction of human experience (development) overlaid on biology, both interacting with the broader canvas of our society and culture. This picture is complicated further by the obvious presence, within people, of masculine and feminine selves: Jung's animus and anima, which often are concealed by the appearance endowed by biology. The assumption that all women are feminine 'all of the time' and men masculine, is questionable. The women's movement – and the Johnny-come-latelys of the men's movement – challenge these stereotypes. Men can be sensitive and vulnerable and women can enjoy talking about sex, even talking dirty. Our prejudices leap to the conclusion that this exemplifies 'cissies' or 'trollops'. Closer examination may reveal that these variations reflect the increasing complexity of sexuality. Our ideas about what sex means generally, what it means to us in particular, are complex. What is our unique sexual identity – indeed do we even have one – are questions which become more complex, the more we talk and write and make films and cross reference all these images, icons, assumptions and tentative conclusions in this intellectual mess we call post-modernity.

When we reflect on these issues, their philosophical basis becomes all-too transparent. Few of us enjoy philosophy, especially moral philosophy, since it leads us ultimately to consider notions such as 'what is right and fitting?' and 'what is right or wrong?'. For most of us, these questions are virtually unanswerable. We resolve the dilemmas they pose by turning to the rules and limitations of social institutions, or become hedonists, anarchists or ostriches. I introduce the ethical dimension merely to provide myself with an easy access to the final dimension of prejudice: its effect on the social construction of sexuality as a spiritual project – part of the ongoing construction of the self.

Much has changed in the past thirty years, but perhaps we have only taken a short step from prejudice to pity and back again. People on the receiving end often describe the experience of prejudice and pity in similarly distasteful terms. John Daniel has written of his experience at a well-known HIV centre where

> 'one afternoon, a group of lads were happily watching television, only to be disturbed by a troupe of volunteers, who had returned from a rather grand funeral, laden with flowers. With suitable solemnity and to the disbelief of the residents, they decorated the sitting room with the funeral bouquets,

modifying the atmosphere from that of an enjoyable social space to that of a chapel of rest. Pedestrians four floors below were no doubt mystified a short while later to find themselves showered with carnations, lilies and chrysanthemums' (Daniel 1997:329).

This represents an update on the pity first expressed towards 'consenting homosexual adults'. The effect of conferring victim status on people with HIV/AIDS is marginalisation: the centre wishing to keep the person at the edge of their social world.

John Daniel's experience in the border country of HIV/AIDS serves as a fine analogy for the spiritual journey many of us take as we drift away from the centre, or even strive to reach the assumed margins of our social world. The mere act of exploring our world, its inherent assumptions and often insane presumptions, may alienate us from those who are comfortable only at the plumb centre. Daniel says that in this border country one is asked to account for oneself: to declare one's assets, show a passport, to *identify* ourselves. However, the process of crossing the border necessitated by HIV/AIDS requires us to establish and realise a new identity: refusing to be labelled, even when our conduct is assessed as beyond the bounds of reason. In Daniel's words:

> 'The mere act of exploring our world, its inherent assumptions and often insane presumptions, may alienate us from those who are comfortable only at the plumb centre'

'In accepting the energy generated in border country, which involves the full realisation of death and disorder and disintegration, one approaches, I believe a state of fullness. Fullness of darkness, of misery and persecution, but also fullness of life and joy. All of us find it hard to be confronted by such fullness' (Daniel 1997).

I conclude with John Daniel's wise words. The threat to our identity posed by all forms of prejudice might also, to the Chinese mind, be seen as an opportunity – an opportunity to review our emerging identity, to return the prejudiced stare with compassion. How we all deal with our own prejudices as well as those of our public is a necessarily complex business. As I noted earlier, the superficial nature of prejudice is misleading, since it is like a thin veneer which covers a host of deeper issues – personal, cultural and social. In addition to recognising this complexity, we might also try addressing – rather than attacking – prejudice on the widest possible front, using the widest possible range of means.

NOTE

This chapter is based on a paper presented to the Third Regional Conference for HIV/AIDS Trainers, Newcastle, Co Down, Northern Ireland, on 27 November 1997.

REFERENCES

Allport G W 1958 The nature of prejudice. Doubleday, New York

Casti J L 1989 Paradigms lost: images of man in the mirror of science. Abacus, London

Cohen S 1973 Folk devils and moral panics: the creation of the mods and the rockers. Paladin, London

Daniel J 1997 Reframing the experience of AIDS, marginalisation, liminality and beyond. In: Barker P, Davidson B (eds) Psychiatric nursing: ethical strife. Arnold, London

Festinger L, Riecken H, Schacter S 1956 When prophecy fails. University of Minnesota Press, Minneapolis

Flew A 1991 Thinking about social thinking: escaping deception, resisting self-deception. Fontana, London

Hamilton D ed 1981 Cognitive processes in stereotyping and group behaviour. Erlbaum, Hillsdale, NJ

Janoff-Bulman R, Schwartzberg S S 1991 Toward a general model of personal change. In: Snyder C R, Forsyth D R (eds) Handbook of social and clinical psychology: the health perspective. Pergamon, Oxford

Levidow L 1989 Witches and seducers: moral panics for our time. In: Richards B (ed) Crises of the self: further essays on psychoanalysis and politics. Free Association Books, London

McLeish K 1994 Key ideas in human thought. Bloomsbury, London

Thomas A 1997 Legal, decent, honest, truthful? Earth Matters 36 (winter) 24–25

Commentary

Steve Jamieson

Sexuality is a highly complex, multidimensional phenomenon in the integration of biological, psychological, social, interpersonal and cultural aspects of our being. It is therefore an important factor in nursing and health care. As with all stereotypes, those which operate in this context are wasteful of men's and women's caring and intellectual capacities and hurtful to their self-concepts. Self expression is curbed and prejudice given free rein. History has led us to the position in which sexuality plays a determining role in health care but, simultaneously, fundamental issues of sexuality are neglected for professionals and patients alike. Holistic care is much discussed but little practised, at least in respect of sexuality.

The victims of prejudice in sexuality are, in my opinion, every member of society. We all have prejudices and we all have felt vulnerable about our sexuality. Sexuality is heavily regulated in all societies. One measure of the strength of this regulation is the extent to which social rules governing sexuality are internalised into public attitudes and opinions. Prejudices are reinforced by beliefs and often attract strong feelings that will lead to particular forms of behaviour.

However, the more knowledge individuals have about sexuality issues, the more open and flexible they are likely to be in their attitudes towards their own and others' behaviour, and their personal development and interpersonal relationships will benefit as well as their professional work.

The exercise of prejudice and sexuality is one which dominates the health care profession and causes many nurses to adopt a state of avoidance when faced with the possibility of talking to a patient about sex. As the chapter highlights, the issue of morality is entwined in all our beliefs around sexuality but do we actually act on them either directly or indirectly? Just because we may not have the same sexual orientation or insight into someone's sexuality does not justify our sometimes dismissive, or in some cases totally unacceptable, behaviour and attitude.

I have had the unfortunate and very distressing task of dealing with a patient in the terminal stage of an HIV illness where his parents had disowned him due to his sexual orientation and, more alarmingly, where an agency psychiatric nurse on a HIV medical ward refused to care for him because she was afraid of contracting the virus. This highlighted two main issues for me:

- The difficulty that sexual orientation and sexuality have on society in relation to acceptance. This paper clearly points out the impact of prejudice as a social phenomenon which focuses mainly on people belonging to social groupings. This patient did not fit into his parents' membership group because of his sexuality, and therefore they acted by demanding that he left his home and did not return to them until 'he had converted to their moral beliefs and standards'.
- Secondly, the nursing profession once again let themselves down by their lack of knowledge about his illness and reacted in a hostile and,

I guess, scared manner. Bor & Watts (1993) suggest that talking to patients about sexual matters is as difficult as addressing death and dying.

Nurses and, in my experience, mental health nurses have a cognitive and behavioural block in this area which includes embarrassment, a belief that it is not relevant to the patient's care, a feeling of being inadequately trained for the task. Part of the reasons nurses experience embarrassment and don't recognise the relevance of addressing sexuality may be to do with their levels of knowledge, attitudes and prejudices towards sexuality. A number of studies have shown that student nurses have low knowledge levels about sexuality and hold conservative attitudes in comparison with other students. There is also a widespread belief among nurses that patients would not think it appropriate for them to initiate discussions about sexuality. In a study by Wilson & Williams (1988), 25% of oncology nurses had never offered sexual counselling to patients, yet 91% would be happy to do so if the patient initiated the discussion.

Bor & Watts (1993) also state that negative attitudes towards some sexual lifestyles and practices, such as homosexuality, are a further barrier to communication. Studies carried out in the context of care of people with HIV and AIDS have shown that many nurses had negative attitudes and prejudices towards gay men and felt them more deserving of their illness than other people with AIDS (Kelly et al 1988). Smith (1992) cites a definition of homophobia as 'irrational fear and hatred of anyone or anything connected with homosexuality, or a fear of one's own real or potential homosexuality'.

Sexuality and sexual health have never been higher on the nursing agenda. This is evidenced by the vast increase in the number of publications on the subject. In addition, statutory bodies such as the English National Board for Nursing, Midwifery and Health Visiting (ENB) have published sexual health learning packs for practitioners and guidelines for good practice in sexual health education and training (ENB 1994).

The increased recognition of nurses' role in health promotion has also drawn attention to sexual health issues whilst many nursing models have specifically identified sexuality as a key area for assessment and intervention. In relation to mental health nurses, Thomas (1989) acknowledges that, historically, psychiatric nurses have only addressed sexuality when it was perceived as a problem, such as a patient masturbating in a public area.

In conclusion, I feel that to examine prejudices in relation to sexuality we must all begin to 'unpack' our own feelings and beliefs and acknowledge that we are all different. This is much easier said than done. However, the acknowledgement of sexuality as an integral component of health and the recognition that we need to be open and willing to learn can only enhance our own value system and in turn our holistic care approach to our patients. I would like to end with a comment from Adam Mars Jones.

Sexuality is like painting a picture.
Today we are starting with a blank canvas.

REFERENCES

Bor R, Watts M 1993 Talking to patients about sexual matters. British Journal of Nursing 2(13):657–660

ENB 1994 Caring for people with sexually transmitted diseases, including HIV disease. English National Board for Nursing, Midwifery and Health Visiting, London

Kelly J A, St Lawrence J S, Hood H V, Smith S, Cook D J 1988 Nurses' attitudes towards AIDS. Journal of Continuing Education in Nursing 19(2):78–83

Smith G B 1992 Homosexual psychiatric patients. Journal of Psychosocial Nursing 30(12):15–21

Thomas B 1989 Asexual patients. Nursing Times 85(33):49–51

Wilson M E, Williams H A 1988 Oncology nurses' attitudes and behaviors related to sexuality of patients with cancer. Oncology Nursing Forum 13:39–43

Postscript: the postcard from Gotham

American Tails

This is a story I never told – a paper I never delivered – a collection of reflections that, perhaps, needed to lie dormant until I had established, more clearly, what they might mean.

The 'postcard' was a set of notes in the journal kept during a trip to the USA in 1994. My old friend Shirley Smoyak from Rutgers University had facilitated the study tour, and I always intended to turn these reflections into a paper for *Psychosocial Nursing*, which Shirley edits. I never got round to it.

I unearthed these afterthoughts when looking for something for Ed Manos, whom I met for the first time on the '94 trip. We were planning to meet up in April '98 in New York, as part of another short study tour. I had just finished editing this book and was thinking of an 'epilogue', when I came across the 'Postcard from Gotham'. I took this with me to New York and … the tale really begins from there.

APRIL 1994

> *'One kid to another: "lets play Patients and Health Care Providers"'*.

This sporting life

I wasn't sure what I expected of New Jersey. My father was a boxing fan who induced in me an awareness of all things American – at least as far as the fight game was concerned. Among his long list of the 'all-time greats' stood one Jersey Joe Walcott – a heavyweight champion, who later became a famous referee and enduring ambassador for the noble art. Needless to say my monochromatic memories of post-war boxing, distilled from nights spent poring over old copies of *Boxing News* or *The Ring* are light years away from contemporary New Jersey; but then I never did get around to visiting Jersey City, birth place of Jersey Joe. I am, however, connecting with the sporting symbolism that permeates, or may be even underpins, American society. It gives me a critical benchmark as I try to get to grips with the nuances of care in the community – US style.

My first adjustment was to the 'game plan', usually framed – like the coding system of American football – as optional moves. Many Americans, at least on the frantic east coast, structure their days, if not their entire lives, like a sporting event. Time is, invariably of the essence. For *Homo Sapiens Americanus*, life is a human *race*. The emphasis upon the pace of life, and the multiplicity of roles and lifestyle dimensions, illustrates neatly the east–west divide. In Zen I learned something of the reverence for the 'here and now':

living in – if not for – the moment. In much of American society – at least in the north east – the reverse is the case: the 'game planner' craves motion and is always going somewhere; and the 'life strategies' are future paced, rather than present set. This may, in part, explain the affection for change: indeed change merely for the sake of change. The restless energy of American society can be exciting. It can also be enervating. At times, however, I wondered what, exactly, was fuelling it and what it might all be *for* at the end of the day.

The power of word-play

This restless headlong rush forward may explain, in part, the pace of American life, although as one moves inland – towards 'Middle America' – the pace slows appreciably. (The New Yorker's nightmare is to wake up on the laid-back shores of the west coast.) It is easy to form the impression that the USA is a collection of countries, rather than states, such is the extent of change from one state to another. These differences might be culturally determined, depending upon which race or culture set the agenda for a town back in the pioneer days. It might also be something to do with the junior status of the 'New World'. The USA is an adolescent society, which may have matured too fast and too soon. The USA may be the symbol for the loss of childhood innocence, which so many contemporary social critics see arising from the 'forced adolescence' produced by the technological transformation of the (post)modern world: what Alvin Toffler called 'future shock' (Toffler 1970). As we develop increasingly sophisticated ways of communicating, McLuhan's global village has shrunk to the size of a hamlet. Increasingly, I get the feeling that we have little to say to one another.

I discovered a few disturbing expressions of this in the American 'sculpting' of the English language, where a new word or phrase seems to be coined every day. Indeed, I felt my 'Olde Worlde' hackles rising as I learned a new vocabulary of flexible epithets – most with a range of different meanings, according to the situation; phrases which would soon achieve 'street cred' back home with anyone aspiring to hipness. The Americans have reframed Lewis Carroll, or maybe even Wittgenstein: words can mean whatever they choose them to mean – neither more nor less. Such anarchic constructivism is, of course, beloved of casuists – or those who reason speciously on ethical or ideological matters (Bennett 1994). This might explain the proliferation of ideologies and methodologies, which the USA has witnessed in recent years. This led me to think of Shakespeare, with a few thousand words at his disposal, fashioning countless memorable explorations and illustrations of the human condition. I wondered then why, with almost ten times as many words, we are often lost for words; drowning in a sea of verbal lifebelts? In community care terms, why are we able to talk so volubly about 'it' yet fail repeatedly to achieve much in the way of consensus?

De-institutionalisation

These reflections on word-games were sparked by informal observations of mental health services in New Jersey.[1] I was intrigued, repeatedly, by the way services were described: by the rhetorical language, both of front-line staff and sophisticated researchers. Here I discovered an important linguistic lesson: those who were most profligate with the language were least likely to be involved in the business of change.

Greystone Park Psychiatric Hospital is a 657 bed public institution outside of Morristown, funded by the State of New Jersey. Greystone Park has provided mental health services to the Northern Region of New Jersey since 1876. The hospital was the result of lobbying by Dorothea Dix, schoolteacher turned pioneering mental health reformer, who prised two and a half million dollars from the legislature to purchase the 450 acres upon which Greystone still stands. Thomas Kirkbride, Superintendent at the Philadelphia Asylum, influenced the design of what became the State Lunatic Asylum at Morristown. Kirkbride believed that a hospital should house no more than 250 patients;[2] should be light and airy with only two patients to a bedroom; and use as little wood as possible, to offset the possibility of fire. The huge stone-built edifice is, as a result, greatly at odds with the largely wooden construction of private homes and public buildings in New Jersey, where stone has always been at a premium.

Kirkbride's design resulted in a 'Main Building' built in sets of three wings, each 140 feet long on five floors. Each wing was set back from the preceding, 'to allow the inmates to view the beauty of the surroundings'. Greystone Park was the largest edifice on a single foundation in the USA until Washington completed the Pentagon in 1943.

The massive 16-foot high oak doors of the Main Building opened for the first time when, on a hot August day in 1876, a train transferred 292 patients from the grossly overcrowded State Lunatic Asylum at Trenton, New Jersey. No major structural changes at Greystone Park were undertaken until the early 1920s when the State Board of Mental Hygiene found it to be overcrowded and in dire need of repair. By then Greystone, which originally had 600 beds, housed more than 2,700 patients. With the end of the Second World War, Greystone Park became home for large numbers of war veterans, suffering from post-war trauma, or 'shell shock'. By then the census showed more than 7,000 patients, and Greystone Park had become a town in its own right, with its own postal address and a Post Office, which remains in operation today.

In 1982, the hospital opened 20 'independent living' cottages, which provide accommodation for eight patients in a normal home-like atmosphere where patients share a bedroom in the tradition first espoused by Dr Kirkbride more than a century ago. Today Greystone Park works in close partnership with a range of Community Mental Health Centers, Screening Centers and local Community hospitals. Patients can only be admitted to Greystone Park by referral from a designated 'Screening Center' or a Court Order signed by a Judge.[3]

My visit to Greystone Park provided a new appreciation of an old psychiatric word and an introduction to a new one – albeit long established in American terms. I had known the term 'back ward' for almost thirty years, since my student days. It was used as a popular, derogatory adjective for any 'long term' facility where patients might spend years or a whole lifetime in 'care'. I did not appreciate that it derived from the 'stepwise' architectural progression designed by Kirkbride, where patients moved through, increasingly, longer-term placements. New patients were admitted to wards at the front of the Main Building. If successfully 'treated', they would be discharged. If not, they would move 'back' to the next level, or wing, for further treatment; and so on until they arrived at the 'back wards' of the institution – where many would end their days. Although from the outside one can walk from the front entrance to the back of the Main Building in about three minutes, in its heyday the internal journey – through double locked doors connecting each wing – took at least 20 minutes. As my footsteps echoed along these corridors, now eerily empty, the sense of stepping back in time, and the kinaesthetic appreciation of making the stepwise progression from admission to 'back ward,' was all-pervasive.

I learned too that State Hospitals are no longer 'warehousing' patients, but emphasise rapid treatment and early discharge. The exact meaning of 'warehousing' remains unclear, since it is distinct from both long-term and custodial care. Again, I 'sensed' the meaning as I craned my neck to see the highest windows on the top floor of each wing. The majestic entrance, like those of many British asylums, was a theatrical sham. After passing through the grandeur of the foyer, with its etched glass windows and oak-panelled walls, Greystone strips down to its bare essentials: the human warehouse. Those patients who entered were stripped down both physically and metaphorically, as they too passed from the sham to the reality. The first shipment of residents had arrived, ironically by freight train. For the majority, this had been a road to nowhere: a human storage system with a very flexible shelf life.

The advanced nurse practitioner

One of my interests was in the development of psychiatric nursing in New Jersey. Staff recruitment ads at Greystone Park boasted 'A New Approach To An Old Tradition'. I met Merle Hoagland, Director of Nursing, who, unlike most of her peers in the UK, was a multidimensional professional: a Psychiatric Clinical Nurse Specialist, a Certified Psychotherapist *and* a Quality Assurance Coordinator. Judging from her jewellery and dress, Merle could have walked out of a movie. Her style of engaging personally with every staff member we met – touching them gently *and* paying each one different compliments – suggested that Merle was the genuine article. If these were 'skills' in 'human resourcing', they were honed to near-perfection.

Clinical nursing support is provided by Clinical Nurse Specialists who function in a consultative, educational role to staff, in addition to working directly with selected patients. Compared with the UK, New Jersey appeared to have been slower to implement any distinct group of community psychiatric nurses. Traditionally, Clinical Nurse Specialists – all prepared to master's level, and all certified psychotherapists of one persuasion or another – were focused on hospitals, or community clinics. Following the heavy deinstitutionalisation programme, driven at an erratic – if not dangerous – speed by the Reagan administration, the spotlight for nursing developments has turned on the natural community.

Nurses in the USA have, for the past forty years, enjoyed a Master's level educational preparation which has focused upon the development of various forms of psychosocial intervention. The emphasis in the 1950s was upon derivatives of psychoanalytic method, which gave way increasingly to a focus upon mileu therapy, family therapy and a range of humanistic and cognitive-behavioural therapies. The Master's-prepared Clinical Nurse Specialist in the USA was, therefore, a well-prepared psychotherapist, who frequently maintained a private practice outside of her involvement as a specialist practitioner or consultant to nurses in hospital or clinic settings. (Unlike the UK, the vast majority of Masters-level psychiatric nurses are women.)

It is also noteworthy that facilities in hospitals like Greystone Park are run by a relatively small number of registered nurses (RNs) supported by nursing technicians – trained to give out medication, for example – and nursing aides. In a huge ward housing about forty men – almost all white – the aides were mainly black men. The ward in 'Cuckoo's nest' is often dismissed as an American fiction, or at least a relic of a bygone era. The ward in the film set was considerably better looking than where I stood this morning, despite Kesey's novel being based on events thirty years ago. I had a long talk there with an 'inmate' (his words) called Bud: a seventy-year old 'runaway' with a grimy baseball cap. For some reason they kept bringing back this old guy who looked as if he had walked straight out of *Grapes of Wrath*. Bud wasn't sure how long he had been in Greystone, or why. He looked as if he could have stepped down from that first train, back in 1876.

The strength of psychiatric nursing in the USA lies in that relatively small group of highly educated Clinical Nurse Specialists – many of whom have Associate Clinical Professor status in nursing faculties. Unlike nurse educationalists in the UK, American nurses who teach – and research – invariably also practice. This might explain the American fascination with theories and models of nursing practice: their diversity issuing from the wide range of clinical and therapeutic environments in which nurses are employed. Maybe we have a 'theory – practice gap' because so many educationalists have cut themselves adrift from the lifeblood of practice.

Although not all nurses in the USA have aligned themselves to particular theories or models of nursing, some University programmes declare very clear assumptions concerning the nature or 'essence' of nursing practice, which guides the development of their curriculum. The University of Medicine and Dentistry, New Jersey (UMDNJ) is New Jersey's 'University of the Health Sciences' and has a faculty of nursing which has an active partnership with Ramapo College of New Jersey and Middlesex County College, both of which also offer nursing programmes. The School of Nursing within UMDNJ offers a wide range of graduate and postgraduate programmes from baccalaureate degrees through a number of master's programmes to taught doctorates and post doctoral programmes.

Nursing at UMDNJ uses the American Nurses' Association definition that nursing involves 'the diagnosis and treatment of human responses to actual or potential health problems'. Nurses facilitate the health of humans through the nursing process. Nursing is a practice-oriented profession based on knowledge derived from nursing research, basic sciences, humanities, and social sciences. The goal of nursing is to assist humans to achieve optimal health.[4] I had difficulty with the repeated use of 'humans' as opposed to people in the UMDNJ literature. I discovered later that this emphasis derived from the School's adoption of Martha Roger's 'conceptual model' – referred to in their literature as the 'Science of Unitary Human Beings'. Within Roger's model, health is perceived as 'a dynamic state manifested by the individual's total pattern or state of being'. As an ideal condition, health is seen as 'the fullest possible realization of human potential'. The model adopts the view that each human being is unique and can be understood only by examining the whole person rather than looking at parts.

UMDNJ, in common with most other universities with a health sciences faculty, offers a range of degree programmes in nursing – including master's level preparation in psychiatric nursing. I got an overview of developments in UMDNJ's master's programmes from Barbara Ann Caldwell, the Associate Professor of Clinical Nursing. UMDNJ is pioneering a Psychiatric -Mental Health Nurse Practitioner programme which is multidimensional in nature. It encompasses the identification, management and/or referral of health and mental health problems as well as their maintenance, prevention and promotion. UMDNJ is taking seriously the concept of holistic nursing by considering what breadth, and depth, of knowledge and skill might be necessary for nurses to respond to the whole person, rather than simply to tinker with parts. Barbara sounded as if she *really* knew about nursing and, more importantly, knew what she was talking about. By contrast, holism is little more than a popular buzzword in the UK – invariably meaning little more than not treating the person as if (s)he were an object.

The UMDNJ nurse practitioner programme is a serious attempt to develop nursing leadership for a small proportion of nurses, locating nursing practice at the centre of health promotion and treatment. Again, the emphasis on leadership is not simple rhetoric. An existing module in the Master of Science in Nursing (MSN) programme is focused upon the 'entrepreneurial' context of nursing. Students are provided in this elective with opportunities to 'explore the fundamental skills and mechanics of entrepreneurial roles in health care'. This elective allows the student to develop an appreciation of his or her future role in 'consultation and education related to *entrepreneurial practice* in the marketplace' (emphasis added).

Expectations for Advanced Nurse Practitioners in Psychiatric and Mental Health Nursing are high indeed. Six functional roles have been outlined to form the basis of this 'supernurse' who will be expected to:

- conduct a comprehensive assessment including complete health history-taking, physical and mental status examination
- make diagnoses of acute and chronic health problems, initiating and evaluating diagnostic tests and developing differential diagnoses
- formulate plans for treatment and management of both physical and mental health problems
- implement nursing care plans using a range of psychotherapeutic

interventions – from brief therapies for individual and families to group psychotherapy. These plans should also emphasise, as appropriate, holistic health management, education and rehabilitation and the prescription of medication under joint protocols

- consult and collaborate with other disciplines in the promotion of team building, case management and organizational consultation
- extend the role of the advanced practitioner through scientific research, education and professional development.

This development appears to fit the expected reforms of Hilary Clinton's Health Bill, although there is much concern as to whether or not these reforms can be delivered. By broadening the role of the nurse practitioner in this way, the need for medical input – at least at a basic level – would be reduced. The American Medical Association is, perhaps not surprisingly, ambivalent about this development. There would be greater freedom to pursue more specialised medical interventions, but also a loss of power over large numbers of patients. On a political front, the AMAs opposition may be too little, too late. In the view of David Mechanic, Director of the Institute for Health Care Policy and Aging Research at Rutgers University, the proposed health reforms have little empirical foundation. The health care sector changes occur so fast that it becomes a 'moving target': those evaluations which have been undertaken emphasise employer savings, rather than patient benefits. Given the emphasis upon using discrete physical illnesses as the benchmark for change, special problems emerge in relation to the severely mentally ill; in particular the threat to all forms of psychosocial intervention. This appeared to mirror my experience of UK health service reorganisation, where confirmatory evidence of the effectiveness of new or 'alternative' systems is conspicuous by its absence, and mental health research becomes increasingly driven by a political agenda.

I was intrigued to discover that the broadening of the role of the advanced nurse practitioner has rung warning bells also for clinical psychologists, who have tried to negotiate prescribing rights, but to no avail. This failed development may indicate the vulnerability felt by psychologists working in a society which, perhaps more than any other, has capitalised upon the psychopathology of everyday life. One dividend of Ronald Reagan's support for the 'decade of the brain' has been the emergence of new, allegedly much-enhanced, neuroleptics. Respiridone and Clozaril have been hailed as virtual miracle cures for some people with schizophrenia, while Prozac is seen not only as effective for 'resistant depressions' but can reconstruct personalities among the jet-setting professional classes. Perhaps clinical psychologists fear that their armamentarium may be viewed as limited in the 'biopsychosocial' 90s.

One important dissident voice who still wishes to be heard above the din of such chattering-class developments is my aging, yet youthful, mentor Hildegard Peplau: Professor Emerita of Nursing of Rutgers University. We met up at Columbus Ohio where she was presenting a review of the nurse's therapeutic role with people suffering from schizophrenia at a huge psychiatric nursing convention. Peplau, commonly hailed here as the 'mother of psychiatric nursing', completed her psychotherapeutic training at the end of the Second World War and was, for a time, a colleague of Harry Stack Sullivan at Chestnut Lodge. It would be no exaggeration to say that Peplau has been the foremost analyst of modern psychiatric nursing. She has been retired for almost twenty years but finds herself, at 86, busier than ever. Finding a realistic successor appears to be a task of classic proportions.

In Peplau's view, the emergence of the 'advanced nurse practitioner' is 'just another example of nurses getting into bed with doctors again'. She noted wryly that 'although these kind of things sometimes just happen' she clearly doubted the wisdom of broadening the role of the nurse to accommodate prescribing and physical assessment skills. These would represent no more than 'hand-me-downs from doctors anyway'. Her main concern focused on her belief that psychiatric nurses had not yet clarified adequately the unique role and function of the nurse. I found this reservation at once admirable and alarming. The Columbus conference boasted plenary review papers of nursing research in the major therapeutic modalities from interpersonal therapy, through milieu, to family systems work – spanning four decades. The research tradition in the UK was kick-started in the 1970s and has enjoyed no more than a spluttering career since. The recent Department of Health Report on psychiatric and mental health nursing – *Working in Partnership (1994)* – asserted that 'mental health nursing' (sic) research should be institutionally based: built upon university departments and formal research institutes. My experience at the Columbus conference confirmed the gulf which exists, attitudinally, educationally and temporally, between British and American psychiatric nursing. Despite the relative infancy of the Diploma-status Project 2000 programme, there have already been numerous calls for 'generic nurse' degree programmes, after which specialisation could be taken, at post graduate level. The development of 'nurse practitioner' schemes, and the imminent addition of prescribing to some nurses' responsibilities, are other examples of accelerated developments which appear to be over-strenuous attempts to keep pace with the American scene. These ambitions ignore, perhaps at our peril, the fact that, in the UK, we do not have forty years of research and higher degree nursing educational experience, upon which to base such heroic professional adventures.

The collaborative support program

The development of the *Advanced Psychiatric Nurse Practitioner* is focused, unashamedly, upon people with severe mental illness. This development dovetailed with the third strand of my tour, which was to explore the role of consumers in the development of mental health services. The *Collaborative Support Program of New Jersey* (CSPNJ) is a statewide, consumer-run, non-profit mental health agency. CSPNJ promotes a variety of drop-in centres, self-help groups, supportive services and supported housing. Its emphasis also is, unashamedly, on people with serious mental illness. However, unlike traditional mental health systems, which emphasise the identification of psychopathology and symptomatology, CSPNJ pays more emphasis to identifying and developing personal strengths and abilities: the core elements of empowerment. The organisation believes that 'positive role modelling' and the person's experience of mental illness represent the key tools and skills. They encourage people with mental illness – including health professionals – to 'come out of the closet'. The best 'persuasion against stigma and prejudice is to offer ourselves publicly by saying who we really are' (Manos 1993).

CSPNJ is the only consumer-run mental health agency in New Jersey, which has a population of around 6 million. The state is slightly smaller than Scotland but with almost one million more inhabitants. The CSPNJ programmes emphasise access to advocacy training, practical coping skills, symptom management and peer natural supports. CSPNJ represents over 89,000 adults with a serious mental illness who have, or are currently using, mental health services. Around 1400 people are active participants in CSPNJ programmes: this includes 36 residents of CSP – supported housing, 400 members of Drop-in Centers in eleven counties, over 300 members of self-help groups, and 600 people who are members of the Coalition of Mental Health Consumer Organizations (COMHCO). CSPNJ has a Board of Trustees, of whom two thirds (20) are consumers or 'survivors' of psychiatric treatment. Their main funding comes from the New Jersey Department of Human Services, Division of Mental Health and Hospitals. This year, of the total budget (over \$1.257M), almost half is allocated to Supported Housing and Peer Support Services. Additional funding is provided by grants from the Washington Center for Mental Health Services (formerly the National Institute for Mental Health, NIMH) and the New Jersey Department of Labor – the latter to fund vocational rehabilitation. A federal NIMH 3-year demonstration grant given in 1990 allowed CSP to develop an innovative supported housing and peer support model which resulted in CSPNJ becoming a leader in housing for mental health consumers in New Jersey, as well as a national leader in the development of consumer programmes.

These developments are all underpinned by a belief that people are entitled to full citizenship: people with mental illness should, therefore, be afforded the opportunity to live, work, learn and socialise in homes and communities of their own choice. I met Ed Manos, who is the Self-Help Co-ordinator of CSPNJ and who has promoted the concept of *prosumers*: a former consumer who has decided to look beyond self and toward the larger work to be done in the mental health field. Although Ed Manos' use of the term was almost intuitive, he has traced its origins to Alvin Toffler's *The Third Wave*, published in 1980. In Toffler's view, the post-industrial society, with its emphasis on information, biotechnology and computers, repaired the gulf between the producer and the consumer – producing the notion of the prosumer. Ed Manos uses the term in a different way, linking professional and consumer – emphasising the potential for people with mental health problems to develop a 'professional' service role: and for professionals to acknowledge their consumption of mental health services, themselves.

Ed Manos cites the development of self-help groups for different kinds of mental health problems, the provision of advice about medication management, and 'buddy systems' as three classic examples of the prosumer function. He believes that the prosumer's advocacy and support role can be best applied in settings where people are still struggling with their illnesses, and have been unable to develop good interpersonal relationships with their professional caregivers. Prosumers offer a credible form of support: 'we've been there and know that there is a way out' (Manos 1993). Further examples of the prosumer role are to be found in their engagement with case management programmes and involvement in planning and programming as members of boards of directors.

The development of organisations such as CSPNJ is not entirely without complication. One notable problem lies in the debate over the extent to which 'consumers' of mental health services should collaborate with official providers. Ed Manos told me that he was viewed by some survivors as 'an Uncle Tom' – that some survivors of psychiatric services remain, perhaps intractably, bitter towards the symbol of their oppressive treatment – brought me down to earth. This also provided a further reflection of recent developments in the UK, where clear distinctions appear to exist between those who are 'giving in' to professional treatment, through collaboration; and those who aspire to develop alternatives – perhaps run and managed wholly by 'survivors'.

To what extent is the health care system of the UK following, blindly, that of our north American cousins'? Ruth Murray a Professor of Nursing at Pennsylvania, argues that the British only imitate the worst aspects of the American experiments. I had countless incredulous encounters as I described how, to the American viewer, we are trying to work towards what they are trying to escape from. This appears also to be true of their mental health services. As Britons become increasingly concerned with psychotherapy (again) and registers of qualified practitioners, etc., the Americans are promoting systems work, natural communities and the 'ordinary living' ethic. President Reagan's assertion that there was 'no society, only the individual' – echoed by Prime Minister Thatcher, at the British end of the 'special relationship' – sounds very dated after a visit to CSPNJ. Even the quasi-medical role of the holistic practitioners of the UMDNJ master's programme can be viewed as a recognition that the psychosocial needs of the person cannot be divorced from the physical factors which either precipitate or follow from mental distress.

My thoughts return to Jersey Joe Walcott as I fly back to the UK. Walcott may have been a good example of the professional boxer: clean living, fair fighting and committed to a noble, if brutal, art. In the increasingly razzamataz, over-hyped entertainment which passes for professional boxing, who remembers him now? I am sure there are still similar fighters around. They are suffocated, however, by the strutting arrogance of over-inflated egos and four different 'versions' of a world title – at every weight; surely a contradiction in terms. The current champion, Mike Tyson, was only an infant when I lay down in the dark to listen in to those crackling commentaries from Madison Square Garden, with my father. Yet Tyson knows the meaning of respect. He is a walking encyclopaedia on the boxing Hall of Fame. His knowledge of the men he respects may have been passed down through the oral culture of grimy gyms, or was drawn from the same dog-eared old magazines that taught me. Tyson knows that he is treading the same path that they trod, and clearly is grateful that they, somehow, lit his path. I felt much the same way about Dorothea Dix, Macalpine, Hilda Peplau, Ed Manos, and the ever-youthful Shirley Smoyak. I am acutely aware that many of my colleagues back home may never have heard of these people, who have been carving their inimitable American Tale on the face of modern and postmodern psychiatry. Some, may even dismiss them as alien to the British tradition, or anachronisms in our present neuroscientific nightmare. As I stand in the shadows of their stature, I have a deep sense of privilege and a conscious awareness of my own need for humility. I hope that, in his own time, 'Iron Mike' may have felt a similar sense of scale and with that, a need to pause for a moment of respect.

All this says, of course, is that sport represents the finest metaphor for life, and the boxing world, often thought to be corrupt rather than noble, is a fine metaphor for mental health and community care. A pill for every ill has been replaced by an ideology for every colour of the political spectrum. The strutting and posturing of the commentators on health care, obscure, rather than explicate, the models of practice. What such models might be for – in human terms – seems increasingly to get lost. To what extent are our experiments in health care reform intellectual exercises: we learn how to do it, or at least we learn the language which describes the action, but have no real lived-experience of doing it.

I am intrigued to find so many records in my notebook of how the use of technical language, jargon and psychiatric nomenclature decreased, progressively, as I moved from Greystone Park, through the UMDNJ experience to CSPNJ. Staff in the old, fascinating but disturbing, institution struggled to construct something like a human identity, but remained trapped by the institutional language, which like a local patois, slipped all too easily back into the dialogue. Ed Manos and several other colleagues of the 'prosumer' ilk seemed content just 'to be' whomever Fate had declared they should be: adopting an almost Zen-like acceptance of their mental illness, but then moving, swiftly and impressively, on to establishing what needs to be done. The aggressive 'New World' of New Jersey seemed to be rediscovering some of the oldest wisdom of the Olde Worlde and was rebuilding a true sense of community in the process.

APRIL 1998

I am reviewing these notes from four years ago as I lie on my bed in a Boston motel. I've just returned from Northampton, Massachusetts, where my colleagues and I were truly feted by Jeff Fortuna and some of his colleagues at the Windhorse project.[5] I had read about Jeff's work about seven years ago, when I reviewed Ed Podvoll's book, *The Seduction of Madness* (1991). Podvoll is a psychiatrist who was heavily influenced by the psychoanalytic work of Ronnie Laing and also the therapeutic community ideas of Maxwell Jones. He committed himself to trying to develop, like Laing, Berke and Schatzman at Kingsley Hall, therapeutic communities for people in psychosis. He was also strongly influenced by Buddhist ideas about the nature of the 'self' and levels of experience:

'From the traditional Buddhist point of view, mind of insanity is a particular journey through the six realms of existence. To give a summary of that journey, we could say the mind in psychosis swings back and forth between the god realm and the hell realm' (Podvoll 1980).

Podvoll recognised the inherent truth of Laing's original work – in which he saw madness not as break-*down*, but break-*through*. Of course Laing is now largely reviled, dismissed as a hapless drunk: worse, a hapless Celtic drunk, perhaps just as disturbed as the patients he was so close too! (I recall reading that American psychiatrists said much the same about Harry Stack Sullivan, back in the 1940s. Maybe those who get close, empathically, to real madness, scare the pants off the rest of us, who try to retain our objectivity – and distance.) I often wondered about the motivation of Laing's detractors, their knowledge of his writings and, more importantly, their direct experience of his work with people in psychosis. Podvoll had the direct experience of Laing and was impressed but not consumed by the experience:

'His [Laing's] ability to reach them, to reach out to them, to contact them and be utterly human with them was very unusual. There's a lot to learn from that. In many ways he was a very charming person, and in many ways he was not, as people know' (Podvoll 1990).

Laing and Podvoll shared an *appreciation* of psychosis, now largely abandoned by institutional psychiatry. Podvoll took the *compassionate* stance a stage further, seeing the manifestation of psychosis as:

'an enormous display of colour and vitality and depth of emotion. When we see this happening in people, we are witnessing a process of murder and resurrection, an attempted transformation of the self' (1980:30).

Podvoll's book is a psychiatric *tour de force*. It not only offers a plausible alternative conceptualisation of the most extreme forms of madness, but articulates carefully a human process for responding constructively, and effectively, to psychosis. It describes in great detail how one might develop a model of compassionate *caring*, and how staff and patients might be fully supported in the development of the model in practice. I had planned this trip to Windhorse for some time. I had been writing to Jeff Fortuna and his wife Molly over the past year, and also had enjoyed a very close (albeit through the Internet) relationship with Sally Clay, who had been one of Podvoll's patients. Sally had experience of working in Windhorse as a team therapist, and had graduated to become key voice of the consumer-advocate movement in the USA. My vicarious experience of Jeff, Molly and Sally stoked the fires of my imagination about Windhorse. The human reality – complete with trials and ordinary tribulations – of their endeavour came through strongly, but most of all Windhorse seemed to be a 'human project'. As Podvoll had said:

'We cannot ask them [the patients] to renounce what they have been through but, rather, somehow to go beyond it, for what they have experienced in this

breakthrough is an alternative to the way they have previously lived their lives ... breaking out into psychosis is an extraordinary event. It is an alternative to suicide' (1980:30).

I recall thinking that I was headed for Northampton with some trepidation. Would this turn out to be a sham, another psychiatric fabrication, an attractive idea, which had failed its own transformation test? I needn't have worried. What I found was – a least to my eyes and ears – the 'genuine nursing of the mind' which Podvoll had described. Jeff Fortuna gave generously of his time, and had arranged for one of the 'patients' in the programme to join us, and tell us about his experience of the Windhorse method. Later we visited one of the houses, where we met another 'patient' and his 'housemate', both of them discussing the programme: how it was focused on developing awareness – like a kind of 'meditation in life'. I particularly liked the way the 'patient' and the 'housemate' talked about their experience of the programme: this was no one-way therapeutic traffic.

The interior of the house was beautiful, and David – the patient – asked us all to remove our shoes as a mark of respect, whilst he turned off the classical CD which was playing, perhaps as a mark of respect for his visitors.

At the end of the afternoon we all returned to the Windhorse base, where Jeff Fortuna led a 'class' – comprising my colleagues and I, Windhorse therapists, housemates, patients, their family members and even some members of the Windhorse Board, who had not direct therapeutic involvement. The discussion began with a consideration of a piece of Podvoll's writing, but then led off into highly personal, and revealing, experiences of the group members. In some ways, it reminded me of experiences of therapeutic communities back in the UK. However, here we were all in this together: it wasn't only the patients who were journeying, we were all journeying. The session began and ended with a 'moment for silence'. The silence was palpable, as was the sense of connectedness. One of my colleagues remarked later that the silence was a 'bit west coast'. Strangely enough, it wasn't any kind of coast. As far as I was concerned, this was heartland: this was the human core. Today I felt that I had joined with a whole roomful of people in a way that I had never done before, at least not under the aegis of psychiatry.

The irony of this visit almost overwhelms me. Our *Need for Nursing* research, completed just before leaving England, had concluded that what patients needed, when most distressed, was validation of their distress, and ordinary relationships which allowed the development of mutual, sharing relations with nurses (Barker 1998). Baseball and mom's apple pie, one might think but, according to our large sample, not much in evidence in our increasingly hi-tech, evidence-based health care system. It does seem ironic that, four years ago, I visited some of the 'great and the good' in psychiatric nursing in the USA, discovering how they were all seriously intent on 'developing' and 'professionalising' nursing. The drive that was warming up, in '94, to justify the need for nursing, to extend the roles of the nurse to cover more medical intervention, and to establish an 'evidence base', have since all been shipped to UK. Yet tonight, my outstanding memory of that trip was of a nursing programme that had no nurses. Today at Northampton it was the same at Windhorse: a genuine nursing of the mind, in action, but only one 'proper' nurse on the staff team.

The figure who towered over everyone in '94 was the amazingly unassuming Ed Manos. We plan to meet up with Ed again in New York in a week's time, and I know that my colleagues will not be disappointed. He is a former policeman and a manic depressive with an amazing life story which he has just written for my next book, *The Ashes of Experience* (Manos 1999). He is also a successful consumer-advocate (prosumer). But to my mind he is none of those things: he is a real nurse. He knows how to use himself therapeutically (as Joyce Travelbee would have put it). He knows how to provide the necessary conditions for the promotion of growth and development, as I said a decade ago (Barker 1989). Just *being* with Ed makes me feel good; the conversation grows and I feel something growing inside me at the same time. Jeff Fortuna has a similar kind of unassuming character. He is a psychotherapist, but if he ever had any aspirations to use his role in a power dynamic, however gently, he appears to have abandoned that. He was generous with his time, he was generous with his attention, he was generous with his organisation, and he gave me a copy of every piece of paper I could find in his little library of reprints. His parting shot was that he hoped we might invite him to England: he wanted to do *more*.

I fear I might patronise the likes of Ed and Jeff by saying that they have a vocation. Nursing once was a vocation, then it became a trade and now it has aspirations to become a profession. Shaw probably wasn't the first to recognise the inherent paradox of professionalism, but at Windhorse I had a sense of people offering a reliable and valid service, with real commitment, but also with great expertise. I suspect that much of the 'expertise' stems from lived experience, and from recognising – as Harry Stack Sullivan wisely observed – that, as far as real madness is concerned, we are all more alike than different.

This is where I should end this book, closing the loop, which seems to be connecting me to my thoughts in the first chapter. That loop connects me with my lived experience of Peplau and Altschul – two people who know a lot about the therapeutic use of self, and who are not afraid just to 'be'. As Podvoll said of Laing, there is much that we might learn from Peplau and Altschul, despite their aged status: perhaps *because* of their aged status. They are not perfect, faultless, god-like, figures. That is exactly why we might learn much from them, for they have modelled the extraordinary craft of making the ordinary meaningful. I wrote in a paper about Peplau's legacy (Barker 1993) that I felt that I could become more knowledgeable, in a human sense, by simply sleeping at the feet of people like Peplau and Altschul. I recall that a journalist friend of mine said that she thought that was the key to the paper. The editor of the journal thought otherwise and, without discussion, edited out that oh-too-personal sentence. I am sure that this isn't only a British disease. I'm sure that lots of professionals in psychiatry are uncomfortable with recognising the true value of human relationships, trust, sharing and true presence and what those qualities might (invisibly) offer us as we journey through life.

The last ten days – added to my 'mislaid' reflections of four years ago – offer me some powerful data to support the hypothesis that nursing is alive as a social, interpersonal, construct, and is a highly effective way of helping people in psychosis to continue their journey of break-through. Fortuna, Podvoll[6] and the Windhorse team proved that, whether or not the people who enact that nursing call themselves nurses, or have a chain of letters which proclaim their 'expert' nursing standing, is unimportant. The efficacy of nursing is determined by its interpersonal enactment, not by charter or diploma, far less by fiat. For that reason, although professionalised nursing may be under some threat, nursing will never die. People need to be cared for and to care. Altruism is probably a biological necessity. All this 'survival of the fittest' is balanced by altruism, even among the so-called lower species. As we rush towards the Millennium, that beacon which we hope will declare the birth of another Golden Age, caring becomes an even more attractive proposition, especially as the world gets more careless and disconnected. When I think about the people I see as 'patients' back home, I struggle to clarify what *exactly* they might need from me that could, definitively, be called nursing. I don't think they need me to diagnose them (like doctors) or to reframe their private experiences (like a psychotherapist) or to structure some cognitive-behavioural intervention to promote change (like a psychologist). Perhaps they need nurses to accept their distress, to validate the journey of breakthrough to some new 'self' or at least the breakaway from self-death. Perhaps they need nurses to share that experience, to acknowledge that I too have been there, in some way, and that when I am ready I might learn something of the experience of my patients, which might enrich me and aid me on my own journey. Perhaps most of all they need me to be and do. Nursing *is* as nursing *does*.

NOTES

1. I am indebted to my dear friend Shirley Smoyak, Professor of Planning at the Institute for Health and Aging research, Rutgers University, New Brunswick, for organising this study tour and, with her husband Neil, for granting me – as always – such wonderful hospitality.
2. I acknowledge the usage of the term patients in the contemporary Greystone Park literature.
3. I appreciate the support of George A Waters Jr, Chief Executive Officer, and Greystone Park Psychiatric Hospital staff in providing information on the history and development of Greystone's present services.
4. Taken from the UMDNJ School of Nursing Catalog 1994–5. With acknowledgements to Barabara Ann Blasi Caldwell.
5. Windhorse Associates, 243 King Street, Suite 41, Northampton, MA 01060, USA.
6. Dr Edward Podvoll is now in lifetime retreat at a monastery in France.

REFERENCES

Barker P 1989 Reflections on the philosophy of caring in mental health. International Journal of Nursing Studies 26(2): 131–141

Barker P 1993 Nursing pioneers: the Peplau legacy. Nursing Times 89(11): 48–53

Barker P 1998 The Newcastle Need for Nursing Studies: a research monograph. University of Newcastle

Bennet C 1994 A prophet and porn: a portrait of Catherine Mackinnon. The Guardian Weekend 28th May pp 20–27

Department of Health 1994 Working in partnership: a collaborative approach to care. Report of the Mental Health Nursing Review Team, London

Manos E 1993 Speaking out: prosumers. Psychosocial Rehabilitation Journal 16:117–120

Manos E 1999 The flight of the phoenix. In: Barker P, Campbell P, Davidson B, Whitehill I (eds) The ashes of experience: reflections on the recovery from psychosis. Whurr, London

Podvoll E 1980 The psychotic journey. Naropa Institute Journal of Psychology 1(1):21

Podvoll E 1990 In memorian: an interview on R D Laing. Journal of Contemplative Psychotherapy 7:114

Podvoll E 1991 The seduction of madness: a compassionate approach to the recovery from psychosis at home. Century, London

Toffler A 1970 Future shock. The Bodley Head, London

Toffler A 1980 The third wave. William Morrow, New York

Index

A

Aboriginal peoples, Australia and
    New Zealand, 40
Advanced nurse practitioner,
    New Jersey, 236–240
'Age of the Individual', Seligman,
    153–154
Aggression in everyday life, 179–180
AIDS/HIV, prejudice, 226–227, 229–230
Aims of psychiatric nursing, 31
Altered states and creativity, 139–141
Altschul, Annie, 4–5, 11–12, 93–94, 246
    interpersonal paradigm, 80
    patient as consumer, 167
    patient/nurse bonding, 68
America, 233–247
    advanced nurse practitioner,
      New Jersey, 236–240
    advanced practice psychiatric-mental
      health nurses, 17, 238–239
    Collaborative Support Program,
      New Jersey, 240–243
    de-institutionalisation, 234–236
    health reforms, 239
    pace of life in north-east, 223–224
    postwar psychoanalysis and
      psychiatric nursing, 8–10, 11
    Windhorse project, 243–247
Andreason, creativity and mood
    disorder, 139
Anxiety and melancholy, 120
Arran relationships model, 172–174, 180
'As Good as it Gets', film, 54
Assessment, 206
Attitudes, changing, 221–222
Authors, creativity and dysfunction, 139
Autonomy, restoration of, 70

B

Beech, research and focus of nursing
    commentary, 53–55
Behaviour therapy, 60
Benson, psychiatric nursing and mental
    health nursing commentary, 93–94
Beuys
    creative experience, 133
    illness as spiritual crisis, 118
Biological
    reductionism, developing role
      of nurses, 13
    sciences, 155
Biomedical
    developments, 99–100
    paradigm, 101, 102
    research, 61–62
Brain-imaging techniques, 62
Brandon, mental health in the new
    millenium commentary, 164–165
Britain
    health system following USA, 242, 245
    postwar psychiatric nursing and
      psychoanalysis, 10, 11
Byron, creativity and altered states, 140

C

Californian self, 153, 154
Campbell, psychiatric nursing, 89
Caras, message to parents, 160
Care
    approaches to, 64–65
    and caring, 50
    development through
      collaboration, 117–127
      commentary, 129–131
    paternalistic view, 31
    physical, 126
    planning, process of, 205–208
    re-emergence, 39
    reification of technology of, 99–100
    research into, 45
    team, diversity within, 207
    value of, 38
Caring
    collaborative, 157
    discovery-based, 123
    experience of, 191
    function of nursing, 120
    human science of, 79–80
    interpersonal context, 87
    the map of, 78–79
    process, 87, 190
    proper focus, 87
    relationship, empowerment in, 208–210
    social context, 88
Cartesian-Newtonian paradigm, 156
Cassel Hospital, psychosocial nursing, 10
Celtic
    art, 89
    origins, psychiatric nursing, 78, 93
Champ, living with schizophrenia,
    129, 131
Change
    people's possibilities for, 118, 119, 120
    process of, 38
Chesterson, care through collaboration
    commentary, 129–131
Clarke, community psychiatric mental
    health nursing commentary, 74–75
Classification see Diagnostic classifications
Clinical nurse specialist
    see also Advanced nurse practitioner,
      New Jersey
    advanced, America, 17, 238–239
    concept, introduction of, 8
Clinical supervision, 183–194
    assumed function, 185–187
    commentary, 196–197
    definition, 183–184
    distinction from preceptorship, 187
    limitations, 193–194
    models, 191–193
    origins, 184–185
    and practice, 189–191
Cognitive therapy, 60
Cognitive-behavioural therapy, 18–19
Collaboration, 84
    developing care through, 117–127
    commentary, 129–131

Collaborative
  approaches, 64
  caring, 157
  Support System of New Jersey, 240–243
Collective consciousness of psychiatric
      nursing, Tyneside study, 86–88
Community, 72
  building of, 162–163
  psychiatric and mental health
      nursing, 57–72
    commentary, 74–75
    CPMH nurses, 61, 63, 65–66, 66–68
Conceptual model, Rogers, 238
Conroy, mental health in the new
      millenium commentary, 162–163
Consumer, patient as, 167
Contextual reality, 220
Cost-effectiveness in care, 68–69
  see also Economic
CPMH (community psychiatric and mental
      health) nurses, 61, 63, 65–66
  wider role bandwidth, 66–68
CPN (community psychiatric nurse)
      as keyworker, 68
Creative
  people, 141
  process, model to explain, 142–143
Creativity, 145
  and altered states, 139–141
  and discipline, 141–143
  and dysfunction, 138–139
  and 'madness', 134, 136
  and psychic distress, 133–145
    commentary, 148–149
  why and how, 140–141, 142
Crick, view of the mind, 144
Cuidad, work with mentally ill, 32, 35–36
Culture
  of care, 40
  customs and beliefs, 39–41
  declining, 32
  traditions and ethical dilemmas, 209–210

D
Daniels, AIDS/HIV
      marginalisation, 226, 227
Darwin, creativity and panic
      disorder, 136–137
Dawson, language of nursing, 86
Dax, Eric Cunningham, 77, 93
Death anxiety and homophobia, 222
Decision-making, everyday, 201–202
Deegan, caring, human condition of, 78
Dementia, 125
Dementia praecox, 170
Depression
  epidemic, 65, 153, 154
  experience of severe, 121
  to psychotic degree, 169
  women with severe, 29, 120, 209
Descartes, 129, 129–130
Developmental
  activity, nursing as, 70, 108, 111, 203

nature of supervision, 189–190
Diagnostic classifications
  reducing people to, 17–18, 28–29,
      35, 71, 85
  segregation into subpopulations,
      27–28, 46, 52
The Dialectics of Schizophrenia, Thomas, 160
Dignity, restoring, 23
Dilthey, science and knowledge, 44
Discipline and creativity, 141–143
Disciplines other than nursing,
      understanding, 115
Discovery-based caring, 123
Disempowerment
  ethnicity, 209–210
  married women and depression, 209
  psychiatric patient, 30, 31, 35
Dossey, power of prayer, 210
Dr Faustus, Mann, 46–47
Durer, image of melancholy, 137–138
Dysfunction and creativity, 138–139

E
Eccentricity, madness and creativity,
      relationship, 134, 136
Economic
  code of ethics, satirical, 211
  imperatives, 51
  pressures, decline of psychotherapy, 18
Education, 124
  therapy as, 58–59
Educative instrument, nursing as, 120, 123
Einstein, theory of relativity, 135
Emancipation in care planning, 206
Emotional needs, and clinical
      supervision, 186
Empowerment, 35, 111, 119
  in the caring relationship, 208–210
  in clinical supervision, 194
  demand for, 69–70
  and patient participation, 99–112
    commentary, 114–115
  through patient-centred care, 107
Enablement, 111
Enlightenment and understanding, 43–45
Environmental sciences, 155
Epictetus, difficult circumstances, 89
Erickson, horstory, 57–58
Ethical conflicts, 199–212
  commentary, 213–215
  nature of, 201–203
Ethics, definition, 201
Ethnicity, disempowerment, 209–210
Everyday
  aggression, 179–180
  decision-making, 201–202
  living, problems of, 27, 61, 88
  psychotherapy, 171–172, 172–174
Evidence-based practice in nursing, 130–131
Existential
  crisis in psychiatric nursing, 21–22
  experience of mental illness see
      Lived experience: of mental illness

problems, mental distress viewed as, 64
Experience, logic of, 117–127
  commentary, 129–131

F
Failure, excuses for, 155
Family
  of psychiatry, metaphor, 24–25
  therapy, 9–10, 60
Farrell, evidence-based practice in
    nursing, 130–131
Feminine nature of caring, 13, 79
Fisher, Dan
  hope, humanity and voice, 151
  self, 161
Formative function, clinical supervision, 185
Fortuna, Jeff, 243, 246
Frame, experience of mental distress, 118
Frankl, Viktor, 51
  anxiety and melancholia, 120
  meanings, 89
  power, 109
  spirituality and religion, 42
Freud
  creativity, 141
  intrapsychic theories, 60, 61
  nature and nurture, psychosis, 171

G
Gay liberation, 222, 223
Gender
  disempowerment, 209
  sex and persuasion, 29–30
Generic or specific services, 67
Genetic transmission, enduring mental
    illness, 144
Genome mapping, 62, 144
Gheyn, melancholy, 138
Goethe, creativity and altered states,
    139–140
Van Gogh, creativity and altered states, 141
Graduate programmes, clinical nurse
    specialists, 17
Greystone Park Psychiatric Hospital,
    New Jersey, 235–236, 237
Group supervision with independent
    facilitator, 192

H
Habermas, lifeworld, 50
Happiness, pursuit of, 83
Hawking, the mind of God, 140
Hays, clinical practice of psychiatric
    nurses, 8
Healing role, psychiatric nurses, 117
Health, 45–48
  definition, Illich, 63, 101
  understanding of, 48
  and wellness, 111–112
Health care
  collaborative approach, 64

humanised approach, 64–65
  managing and damaging, 210–212
  spirituality in, 41–42
Heterosexuality, 29
Historical aspects, psychiatric nursing,
    78, 93
History taking, 57
Holism, 26–27, 156
  holistic caring, 45
  holistic focus, 90
  or neuroscience, 143–145
  and nursing practice, 100–101, 117, 145
  and spirituality, 41–43
  in USA, 238
Holmes, research and focus of nursing
    commentary, 50–52
Homophobia, 29–30, 222, 223
Homosexuality, 29–30
  attitude of pity towards, 222, 226–227
  gay liberation, 222, 223
  and prejudice, 222–223
Hughes, paradox of certainty, 158–159
Human
  genome mapping, 62, 144
  issues, need to focus on, 80
Humanised approach, health care, 64–65

I
Illich, definition of health, 63, 101
'Illness' model of mental disorder, 26
Illness or wellness, 107–110
Immoral action, 202
In-group and out-group membership,
    219, 222, 223
Individual supervision
  by another clinician, 192
  with practitioner from different
      discipline, 193
Individualism, 65, 152–153, 153–154, 164
Information-exchange, 85
Inherent power and inherent values, 106
Internal dialogue, 60
Interpersonal
  activity of nursing, 105
  collaboration, 157–158
  context of caring, 83–84, 87
  methods see Socratic inquiry
  nursing roles and ethical dilemmas,
      213–214
  paradigm, Altschul, 80
  relations
    of caring, 118, 126, 127
    nurse/patient relationship, 122, 200, 247
    schizophrenia, 5, 6, 7
    to illness, 64
  situations and biological changes, 18
  theory, 5–6, 6–7, 80, 172
Interviewing technique, focused, 174–175

J
Jamieson, prejudice and sexuality
    commentary, 229–230

Japan, nursing administration, 196, 197
Jung, physics and psychology, 157

K
Kayama, clinical supervision
    commentary, 196–197
Kekulé, benzene ring, 135
Kelly, house-garden-wilderness
    metaphor, 104–105
Keyworkers, 13–14
Klein, definition of community, 72
Knowledge, 82
Kuhn
    paradigm shift, 82–83
    paradigm-based science, 101
Kundalini, emergence, 179
Kushlick, 'hit and run' psychiatry, 82

L
Labels, obfuscation by, 28–29
    see also Diagnostic classifications
Laing, R D, 4, 244
    power, role in relationships, 171
    The Divided Self, 54
Lakeman, ethical conflicts commentary,
    213–215
Language
    American use of, 234
    and experience, 121, 125
    and growth process, 122
    nursing theory, 86
    personhood and patienthood, 22–24
    redefining nursing, 121
    understanding of, 34
    within medicine, 111–112
        fight metaphors, 38
Learning from the patient, 119
Lego
    psychoanalysis and psychiatric nursing
        commentary, 17–19
    psychoanalytic theory in nursing
        practice, 8
Life review, 108, 110, 118, 121–122, 131
Life story, person in psychosis, 171
Lifeworld, colonisation by science, 50–51
Lived experience, 122–123
    Arran relationships model, 172–174, 180
    of mental illness, 62, 71, 85, 118, 130
        psychosis, 169, 171, 173, 174, 177
        schizophrenia, 129, 131
    and metaphor, 104
Loewi, autonomic system, 135

M
McDonaldization, 42, 51–52
McKenna, philosophy of psychiatric
    nursing commentary, 34–36
McNeill, tapeworm metaphor, 124
Main, psychosocial nursing, 10
Male and female stereotypes,
    challenging, 226

Managed care, demand for, 68–69
Manic depression
    nature and nurture, 170–172
    psychosis, 144
Manos, 246
    collaborative support programme,
        241–242
Market culture, NHS, 64, 107–108
Marriage and disempowerment,
    depressed women, 209
Masculine principle of medicine, 79
Massachussetts, Windhorse project, 243–247
Masters-level psychiatric nurses,
    New Jersey, 237
Meaning
    attribution of, 105–106
    of experiences, establishing, 89, 118
        severe depression, 121
    in life, 43
    in mental distress, 85–86
    in psychosis, 177
    as research question, 44–45
    search for, 138
Medical economists, satirical 'code of
    ethics', 211
Medical model of psychiatry, 35
Medical-expressive tradition, 82
Medicalization of nursing, 239–240
Medication, 162, 239
    reliance on, 54
    side-effects, 114
Medicine
    dominance of, 114–115
    and psychiatric diagnosis, 114
Melancholy
    and anxiety, 120
    and transcendence, 137–138
Men as carers, 78–79, 93
Mental distress, 61
    amongst older and younger people, 154
    and creativity, 133–145, 148–149
    lived experience of see Lived experience
    meanings in, 85–86
Mental handicap, 27, 28
Mental health, 71–72, 157
    concept of, 22, 24, 83–84, 154
    implications of paradigm shift, 156
    and mental illness, care plans, 207
    in the new millenium, 151–161
        commentary, 162–163, 164–165
    nursing, 199–200
        and psychiatric nursing,
            distinction, 79–80
        transformation of psychiatric
            nursing into, 199–200
    service users, 63–64, 67
        experiences, nursing by
            psychiatric nurses, 53–54
    workers, psychiatric nurses becoming, 22
Mental Health Nursing Review Group
    (DoH 1994), 107
Mental illness
    concept of, 24
    genetic transmission, 144

lived experience of, 62, 71, 85, 118, 130
  psychosis, 169, 171, 173, 174, 177
  schizophrenia, 129, 131
  and mental handicap, distinction, 27
Mentor, role of, 187–189
Mentor-protégée relationship, 188
Mentoring and preceptorship, 187–189
Metaphors, 103–106
  being lost as, 108
  family of psychiatry, 24–25
  fight metaphors in medicine, 38
  house-garden-wilderness, 104–105
  of life path, 112
  and lived experiences, 104
  tapeworm, 124
  yurodivy, 109
Midwifery, clinical supervision in, 185
Milieu therapy, 9
  decline of, 18
Mind, 88, 129
  changing views of, 143, 144
  concept of, 117
  as function of society, 26
Mind-body split, 100
Miro
  creative process, 134
  symbolic ladder, 138
Models
  clash of, 26–27
  of nursing practice, 121
  in psychiatry, 35
Moral panics, 223, 224
Multidisciplinary
  collaboration, 51
  team, ethical conflicts, 214–215

N
Narrative self, 52
Nature and nurture, psychosis, 170–172
Needs
  of individuals, 40
  nursing's attempts to meet, 106
  personal and high-tech care systems,
    206
  therapeutic relationship, 109
  what patients need from nurses,
    70, 158, 247
Needs-led service, demand for, 70–72
Neo-Darwinian views, 143–144
Neuroleptics, 239
Neuroscience ,17, 19, 134, 143–145
  creativity, 142
  orthodoxy, 156
  psychosis, 170
'Neurotic' depression, 169
'New Age', 90, 110
New Jersey
  advanced nurse practitioner, 236–240
  clinical nurse specialists, 236–237
  Collaborative Support Program, 240–243
  de-institutionalisation, 234–236
  notes from, 233–243
New physics, 156, 158, 163

Newnes, definition of mental health, 71
Newton, creativity and altered states, 140
NHS, market culture, 64, 107–108
Nightingale
  nursing, modern concept, 78–79
  philosophy of nursing, 32, 35–36
  postmodern update on, 40
Nihilistic attitudes, 42
Nomenclature, psychiatric nursing, 94
Normalisation of subclasses, 28
Normative
  function, clinical supervision, 186–187
  terrorism, 221
Novel, nurses psychotherapeutic role
    in psychosis commentary, 179–181
Nurse
  education programmes, New Jersey,
    237–238
  practitioner schemes, Britain, 240
  preparation for practice, 174–175
  psychotherapeutic role, future, 176–177
  psychotherapists, America, 17
The Nurse and the Mental Patient,
    Schwartz and Shockley, 7–8
Nurse/patient relationship, 88, 105
  interpersonal collaboration, 157–158
  learning from, 119
Nurse's role see Role of nurse
Nursing, 246
  see also Proper focus of nursing;
    Psychiatric nursing
  as craft, 105
  as developmental activity, 70, 108, 111, 203
  as educative instrument, 120, 123
  experiences of in psychiatric and
    surgical settings, 39
  and holism, 100–101
  metaphors of, 103
  nature of, 200, 202–203
  nurses attempts to define, 54–55
  phenomenological focus, 81
  redefining, 121
  science, research, 37

O
Obiols, creative process, 142–143
Objective reality, 220
One-to-one relationship, 6, 7, 8, 9
  see also Interpersonal:
    nurse/patient relationship
Optimism, 126
Originality and the creative malady,
    136–137
Outreach support, 67–68

P
Panic disorder, Darwin, 136–137
Paradigm shift, 44, 82–83, 101–103,
    110, 154, 159
Paradigm shift (cont'd)
  implications for mental health, 156
  new physics, 156

Paradigm-based science, Kuhn, 101
Partnership, 205–206
  working in, 103
Paternalistic view of care, 31
Patient
  as consumer, 167
  disempowerment, 30, 31, 35
  participation and empowerment, 99–112
    commentary, 114–115
  as person, need to recognise, 102
  as term, 34
Patienthood, concept in psychiatry, 23
Peer group supervision, 191–192
People, patients and populations, 27–28
Peplau, Hildegard, 8–9, 71, 79–80, 93–94, 246
  focus of nursing, 46
  influence, American psychiatric
    nursing, 11
  internal dialogue, 60
  interpersonal theory, 5–6, 6–7, 172
  medicalization of nursing, 239–240
  method, 7, 18
  nursing as developmental and
    educative activity, 108, 120
  paradigm shift, 102–103
  research, brain and mind, 171
  schizophrenia, 81, 176–177
  talk, expressing feelings, 122
Personal
  dimensions, mental health problems, 64
  identity, 52
Personality, changing views of, 143
Personhood and patienthood, 22–24
Perspectives, development of alternative, 121
Phenomenological focus of nursing, 81
Philosophy of psychiatric nursing, 21–33
  commentary, 34–36
Physical basis for mental illness, 170, 171
Physical care, 126
Physics, new, 156, 158, 163
Picasso, creativity, 134, 142
Pirsig
  forms of reasoning, 46
  Zen and the Art of Motorcycle
    Maintenance, 125
Plato, the unexamined life, 118
Podvoll, Edward, 243–244, 244–245
  compassionate environment, 125
Poincaré, Fuschian functions, 135
Political correctness, 221
Polkinghorne, view of the mind, 144
Postmodern direction, psychiatric
  nursing, 159–160
Power, 34, 109
  disempowerment see Disempowerment
  inherent, 106
  of prayer, 210
  and professionalism, 111–112, 115
Preceptorship and mentoring, 187–189
Preference, expression of, 218
Prejudice
  adoption of, 218–219
  challenge to, 221–222
  counteracting, 221

impact of, 219–220
nature of, 217–218
and sexuality, 217–227
  commentary, 229–230
  effects on victims, 220
  as form of terror management, 223
  homophobia, 29–30, 222, 223
PREP, 193–194
Preparation for practice, 174–175
Pride and prejudice, 219
Primary care nurse, 17
Primary nursing, 13–14
Problem-focused therapies, 60
Problems of everyday living, 27, 61, 88
Process of nursing, ethical issues, 203
Professionalism, 77–78
  and power, 111–112, 115
Proper focus of nursing, 75, 82, 87,
    107, 174, 200
  appropriate care systems, 62–63, 64
  and biomedical developments, 99
  depression or psychotic disorder, 124
  failure to clarify, 108
  needs-led, 70, 71
  Peplau, 80, 81
  rediscovery, 13, 115, 125
Prosumers, 241, 242
Psychiatric nurse practitioners, America, 17
  advanced, 238–239, 240
Psychiatric nursing
  see also Proper focus of nursing;
    Role of nurse
  definition, 94
  development of, New Jersey, 236–240
  existential crisis, 21–22
  holism or neuroscience, implications
    for practice, 143–145
  and mental health nursing, 62–63,
    77–90, 89, 199–200
    commentary, 93–94
    distinction between, 79–80
  postmodern direction for, 159–160
  postwar, 8–10, 11
  and psychoanalysis, 3–17
    commentary, 17–19
  psychotherapeutic work, psychosis,
    169–177, 179–181
Psychiatric nursing papers,
    50s and early 60s, 9
Psychiatric survivors, 84
Psychiatric-Mental Health Nurse
    Practitioner programme,
    New Jersey, 238
Psychiatry as 'hit and run' activity, 82
Psycho-technologies, 63
Psychoanalysis and psychiatric
    nursing, 3–14
  commentary, 17–19
  postwar, 8–10, 11
Psychoanalytic concepts
  influences in nursing
Psychoanalytic concepts (cont'd)
  decline, 18
  development, 8–10, 11

integration into psychiatric nursing, 17
introduction, graduate nurse education, 3
Psychopharmacology, 54, 62, 114, 162
  neuroleptics, 239
  'Star Trek school of nursing', 54
Psychosis
  see also Manic depression; Schizophrenia
  classification, history of, 170
  interpersonal relations theory, 172
  lived experience, 169, 171, 173, 174, 177
  as major psychiatric disorder, 169, 179
  manic depressive, 144
  nature and nurture, 170–172
  nurses' therapeutic role, 169–177
    commentary, 179–181
  Podvoll and Laing, 244
  severe, Altschul, 12
Psychosocial Intervention (PSI), 63
Psychosocial problems, 28
Psychotherapeutic role, psychosis ,169–177
  commentary, 179–181
  preparation for, 174–175
Psychotherapy
  everyday psychotherapy,
    171–172, 172–174
  'waves' of, 60, 61, 72

Q
Quality of life, 42
Questions, asking, 123, 124

R
Radcliffe, creativity and psychic
    distress commentary, 148–149
Rapid assessment team, 68
Rapprochement, searching for, 88–90
Reality, 180
  objective and contextual, 220
  and psychosis, 169
Reductionist approaches, 35, 41, 100–101
Reflective
  practice, 43
  practitioner, 215
  processes, 120
  see also Life review
Relationships and interactions,
    person in psychosis, 173
  see also Interpersonal: relations
Report of the Mental Health Nursing
    Review Team (DoH 1994), 62, 64
Research
  goals, 45
  and the proper focus of nursing, 37–48
    commentary, 50–52, 53–55
  within nursing, 37
Resources, availability and demand, 206–207
Response to mental illness, 64, 107
Restorative function, clinical
    supervision, 186
Restriction by legal mechanisms, 111
Rights, sufferers of mental illness, 69
Rogers, conceptual model, 238

Role of nurse, 115, 117–118, 119, 203–205
  see also Proper focus of nursing;
    Psychotherapeutic role, psychosis
  biological reductionism, 13
  conflicts, 204, 213–214
  CPMH nurses, 65–66
    wider role bandwidth, 66–68
  extension and development, 82, 205
  support for doctors, 82
Role theory, 23
Russell, modern societies, progress, 38

S
Schizophrenia, 101, 129, 143, 144, 170,
    176–177
  concept of, 84–85
  Dialectics of Schizophrenia, Thomas, 160
  experience of, 129, 131
  interpersonal relationships, 5, 6, 7
  nature and nurture, 170–172
  social explanations, 25
  WHO study, 1973 and 1979, 25
Science, 50
  science-as-process, 44
  and technology, faith in, 53
Scientific
  approach to mental illness, paradoxes, 54
  discovery and lapses in rational
    thought, 134–136
  paradigms, 155
  reductionism see Reductionist approaches
Self-determination, right to, 69
Self-fulfilling prophecy, 220
Self-improvement, fashion for, 47
Seligman, individualism, 152–153, 153–154
Sense of self, fragmentation, 52
Serious mental illness, concept, 84
Service provision, standards, 193
Sexual health and health promotion role, 230
Sexuality, 221, 222
  see also Prejudice: and sexuality
  nurses' embarrassment in addressing, 230
  preference and orientation, 224–227
Shingler, creative process, 133
Skellern, psychodynamic approach to
    nursing, 11
Skills in CPMH nursing, 63
Smoyak, family therapy, 9–10
Social
  anxiety and the media, 154–155
  construction of sexuality, 226
  context of caring, 88
  explanation, schizophrenia, 25
  grouping, 219, 222, 223
  sciences, 155
  support systems, erosion, 65, 66
Society
  and the individual, 212
  mind as function of, 26
Socratic inquiry, 7, 172, 174–175, 175–176
Spiritual
  activity, nursing as, 117–118
  distress in mental illness, 90

Spirituality, 89
   and holism, 41–43
   in nursing, 51
'Star Trek school of nursing', 54
Stories
   life review, 121–122
   of lives, 118
   and the mind, 117
   rewriting to re-author life, 125
The Stormy Search for Self, Grof and Grof, 179
Stress creation, individualism, 164
Subpopulations, segregating people into,
      27–28
Sullivan, Harry Stack, 5, 80
   interpersonal dimension of loving
      and giving, 83–84
Supervision *see* Clinical supervision
Supervisor
   characteristics of, 187
   roles, 189
Szasz, metaphors, 103–104

T
Taoism, 101, 145
Technological change, 61, 62
   therapeutic innovations, 63
Technology of care, reification, 99–100
Teirney, use of research, 43
Theoretical base, weak, 86, 94
Therapeutic relationships, 6, 162
   see also Interpersonal: relations
Therapy, 123
   as education, 58–59
Thomas, *The Dialectics of Schizophrenia*, 160
Titanic, James Cameron's, 53
Transcendence and melancholy, 137–138
Transcultural nursing, 40–41
Trends and influences, 66
Trephotaxis, 70, 108, 121
Truth, construction of personal, 124
Tyneside study, 86–88
Tyson, Mike, 242–243

U
UK health system, following USA, 242, 245
University of Medicine and Dentistry,
      New Jersey, 237–238
USA *see* America
Users, mental health services, 53–54, 63–64, 67

V
'Value for money', concern with, 51
Values
   attitudes and belief systems, 221–224
   ethical conflicts, 213–215
      discarding to resolve, 214–215
   inherent, 106
Da Vinci, Leonardo, 97–98, 133
Vulnerability and hostile responses, 39

W
Waters, patient participation and
      empowerment commentary, 114–115
Webb, nursing research, 45
Wellness, or fixing illness, 107–110
Wheel, invention of, 134–135
Windhorse project, Massachussetts, 243–247
Winship, psychoanalytic influences in
      nursing, 11
Women
   needs as service users, 67
   severe depression, 29, 120, 209
Worldview, 34
'Worried well', the, 28–29, 65

Y
Yurodivy, metaphor of, 109

Z
*Zen and the Art of Motorcycle
      Maintenance*, Pirsig, 125
Zukav, new physics, 156, 158